(16.35 The
Set)

CLINICAL BIOCHEMISTRY
OF
DOMESTIC ANIMALS

Second Edition
VOLUME II

Contributors

George H. Cardinet, III
Embert H. Coles
Charles E. Cornelius
W. Jean Dodds
G. O. Ewing
J. J. Kaneko
Jack R. Luick
George W. Osbaldiston
Victor Perman
John B. Tasker
B. C. Tennant

CLINICAL BIOCHEMISTRY
OF
DOMESTIC ANIMALS

Second Edition
VOLUME II

Edited by

J. J. KANEKO

Department of Clinical Pathology
University of California
Davis, California

and

C. E. CORNELIUS

Department of Physiological Sciences
Kansas State University
Manhattan, Kansas

ACADEMIC PRESS   1971   **New York and London**

ACADEMIC PRESS, INC.
111 Fifth Avenue, New York, New York 10003

United Kingdom Edition published by
ACADEMIC PRESS, INC. (LONDON) LTD.
Berkeley Square House, London W1X 6BA

LIBRARY OF CONGRESS CATALOG CARD NUMBER: 72-117089

PRINTED IN THE UNITED STATES OF AMERICA

Contents

1. THE KIDNEY: ITS FUNCTION AND EVALUATION IN HEALTH AND DISEASE

George W. Osbaldiston

2. FLUIDS, ELECTROLYTES, AND ACID–BASE BALANCE

John B. Tasker

3. GASTROINTESTINAL FUNCTION

B. C. Tennant and G. O. Ewing

4. SKELETAL MUSCLE

George H. Cardinet, III

5.   HEMOSTASIS AND BLOOD COAGULATION

W. Jean Dodds and J. J. Kaneko

6.   CEREBROSPINAL FLUID

Embert H. Coles

7.   SYNOVIAL FLUID

Victor Perman and Charles E. Cornelius

8.   TRANSUDATES AND EXUDATES

Victor Perman

9.   USE OF RADIOACTIVE ISOTOPES IN VETERINARY CLINICAL BIOCHEMISTRY

Jack R. Luick

List of Contributors

Numbers in parentheses indicate the pages on which the authors' contributions begin.

George H. Cardinet, III (155), Neuromuscular Research Laboratory, Department of Physiological Sciences, College of Veterinary Medicine, Kansas State University, Manhattan, Kansas

Embert H. Coles (207), Department of Infectious Diseases, College of Veterinary Medicine, Kansas State University, Manhattan, Kansas

Charles E. Cornelius (233), Department of Physiological Science, College of Veterinary Medicine, Kansas State University, Manhattan, Kansas

W. Jean Dodds (179), Division of Laboratories and Research, New York State Department of Health, Albany, New York

G. O. Ewing (111), Department of Clinical Sciences, School of Veterinary Medicine, University of California, Davis, California

J. J. Kaneko (179), Department of Clinical Pathology, School of Veterinary Medicine, University of California, Davis, California

Jack R. Luick (271), Institute of Arctic Biology, University of Alaska, College, Alaska

George W. Osbaldiston (1), Department of Infectious Diseases, Kansas State University, Manhattan, Kansas

Victor Perman (233, 255), Department of Veterinary Pathology and Parasitology, College of Veterinary Medicine, University of Minnesota, St. Paul, Minnesota

John B. Tasker (61), Department of Pathology, New York State Veterinary College, Cornell University, Ithaca, New York

B. C. Tennant (111), Department of Clinical Sciences, School of Veterinary Medicine, University of California, Davis, California

Preface to the Second Edition

The marked expansion of knowledge in the clinical biochemistry of animals since publication of the first edition of this book seven years ago has necessitated this major revision. In this period, a wealth of new information on clinical biochemical aspects of disease in animals has become available. This has been made possible by the continued rapid advances of modern biochemistry, the increasing awareness of the usefulness of animal models of human disease in biomedical research, and the ever increasing growth of both veterinary and human medicine. In keeping with this expansion of knowledge, this edition is comprised of two volumes. Chapters on the pancreas, thyroid, and pituitary–adrenal systems have been separated and entirely rewritten. Completely new chapters on muscle metabolism, iron metabolism, blood clotting, and gastrointestinal function have been added. All the chapters of the first edition have been revised with pertinent new information, and many have been completely rewritten.

Emphasis continues to be placed on the interpretation of biochemical findings in disease of the domestic animal species. A notable exception is the inclusion of information on subhuman primates in the chapter on liver function. We can already anticipate a marked expansion of biochemical knowledge on primates as well as on laboratory animal species that will be included in subsequent editions.

Keeping pace with the explosive expansion of new biochemical knowledge among a variety of animal species is a formidable task for the veterinary student, his teachers, the veterinary practitioner, the biomedical researcher, and the experimental biologist. It is our hope that this treatise, primarily devoted to the interpretation of biochemical findings in diseases of animals, will contribute to the accomplishment of this task.

We are deeply indebted to the contributors for their dedicated efforts and perseverance. Thanks are also due to the users of the first edition whose many helpful suggestions have guided this revision. Finally, we extend our greatest appreciation to our wives, Frances and Bette, and our families who have cheerfully persevered through this second edition.

J. J. Kaneko
C. E. Cornelius

November, 1970

Preface to the First Edition

Interest in the clinical biochemistry of animals has increased rapidly in the past decade owing to the expansion and growth of veterinary science as well as the increasing use of domestic animals in comparative medical research. Selected data concerning the changes which occur in the chemical constituents of the blood and tissues can provide for a better understanding of the disease process as well as supply information helpful in differential diagnosis, therapy, and prognostication. This book represents a first attempt to provide the veterinary student, the practitioner of veterinary medicine, and the experimentalist with a specific volume of information concerning the interpretation of biochemical findings in diseases of domestic animals, and it does not purport to be a laboratory manual. Methods, however, are included whenever their understanding is believed to greatly enhance the interpretation of the blood chemical findings. The normal values of the various blood constituents as determined by more recent methods should be of help to all experimental biologists. The information has been gathered from the internationally available scientific literature and, in addition, includes original data obtained in the laboratories of the Department of Clinical Pathology, University of California.

Experience in the clinical laboratory has impressed the editors with the difficulty students and practicing veterinarians encounter in bridging the gap between the fundamental sciences and the practice of clinical animal medicine. It is the hope of the editors that this volume will be of help in the application of some of this highly specialized basic knowledge to animal diseases. The topics included in this volume reflect the diagnostic areas of emphasis presently taught in the second semester of a year course in clinical pathology at the School of Veterinary Medicine of the University of California. The editors welcome suggestions for topics to be added in subsequent editions.

C. E. Cornelius
J. J. Kaneko

March, 1963

Contents of Volume I

1 _____ # The Kidney: Its Function and Evaluation in Health and Disease

George W. Osbaldiston

I. PHYSIOLOGICAL FUNCTIONS PERFORMED BY THE KIDNEY

Urinary excretion is the major avenue for the passage of soluble products from the body, and the kidney performs an important function in maintaining the normal composition and volume of body fluids. The kidney differentiates between waste and essential substances, the latter being excreted in response to blood plasma and renal cell concentrations. It also recognizes foreign substances, and in practicing this selective secretion the kidney attempts to correct the deficiencies or excesses of the other excretory pathways of the body.

The kidney achieves control of the milieu interior by regulating or assisting in the regulation of (1) excretion of waste metabolic products such as urea, phosphate, creatinine, and sulfate; (2) water and electrolyte balance; (3) acid–base balance and hydrogen ion excretion; and (4) metabolic functions such as the production of the hormones renin and erythropoietin, the excretion of ammonia, and the production of glucose by gluconeogenesis.

A. URINE FORMATION

Three processes are involved in urine formation: (1) removal at the glomerulus of plasma water and most of its soluble constituents, (2) selective reabsorption within the tubules of substances necessary for the maintenance of homeostasis in the body, and (3) secretion by the tubular cells.

Because the solution passing into the proximal tubule resembles an ultrafiltrate in composition, the transfer process occurring at the glomerulus is referred to as filtration. By precise definition, filtration means the separation of insoluble material from solution. The glomerulus does not perform entirely in this manner because cells and many molecules which are in solution in plasma do not cross this membranous barrier.

The epithelial cells lining the renal tubules have the ability to modify the composition of the glomerular filtrate, and consequently the kidney becomes a prime organ in assisting in the maintenance of homeostasis of the body. This is the context in which one should clinically consider renal function, as the diseased kidney may be unable to make the necessary adjustments for homeostasis and hence affects the function of many organs and tissues.

Filtration is dependent upon the unique properties of the glomerular capillaries: (1) They are anatomically situated between two arterioles; blood enters from the afferent arteriole and leaves via the efferent arteriole. Because of this arrangement, their hydrostatic pressure is 50–60 mmHg, which is twice that in capillaries elsewhere in the body. (2) They are architecturally different in having a double membrane with an inner vascular endothelium and an external capsular epithelium. Sandwiched between these two layers of cells is a basement membrane (lamina densa). The basement membrane is 100 Å in thickness and has a fibular, reticulating, homogeneous structure; it is permeable but not perforated, unlike the multiperforated endothelial and epithelial cell layers on either side. (3) These capillaries, in contrast with other capillaries in which filtration is followed by reabsorption, have unidirectional fluid movement with exclusively outward transfer of water and solutes.

The fluid passing from the glomerulus into the lumen of the tubule contains all of the soluble constituents of the plasma with the exception of the plasma proteins, most enzymes, and hormones which have molecular weights larger than 70,000. The mechanism of the transport process of the soluble plasma constituents which cross the basement membrane to form the ultrafiltrate is not known. It is generally assumed, although not unequivocally demonstrated, that microscopic pores 75–100 Å in diameter (Pitts, 1968) exist in the basement membrane. Whether pores exist or not, the basement membrane behaves as the selective sieve rejecting large molecules and allowing easy transport of the small ones. The molecular weight of 70,000 is based on the observations that free hemoglobin (MW 68,000) and some albumin (MW 69,000) undoubtedly pass into the Bowman's space and that these substances are reabsorbed in the tubules. One would expect pores of 100 Å to allow easy passage of albumin, but its passage is retarded due to viscous drag as well as steric and electrical hindrance (Searcy, 1969). Proteins of molecular weight larger than 70,000 are not normally found in the urine of healthy animals, and (as far as it is known) there is no barrier to proteins of smaller molecular weight. As a guide to damage of the glomerular membrane, it is of no clinical importance to identify large protein molecules in the urine. Although the basement membrane may have no pores, it does not allow selective permeability to ions or solutes of low molecular weights, a feature characterizing all other cell membranes. The size selectivity of this structure is surprisingly precise, however. For all practical purposes the fluid that passes into the Bowman's space is an ultrafiltered solution, whatever the mechanism of selection.

The outward transfer of fluid at the glomerulus depends on the hydrostatic pressure of the blood in the glomerular capillaries, which is ultimately derived from the contraction of the myocardium. Blood pressure measurement is rarely made in veterinary medicine; however, one should be aware of the consequential effects on renal function of those diseases which alter cardiac output either by altering heart rate or stroke volume. Within the arterial blood pressure range of 100–180 mmHg, renal blood flow (RBF) and glomerular filtration rate (GFR) are almost constant. Under these circumstances, glomerular capillary pressure remains in the range of 70 mmHg. This hydrostatic pressure of the capillaries which is responsible for filtration, is opposed by two other forces which are (1) the hydrostatic pressure of the proximal tubule fluid of approximately 15 mmHg (Gottschalk and Mylle, 1956), and (2) the oncotic pressure of the plasma proteins of approximately 25 mmHg. The net filtration pressure is of the order of 30 mmHg [70 − (15 + 25) = 30]. Thus, if arterial blood pressure falls below 90 mmHg, filtration ceases because no energy is available for the outward transfer of the plasma water. At normal physiological concentrations, the osmotic pressure of the plasma proteins (oncotic pressure) of most mammals exerts a pressure of approximately 25–30 mmHg (Bard, 1961). As oncotic pressure depends upon the molecular size, albumin exerts a greater effect than the various globulins or fibrinogen. Consequently a large decrease in albumin concentration influences filtration dynamics.

B. DISTRIBUTION OF CIRCULATION WITHIN THE KIDNEY

Blood is not evenly distributed throughout the entire kidney tissue. An understanding of the distribution of the circulation within the kidney is essential for the explanation of many of the functional changes observed in renal disease.

The anatomical subdivision of the kidney is into cortex and medulla. Within these areas the functional unit is the nephron and the structural unit is the lobule, which is comprised of many nephrons. The renal artery progressively subdivides within the kidney to become the interlobular artery and hence into afferent arterioles to supply glomeruli in neighboring lobules. By this arrangement, blood is not discretely distributed, because an individual lobule can receive blood supply from several interlobular arteries. The efferent arterioles from the glomerules break into capillaries which supply the convoluted tubules (peritubular capillaries) or the loops of Henle (vasa recta vessels). These vessels do not necessarily perfuse either the tubule or the loop of Henle of their respective glomerulus. This efferent blood is uniformly distributed to all areas. Most of the efferent blood supplies convoluted tubules with the result that the medulla has a very much lower blood flow than the cortex (Trueta et al., 1947; Kramer et al., 1960). In unanesthetized dogs, the blood flow in ml/100 gm-min was 74.2 for the cortex, 13.2 for the outer-medulla and 1.7 for the inner-medulla region (Thorburn et al., 1963). The low blood flow to the medulla assists in the maintenance of the osmotic gradient necessary for the functioning of the countercurrent mechanism which is responsible for the concentration and dilution of the tubular fluid. The medulla is an oxygen-poor tissue because of the low blood supply, and this probably explains several anatomical and functional observations. The mitochondria are either absent or few in number (Rhodin, 1958), and cell metabolism is primarily anaerobic (Kean et al., 1961). The low blood flow to this area causes both an osmotic and oxygen gradient from the corticomedullary junction to the tip of the papilla. Because of the free diffusibility of oxygen, urine oxygen concentration is the same as that at the papilla of the medulla. Factors which alter the blood flow through the medulla and reduce the oxygen gradient can therefore be monitored by changes in urine oxygen tension.

Unlike the glomerular capillaries, the peritubular capillaries have bidirectional fluid movement, supplying oxygen and nutrient to the metabolically hyperactive tubule cells, as well as accommodating the fluid absorbed by the tubule cells from the glomerular filtrate.

The production of osmotically concentrated urine depends upon the maintenance of high renal medullary osmolality and antidiuretic hormone (ADH) activity, and it has been suggested that one effect of ADH may be the reduction of medullary blood flow by selective vasoconstriction of the medullary vessels. Recently Aukland (1968) has demonstrated that ADH has no effect on total renal perfusion or medullary blood flow. Factors influencing the regulation of medullary blood flow have not been fully identified. Jick et al. (1963) have suggested that glucocorticoids may be essential for the maintenance of the low medullary blood flow. Renal intraarterial perfusion of bradykinin caused "washout" of the medulla leading to failure of urinary concentration which could not be corrected by ADH (Barraclough and Mills, 1965). Other renal vasodilators, choline, kallidin, and acetylcholine, produce similar effects. Studies with isolated perfused kidneys (Mills et al., 1966), in which increased blood flow was not reflected by a rise in GFR, demonstrate that the medullary vasculature does not have autoregulation and therefore can accommodate a greater blood flow. The medullary capillaries are conspicuously thin-walled (Spargo, 1966), and it is possible that they are easily occluded and dilated with corresponding changes in the medullary blood flow. The circulation time through the medulla has been found to be 30 seconds as compared with the normal cortical circulation time of 3 seconds (Ullrich et al., 1961).

C. RENAL BLOOD FLOW

The normal cardiac output of the dog ranges from 2500 to 4500 ml/min, and the rate of blood flow through the kidneys varies from 200 to 400 ml/min. That fraction of the cardiac output which passes through the kidneys is of the order of 8–9%. This is in striking contrast to the blood supply of human kidneys to which 20–25% of the cardiac output is supplied. Renal perfusion is dependent on several factors, the most important of which are arterial blood pressure, vicosity of the blood, the diameter or resistance of the arterioles, and the length of the renal capillary bed. At arterial blood pressures between 100 and 160 mmHg, the rate of blood flow through the kidney remains essentially constant. The ability to maintain constant blood flow is known as autoregulation. This property is perhaps best demonstrated in the kidneys, but it is also exhibited by cardiac and skeletal muscles. In muscle tissues, autoregulation is determined primarily by oxygen tension. In the kidney, however, even though oxygen consumption of renal tissue is high, renal venous blood is only slightly less saturated with oxygen than arterial blood because of the large flow rate. Robinson (1967) has suggested that the large circulation seems related to the services rendered by the kidneys rather than to respiratory needs. Oxygen consumption, therefore varies with GFR (Thurau, 1961). Autoregulation of the renal circulation depends entirely upon intrarenal control mechanisms which regulate the tone of the afferent arteriole. Perhaps the pressure perceived at the juxtaglomerular apparatus in some way monitors the blood flow through this organ (Thurau, 1964). The integrity of the nervous system is not essential for autoregulation, since this phenomenon has been exhibited by intact, denervated, and isolated perfused kidneys.

D. Alteration in Renal Blood Flow

Decreased renal perfusion occurs under any condition producing intense sympathetic activity, such as constriction or occlusion of the common carotid arteries, asphyxia, emotion, pain, or fear. Physiological concentrations of adrenaline, noradrenaline, renin, angiotensin, and serotonin all decrease blood flow rate. Most anesthetics have no effect, but cyclopropane, ether, and urethane all decrease renal perfusion. In man, postural hypotension can lead to renal ischemia. Horses kept in slings for long periods are the only animal counterpart to this. Renal blood flow may be limited to such an extent that filtration ceases when (1) cardiac output is decreased as may occur with right atrial dilation during venous engorgement, or (2) when extracellular fluid volume is decreased due to dehydration or hemorrhage. On the contrary, increased cardiac output due to overtransfusion will increase renal perfusion. This is one reason why blood transfusion for small animals at the surgical standard unit of 7 ml/lb body weight should be given no faster than 2 ml/lb-hr. The concept that the kidneys will make rapid compensation by excreting excess plasma water if transfused more quickly is erroneous. Increased renal blood flow will also occur in response to acetate and lactate infusions. Aminopyrine, an antipyretic, will also cause this change when given intravenously. Alterations in renal blood flow under pathological conditions will be discussed later.

E. Perfusion Pressure Changes within the Kidney

Mean renal arterial pressure in the dog is 120–130 mmHg. The first major change in resistance within the kidney occurs at the afferent arteriole at which site the perfusing pressure reduces to 70–80 mmHg. A small fall in perfusion pressure occurs across the glomerular capillaries, but the major alteration occurs at the efferent arteriole where the pressure reduces from 70 to about 20 mmHg. There is a small fall in pressure along the peritubular capillaries and within the interlobular veins so that in the renal vein the pressure is of the order of 7 mm Hg. The two major changes in resistance occur at afferent and efferent arterioles. Pressure distribution within the urinary system is summarized in Table I.

TABLE I   PRESSURE DISTRIBUTION WITHIN THE KIDNEY IN THE DOG[a]

Vascular system	Excretory system
Renal artery (mean), 120	Proximal tubule, 15
Afferent arteriole, 120–70	Loop of Henle, 15–8
Glomerular capillaries, 70	Distal tubule, 8
Efferent arterioles, 70–20	Pelvis, 5
Peritubular capillaries, 20–10	Bladder, 0–5
Renal vein, 6	

[a]All pressures, mmHg.

Gertz et al. (1966) have shown that within the arterial blood pressure range in which autoregulation occurs, the change in resistance of the afferent arterioles is such that it always provides a similar initial pressure at the glomerular capillaries. The concept that the alteration in the afferent arteriolar tone controls autoregulation is widely accepted.

Whe systemic blood pressure falls below 100 mmHg (lower limits for autoregulation in the dog), RBF, GFR, and urine flow all deteriorate. One explanation for these changes has been that as arterial blood pressure falls, there is a corresponding decrease in the glomerular capillary pressure and the net filtration pressure. Filtration ceases ultimately when the net filtration pressure equals the opposing pressures. At presures below 90 mmHg in the rat, the afferent arteriole fails to act as resistance, and the glomerular capillary pressure is essentially equal to the arterial pressure (Gertz et al., 1966). Theoretically, some degree of glomerular filtration must be maintained until systemic blood pressure falls to 45 mmHg, which is below the limits compatible with life. For all practical purposes, GFR ceases in the dog when the systemic blood pressure falls below 100 mmHg, while RBF is maintained at 60 or 70% of its normal level at blood pressures over 80 mmHg. At low levels of perfusion, there is no correlation between renal oxygen consumption and either renal function or urine flow, which suggests that renal ischemia does not cause the functional deterioration (Brun and Munck, 1966).

Although autoregulation implies consistency of perfusion, corollary to this is consistency of GFR. In animals receiving regular feeding, GFR is probably constant, with some allowance for a small diurnal variation. In animals with irregular food intake, GFR fluctuates in accordance with metabolic necessity. As mentioned above, consistency of GFR is constant only if the afferent and efferent arterial pressures remain in balance and the pressure difference across the glomerular capillaries remains small. Besides depending on the hydrostatic pressure at the glomerulus, GFR also is affected by the interplay of the pressures of the afferent and efferent arterioles. Five circumstances could possibly occur:

1. Normally, reduction in pressure across the glomerular capillaries is small, with afferent and efferent arterioles in balance.

2. Constriction of the afferent arteriole may occur with the net result of a fall in GFR and RBF.

3. With dilation of the afferent arteriole, more pressure is transmitted to the glomerular capillaries and the efferent arteriole remains normal, resulting in increased GFR with little change in RBF.

4. With dilation of the efferent arteriole and the afferent arteriole remains normal, there is a large pressure reduction across the glomerular capillaries resulting in a fall in GFR and RBF.

5. Constriction of the efferent arteriole may occur with resulting increased GFR and decreased RBF.

Circumstances 3 and 5 probably do not occur. Apparently there has been no experimental demonstration of increased GFR without concomitant increase in RBF. Included in circumstance 1 is normal afferent and efferent arteriole pressure, or constriction or dilation of both afferent and efferent arteriole; in both cases a small pressure drop across the glomerular capillaries is maintained. With constriction of both arterioles RBF decreases and with dilation of both, RBF increases; in both instances GFR remains normal because it is dependent on the pressure difference and not on RBF.

Both afferent and efferent arterioles are under sympathetic control. If the distribution of α and β adrenergic receptors were such that the efferent arteriole had more β receptors, alterations in GFR and RBF would occur depending on the relative concentrations of adrenaline, noradrenaline, and isopropyl noradrenaline.

F. Tubular Reabsorption

Renal tubule cells selectively reabsorb those substances which are essential to the health of the body. Almost all naturally occurring soluble constituents of the plasma which are filtered at the glomerulus are reabsorbed to some extent. The conspicuous exception is the excretion of creatinine in the dog, which is neither reabsorbed nor secreted. In the horse there is evidence supporting the reabsorption of creatinine (Knudsen, 1959), but in most other animal species, creatinine is secreted.

Tubular reabsorption must have occurred if urinary excretion is less than simultaneous GFR. Reabsorption may be complete or partial, involving either active or passive transport mechanisms. Active transport occurs when a substance is transported against a concentration or electrical gradient. Such a process is energy-dependent, and therefore can be abolished by anoxia or metabolic inhibitors. Passive reabsorption occurs when a substance diffuses along the concentration gradient from the tubular lumen into the peritubular fluid. Both transport mechanisms are time rate-limited and therefore are more complete when the minute urine volume is low.

G. Tubular Secretion

The evidence for tubular secretion is the converse of that for reabsorption, i.e., the urinary excretion of the substance is greater than its simultaneous GFR. Secretion, like reabsorption, occurs in both the proximal and distal tubules. Many substances undergo bidirectional transport; for example, potassium which is reabsorbed in the proximal tubule is secreted from distal tubular sites. Uric acid transport in the Dalmatian dog is very unusual in that reabsorption and secretion both take place in the proximal tubule (Kessler et al., 1959), and it has been suggested that a similar process may occur in man (Gutman and Yü, 1957). There is no evidence to suggest that breeds of dogs other than the Dalmatian secrete uric acid. That which appears in the urine is derived from glomerular filtration.

II. ELECTROLYTES AND NONELECTROLYTES

A. GLUCOSE

Glucose is one of the few plasma components which is completely reabsorbed under normal circumstances; glucosuria is always associated with abnormal renal function. Glucose is freely filtered and actively reabsorbed in the proximal tubule. The transport mechanism depends on a carrier substance within the luminal cell wall and with a high affinity for glucose, joining with the glucose in the tubular fluid. The resulting complex migrates to the cytoplasmic surface of the lumenal membrane where the glucose is cleaved off and delivered to the cytoplasm, and the carrier substance then migrates back to the lumenal surface of the cell membrane (Shannon, 1939; Beyer, 1950). This carrier system illustrates in general terms the active transport of electrolyte and nonelectrolyte. The specific biochemical mechanisms of these systems has not been elucidated. By mechanisms which are not precisely understood, the active transport of glucose can be prevented by phlorizin, a metabolic inhibitor, or by circulating endotoxin (Lotspeich, 1959). Glucosuria occurs when the transport mechanism is saturated because insufficient carrier is available to combine with the quantity of glucose filtered; i.e., more glucose is delivered to the proximal tubule than the carrier system can transport. Under these circumstances, the quantity of the carrier does not increase, and once the reabsorption process is fully saturated, the rate of reabsorption becomes constant regardless of the concentration of glucose delivered to the tubule. The tubular maximum (Tm) varies from animal to animal, but in any one individual, it is remarkably constant. The major factor affecting Tm_G is the number and surface area of functioning proximal tubules. It is not customary to think in terms of tubular maxima in relation to kidney weight. If use is to be made in veterinary medicine of this important measurement as an assessment of proximal tubular activity, it would be best to discuss tubular maxima per unit of body weight. Tm_G is not affected by alternations in GFR and thus provides a reasonable assessment of the number of functioning nephrons.

The quantity of glucose (mg/min) delivered to the proximal tubule is derived from the product of GFR and the plasma glucose concentration. There is only one plasma glucose concentration when the quantity delivered to the tubules exactly equals the Tm_G. That concentration is referred to as the renal glucose threshold and above this concentration, glucosuria occurs. Therefore, to determine the Tm_G it is necessary to know the GFR, the urine volume (ml/min) and plasma and urine glucose concentrations (Shannon et al., 1941). The procedure requires the intravenous infusion of glucose to the extent that the plasma concentration rises to approximately

600 mg/100 ml. Tm_G is the difference between the glucose filtered and the glucose excreted per minute. The relationship between the renal glucose threshold and glucosuria is obviously dependent on the GFR. For this reason, many diabetic dogs with plasma glucose concentrations of the order of 600 mg % may not show glucosuria simply because the GFR is tremendously depressed with the result that the absolute amount of glucose delivered to the proximal tubule does not exceed the reabsorptive capacity.

B. *p*-AMINOHIPPURATE, DIODRAST, AND PHENOL RED

Each of these substances is partially filtered at the glomerulus, the main bulk of their excretion coming from proximal tubular secretion (Brown *et al.*, 1961). These organic acids are secreted by a transport system which is the reverse of that employed for reabsorption. Independent active transport systems operate for the passage both into and out of the tubule cells. None of these organic acids are stored in the tubule cells. The transport mechanisms responsible for transfer into the tubular lumen from the peritubular fluid requires the presence of potassium and calcium ions, neither of which are likely to be limited in a living animal. The effects of calcium and potassium are independent; potassium activates transport at the peritubular membrane, and calcium activates the transport at the luminal membrane (Puck *et al.*, 1952).

Mudge and Taggart (1950a) showed that 2,4-dinitrophenol (10 mg/kg body weight) administered as a single injection caused marked reduction in the tubular secretion of PAH, Diodrast, or phenol red, but had no effect on glucose reabsorption or on renal hemodynamics. This demonstrates that oxidative phosphorylation was specifically involved in tubular secretory transport. In acute experiments, the maximum tubular transport of PAH (Tm_{PAH}) can be increased by infusions of acetate and lactate and decreased by succinate and fumarate. All of these substances were shown to have no effect on Tm_G (Mudge and Taggart, 1950b). The increase in Tm_{PAH} implies that certain cellular components of the secretory transfer process are available in limited quantities. Long-term administration of testosterone (Welsh *et al.*, 1942), thyroxin (Eiler *et al.*, 1944), vitamin A (Bing, 1943), and anterior pituitary extract (Heinbecker *et al.*, 1943) will cause an increase in Tm_{PAH} in the dog. This effect is probably due to hypertrophy of the renal tissue rather than to a specific effect on transport.

C. PROTEIN

The glomerular filtrate is essentially a protein-free liquid. This generalization is true when it is considered that the glomerular filtrate contains approximately 30 mg/100 ml as compared with the plasma protein concentration of 5–8 gm/100 ml (Pitts, 1968). It has been suggested that this concentration of protein in the glomerular filtrate may be an overestimate. With very sensitive immunological methods, no detectable albumin was found in 90% of samples collected from dog proximal tubules under conditions in which 2 or 3 mg/100 ml would have been detectable by other procedures (Berliner, 1966; Dirks *et al.*, 1964). The urine of most healthy dogs contains no detectable protein. The lowest concentration of detectable protein in the urine obtained by the usual chemical methods is between 20 and 30 mg/100 ml.

Normally only 2% of the water filtered at the glomerulus is excreted as urine. Small quantities of protein in normal concentrated urine do not represent any serious disturbance of the renal handling of protein. It is frequently implied that a trace of protein in dilute urine is significant. As a large urine volume of low specific gravity constitutes only 4% of the filtered water being excreted as urine, a small amount of protein in the urine therefore implies 2% of the filtered protein is being excreted, which is insignificant. Under normal circumstances, the reabsorption of protein is complete or almost complete.

Proteins are reabsorbed intact from the tubular fluid either by pinocytosis into the tubule cell, where they are broken down into component amino acids and then transported into the peritubular fluid, or by arthrocytosis, by which they are transported intact to the peritubular fluid. Hyaline or colloid droplets (protein reabsorption droplets) may be seen histologically in tubular epithelial cells (Mendel, 1959). It has recently been argued that these acidophilic granules are not pinocytosed material but oncotically swollen, intrinsic cellular organelles, including mitochondria (Allen, 1966). The reabsorption mechanism has limited capacity, and therefore Tm for protein probably exists; proteinuria occurs only when this is exceeded. From the evidence of Terry et al. (1948), the renal plasma threshold for persistent proteinuria is a plasma protein concentration of 10 gm/100 ml (albumin 6 gm/100 ml), which is not likely to be exceeded. Proteinuria is frequently observed in the osmotic diuresis occurring in chronic interstitial nephritis. Under these circumstances it is the washout effect of the diuresis and not the inability of the tubule to reabsorb protein or excessive leakage at the glomerulus.

At normal plasma concentrations, hemoglobin is 100% globulin-bound, and it is not until its protein-binding capacity is exceeded at approximately 130 mg/100 ml that free hemoglobin is present in the plasma (Lathen, 1959). Hemoglobin is reabsorbed in the proximal tubule (Lathen et al., 1960); whether a Tm exists for hemoglobin is not known, but the amount that is reabsorbed is comparatively small.

D. Amino Acids

The kidney has no regulatory function in amino acid metabolism, because, like glucose, the reabsorption capacity greatly exceeds the quantity of amino acids normally filtered. Active amino acid reabsorption against the concentration gradient occurs in the proximal tubule at the site where the secretion of p-aminohippurate (PAH) is greatest (Brown et al., 1961). Several transport mechanisms are involved, one for each of the following groups: dibasic amino acids (lysine, arginine, ornithine, and cystine); dicarboxylic amino acids (glutamic, aspartic); the glycine group (proline, hydroxyproline, and glycine); and the monoamino-monocarboxylic amino acids (alanine, valine, trytophan, and cystine). There is probably not a single transport mechanism for each group of amino acids; however, there must be some common factor in individual transport mechanisms because glutamic acid partially depresses the reabsorption of most other amino acids. There has been no demonstration of a Tm for amino acids. With increased concentrations of plasma amino acids as may occur in liver failure, quantity filtered exceeds the capacity of the tubules for reabsorption, and under these circumstances aminoaciduria occurs. Proximal tubular defects may also cause aminoaciduria. These may be hereditary (Harris and

Milne, 1964). Aminoaciduria may also occur when plasma amino acid concentrations are normal or reduced, due to defective proximal tubular function (Dent and Harris, 1951; Treacher, 1964). Defects or absence of these transport systems may be congenital (Harris and Milne, 1964), but this has not been established for domestic animals.

E. Creatine

Human urine contains little creatine; and by comparison, urine from most animals contains large quantities of this substance. Pitts (1934) has shown that plasma clearance of creatine rises sharply with increasing plasma concentration and that there is competitive interaction between glycine, alanine, and creatine reabsorption. It is not known what mechanism is responsible for increased urinary creatine in animals.

F. Ammonia

Although the plasma concentration of ammonia is very low, urinary excretion can be considerable, dependent on the metabolic status of the animal. Ammonia is derived primarily from glutamine, but other plasma amino acids also contribute. The distal tubule cells are particularly rich in glutaminases and other enzymes which deaminate amino acids to ammonia (Pitts, 1964). Ammonia diffuses from the cell into the lumen where it is trapped as NH_4^+ from combination with H^+. This creates a diffusion gradient which is dependent upon hydrogen ion concentration (pH) of the tubular fluid.

G. Urea

Urea is a freely permeable molecule. Because of this, the amount passively reabsorbed in each segment of the nephron depends upon both the area of the absorbing surface and the concentration gradient from the tubular lumen to the peritubular fluid. Creation of a concentration gradient for urea depends exclusively on water movement. The proximal tubule, although it has 80% of the surface area of the tubule system, develops only a comparatively small concentration gradient (a urine to plasma ratio (U/P) with maximal value 3) with the result that 20% of filtered urea is reabsorbed. In the ascending limb of the loop of Henle, urea enters the tubular fluid (Ullrich et al., 1963). Variation in urea excretion results from changes in water reabsorption in the distal tubule and particularly the collecting ducts. When moderately concentrated urine is produced, about 20% of the filtered urea is reabsorbed by the distal system and U/P is about 25–30. Under normal circumstances, therefore, approximately 40% filtered urea is reabsorbed. With highly concentrated urine, U/P ratio can be as high as 100, and the percentage of filtered urea reabsorbed by the tubules will be greater. Alternatively, during diuresis, urea reabsorption by the distal system will be minimal, and U/P ratio may be as low as 4. In all animals except ruminants, urea reabsorption and excretion (mg/min) by healthy kidneys varies in direct proportion to plasma concentration. On low-protein diets, sheep conserve urea, but other species do not (Schmidt-Nielsen, 1958).

H. SODIUM

Sodium is reabsorbed by the proximal and distal cells, as well as by cells of the ascending limb of the loop of Henle; sodium enters the tubular fluid in the descending limb of the loop of Henle. Transport of sodium from the lumen to the peritubular fluid across the proximal tubular cell involves two and possibly three transport systems. The interior of the proximal tubular cell is electrically negative and has a low sodium concentration. The luminal membrane is freely permeable to sodium, which enters the cell by passive diffusion along an electrochemical gradient or by carrier-mediated passive transfer (Pitts, 1968). At the peritubular membrane, sodium is actively pumped out of the cell into the peritubular fluid. Transfer of sodium at this membrane is intimately connected with entry of potassium into the cell from the peritubular fluid. These two transport systems are coupled through their interdependence on a membrane carrier. The detailed biochemistry of the sodium pump has not been elucidated. Its energy is probably derived from high energy phosphate bonds, because inhibitors of phosphoralative oxidation, i.e., dinitrophenol or cyanide, block sodium reabsorption. It is the active process for extrusion which determines the net transfer of sodium. As the tubular fluid is electrically negative, approximately 20 mV as compared with the peritubular fluid, net transfer of sodium is against an electrical gradient and is therefore an active process.

The precise mechanism of sodium reabsorption in the distal tubule, which is under the control of aldosterone, has not been established. Increased aldosterone activity results in retention of sodium and increased potassium excretion.

The excretion of sodium into the lumen of the descending loop of Henle is exclusively by passive diffusion across the luminal membrane of the tubule cells, down an electrochemical gradient.

I. POTASSIUM

Filtered potassium is completely reabsorbed in the proximal tubules; that which appears in the urine is secreted by the distal tubule cells (Berliner, 1960). The major factor influencing potassium secretion is the relative concentration of potassium and hydrogen ions in the tubule cells. In common with all cells, those of the proximal and distal tubules actively transport potassium intracellularly. At the distal tubule sites, sodium ions are exchanged for potassium ions. The electrochemical gradient is such that for this process to occur, potassium ions are only passively secreted into the lumen (Malnic et al., 1966; Giebisch et al., 1966). There is some doubt that the potassium secretory process is simply a matter of diffusion down an electrical gradient (Berliner, 1966), because it can be shown at times to be independent of the concentration gradient and is subject to specific inhibition, particularly by mercury (Berliner, 1960; Orloff and Davidson, 1959).

J. HYDROGEN

Hydrogen ions are actively secreted from the tubular fluid into the lumen throughout both the proximal and distal tubules. There is an unlimited pool of hydrogen ions within tubular cells from dissociation of carbonic acid. Hydrogen ions are secreted by all cells in a one for one exchange with reabsorption of sodium ions. Within the proximal tubule, the hydrogen ions are only momentarily present. They immediately combine with bicarbonate ions to form carbonic acid, which dissociates into carbon dioxide and water, both of which are reabsorbed. The availability of bicarbonate ion is limited, and there are usually no bicarbonate ions available at the distal tubule. At this site, hydrogen ion combines with ammonia to form the ammonium ion; or if no substrate is available, they are excreted as such and contribute to the acidity of the urine. Secretion by the distal tubule cell is dependent on intracellular hydrogen ion concentration and like potassium, is exchanged on a one to one basis with sodium. There is usually no competition between the hydrogen and the potassium ion for exchange with sodium because of the extensive availability of sodium ions in the distal tubular fluid.

K. CALCIUM AND MAGNESIUM

These divalent ions are reabsorbed in the proximal tubule and probably share a common intratubular transport mechanism because both are affected by the concentration of circulating parathormone. There is no evidence for their secretion, and the amount which appears in the urine is the net result of reabsorption in relation to the amount filtered. Tubular maxima for calcuim transport probably exist (Copp *et al.*, 1960). At plasma calcium concentrations less than 7 mg/100 ml, no calcium is found in the urine. This observation has formed the basis for a simple laboratory test for hypocalcemia in humans, the Sulkowitch test, which has been found unsuitable for clinical use in animals. There are interesting species differences in the proportions of calcium and magnesium in the urine. While the plasma concentrations in the various species are similar, the cat's urine differs in having relatively little calcium and large amounts of magnesium. Species differences in the sensitivity of the proximal tubule to parathormone probably occur and therefore explain these observations.

L. BICARBONATE

When animals are fed either a carnivorous or mixed diet, the urine is almost devoid of bicarbonate, whereas urine from animals receiving a herbivorous diet contains large quantities of this ion. Bicarbonate reabsorption has been extensively studied in the dog, but little is known about how it is handled by the ruminant kidney. In the dog, bicarbonate is almost completely reabsorbed in the proximal tubule by a mechanism which is *Tm*-limited. The renal threshold for plasma bicarbonate is of the order of 27–28 mEq/liter. Bicarbonate ions are not reabsorbed as such; present evidence suggests the lumenal membrane of the proximal tubule cell is completely impermeable to them. Bicarbonate reabsorption requires the presence of hydrogen ions and the enzyme, carbonic anhydrase. The hydrogen ions are available because they are extruded into the lumen by the proximal tubule cell. Carbonic anhydrase being a small protein (MW 30,000) could be filtered at the glomerulus but it is generally thought to be in very low concentration in the plasma. The more probable source of this enzyme is the proximal tubule cells which have a particularly high concentration along their luminal brush border. The chemistry of bicarbonate reabsorption is exactly the same as that of the bicarbonate buffer system acting in any body cell; the following reaction takes place

$$HCO_3^- + H^+ \rightleftharpoons H_2CO_3 \rightleftharpoons CO_2 + H_2O$$

carbonic anhydrase

The mechanism of bicarbonate reabsorption is that the reaction is driven to the right because CO_2 freely diffuses into the cell along a concentration gradient. The pH at which this reaction occurs influences the dissociation of carbonic acid. At normal physiological pH 7.4 the carbonic acid/bicarbonate equilibrium is such that 95–99% is dissociated, and the carbonic acid/CO_2 equilibrium is only 5–10% in the dissociated form so the overall effect is that the reaction is strongly driven to the left. The pK for carbonic acid occurs at pH 6.1. Thus for bicarbonate reabsorption to occur, the pH of the proximal tubular fluid must be of the order of one pH unit less than normal physiological pH. The extrusion of hydrogen is necessary not only for the combination with bicarbonate, but to provide the necessary acidic conditions for the reaction to be driven to the right. The CO_2 entering the proximal tubule cell at pH 7.4 is therefore in an environment in which the reaction is driven to the left, and bicarbonate and hydrogen ions become available. The hydrogen ions are actively transported back to the lumen (see Section II, J), leaving potential accumulation of bicarbonate within the cell. Unlike the luminal membrane, the peritubular membrane is freely permeable to bicarbonate, which diffuses out of the cell along a chemical gradient. In the absence of carbonic anhydrase, the reaction between CO_2 and carbonic acid is very slow, taking a long time to come to equilibrium. Thus when the action of carbonic anhydrase is inhibited, urine becomes alkaline and contains a substantial fraction of filtered bicarbonate (Gilman, 1958).

M. PHOSPHATE

Although phosphate exists in several forms within the body, only inorganic phosphate is found in the urine. Renal handling of phosphate is similar to that for calcium and magnesium, as it is under the control of circulating parathormone, calcitonin, and thyroxine. A tubular maximum exists for the reabsorption of phosphate, but unlike that for glucose, it is not constant for an individual and shows wide variation over a large population. Like glucose, the tubular maximum for phosphate is independent of GFR, being primarily affected by the filtered load of phosphate (Pitts and Alexander 1944). Increased phosphate excretion is not due to decreased tubular maxima phosphate, but to increased filtered load as parathormone also has a significant effect on GFR. Tubular maxima of phosphate for the ruminant are not known, but are probably greater than those for dog or man, because at normal plasma phosphate concentrations urinary phosphate excretion is minimal. However, the ruminant kidney is very sensitive to increased levels of circulating parathormone. Glucose and phosphate reabsorption are interdependent; it is probably that they share part of a common transport system. Pitts and Alexander (1944) showed that an infusion of glucose sufficient to saturate the reabsorption transport system also reduced the *Tm* for phosphate. Administration of phlorizin increased the tubular maxima of phosphate and inhibits glucose reabsorption.

N. Bilirubin

Both conjugated and unconjugated bilirubin may be found in the urine of icteric patients; there is usually a far greater proportion of conjugated bilirubin (Gries and Gries, 1957). Although bilirubin is strongly bound to plasma proteins, urinary bilirubin excretion is probably by glomerular filtration (Ali and Billing, 1968). Earlier investigations had suggested an active distal tubular secretion process (Barac, 1951; Laks et al., 1963). What remains to be explained is why bilirubin is precipitated in the tubule cells of the proximal tubule and the ascending limb of the loop of Henle in kidneys of icteric animals. The only known exception to this observation is in Dubin-Johnson sheep, in which precipitated bilirubin is found in both the proximal and distal tubule cells. Because conjugated and unconjugated serum bilirubin are firmly bound to serum albumin, only small traces of bilirubin could possibly pass the glomerulus by filtration to enter the proximal tubule. Conventional inhibitors and competitors of tubular secretion do not interfere with bilirubin secretion (Fulop and Brazeau, 1964). There is species variation in the kidney threshold to bilirubin excretion. Sheep are particularly low and the cat particularly high, with dogs and horses intermediate between these species.

O. Mucoprotein

Stopflow studies suggest that the collecting ducts are the site of excretion of mucoproteins (McQueen, 1962; Maxfield, 1961). Although mucoproteins are scarce in plasma, under certain conditions they can be excreted in quantity and are important because of a possible role in cast and calculus formation.

P. Water

Figure 1 shows the functional organization of the nephron in relation to reabsorption of sodium and water and formation of diluted and concentrated urine. The cell wall of the proximal tubule is freely permeable to water. At this site, 80% of the glomerular filtrate is reabsorbed due primarily to the reabsorption of sodium and maintenance of isotonicity of the tubular fluid. The cells of the descending limb of the loop of Henle are also freely permeable to water and at least relatively permeable to sodium; the tubular fluid at this site quickly comes into osmotic equilibrium with the hypertonic interstitial fluid of the medulla. In the ascending limb of the loop of Henle and the initial portion of the distal tubule, cells are impermeable to the transfer of water. Sodium, and possibly urea, are actively pumped out into the interstitial fluid with the result that sodium chloride is trapped helping to establish the hypertonic gradient in the medulla. The permeability of the cells lining the posterior distal tubule and the collecting ducts is dependent on the ADH activity. In the absence of ADH, little or no water is reabsorbed; with increasing ADH concentrations, water transfers from the collecting duct fluid and the urine becomes increasingly hypertonic.

The degree of urine concentration is dependent both on the permeability of the collecting duct and the extent of the osmotic gradient in the medulla. The renal cortex is isotonic with plasma; the osmotic gradient becomes progressively hypertonic,

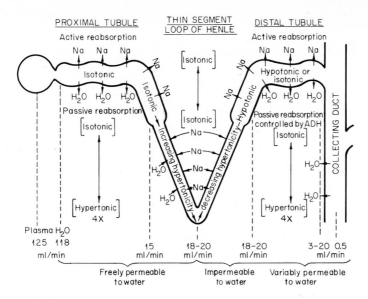

Fig. 1. The functional organization of the nephron in relation to reabsorption of sodium and water and formation of dilute and concentrated urine. The diagram incorporates the views of Wirz, Hargatoy, and Kuhn, and Gottschalk and Berliner. (From Pitts, 1959.)

reaching maximum osmolarity at the renal pelvis. The pattern of this gradient is maintained by the high sodium and urea concentration and the low medullary blood flow in the interstitial tissue fluid in the medulla. Sodium chloride is the major solute in the loop fluid, and urea is the predominant solute in the final urine (potassium is the predominant electrolyte in the urine of domestic animals). The loop fluid becomes hypertonic by the diffusion of water out of the descending limb into the hypertonic medullary interstitium, but inward diffusion of urea also occurs and contributes to the increase in the osmolarity of the loop fluid. The osmotic gradient in the medullary interstitium results from the continuous movement of sodium out of the ascending limb of the loop of Henle without an accompanying water loss. The gradient would be destroyed if it were not for the unique long loops of the vasa recta which double back on themselves. The plasma in the descending vascular limb receives small increments of sodium and becomes more concentrated as it passes deeper into the medulla where the surrounding fluid in turn has an increasing concentration. As the vessel returns to the cortex, it loses small quantities of sodium to the interstitial fluid, which is gradually decreasing in concentration. The net movement of sodium out of the interstitial fluid by way of the capillary loop is small, and the osmolar gradient of sodium can thus be maintained.

Potassium is secreted by the distal tubule cells and in most domestic animal species, particularly herbivores, potassium becomes the predominant ion in the tubular urine. In the presence of ADH, water leaves the tubular urine in the latter portion of the distal tubule and collecting ducts to enter the interstitial fluid, with the result that the urine becomes more concentrated. Urea moves out of the tubular urine into the interstitial fluid, and the same countercurrent exchange by the capillaries results in building up a gradient of urea in the medulla. This recirculation of urea in the nephron from the collecting ducts to the medullary interstitium to the descending limb of the loop of Henle is essential for the maintenance of the maximum medullary osmotic concentration gradient. In prolonged diuresis, the concentration gradient is "washed out" due to the loss of urea for recirculation.

III.   TECHNIQUES USED IN TRANSPORT STUDIES

Stop flow technique pioneered by Malvin *et al.* (1957, 1958), has been widely used to study the spatial sequence of transport of individual substances and relation between substances.

The following is their description of the method (Malvin *et al.*, 1958):

> The method depends upon the concentration pattern derived from urine samples caught serially from a catheter following a brief period of ureteral occlusion. If a dog is infused with a high load of osmotic diuretic, such as mannitol, the urine to plasma concentration ratios (U/P) for most substances approach 1.0. If now the ureteral catheter is occluded, filtration at the glomeruli will stop when the tubular pressure becomes equal to the net filtration pressure. The urine in the tubules which had been relatively unchanged from that of glomerular filtrate will now be exposed to the action of the various nephron segments for as long as the ureteral occlusion lasts. Previous administration of the osmotic diuretic provides a watery menstrum against which electrolytes may be reabsorbed. The various substances will not be reabsorbed or secreted more completely, and new U/P ratios developed which will differ from the control U/P ratio. Also, the concentration of any substance will vary along the nephron depending upon how the individual segments handle that substance. Creatinine concentrations might be expected to vary along the entire nephron only as a result of water movement, secreted substances would show an increase in concentration in the nephron areas which secrete that substance, while the concentration of reabsorbable solutes would fall in those areas responsible for reabsorption. After ample time has been allowed for the concentration patterns to develop during stopped flow the ureteral occlusion is released. Rapid serial urine samples are taken from the new flow. The concentration pattern is caught in these samples collected rapid fire from the polyethylene ureteral catheter after the brief occlusion is released. Thiry to thirty-five samples are collected within about 2.5 minutes, each sample averaging about 0.5 ml. The pattern of concentration is oriented along the column of fluid moving out of each nephron. Serial urine samples segment this into an ordered array which is best caught on a graph if plotted as concentration against the accumulated volume of fluid which has appeared between reinstatement of flow and the appearance of the sample. Plots against time show a distortion due to variable flow rates.

The common modification of the method is the use of inulin concentrations as an indicator of water movement. The technique has the limitation that it can define only grossly the site of reabsorption of secretion (Pitts, 1968). It is, however, the only technique applicable to domestic animals for the study of transport within the nephron. There are many species peculiarities in the renal handling of substances and this technique provides a method for their investigation.

The most exciting technical development in renal physiology has been that of micropuncture of the glomerulus and tubule. The feat was first performed in 1921 by Dr. J. Wearns, who worked in collaboration with Dr. N. Richards, on frog glomeruli. The first major studies on mammalian kidneys were reported by A. M. Walker *et al.* (1941), and the first in dogs were by Clapp *et al.* (1963). Most micropuncture studies involving proximal and distal tubules have been performed on rats; in dogs only the proximal tubule can be punctured. Studies involving the loop of Henle have been performed mostly on hamsters.

The early studies were concerned with fluid composition in the proximal tubule. In the late 1950's, the technique was refined and with the use of sophisticated apparatus, it has yielded detailed knowledge of the magnitude and mechanisms of absorption and secretion by segments of the nephron. Gottschalk and Lassiter (1967) in their review of micropuncture studies of salt and water reabsorption in the mammalian kidney show the impressive data that has been obtained using this technique.

More recently, micropuncture techniques have been used to study functional changes in acute renal damage and have demonstrated some unexpected findings. The experiments demonstrated (1) the formation of urine by morphologically damaged kidneys, (2) functions of such nephrons was not normal, and (3) that the structurally normal parts of the nephrons and collecting ducts partially compensate for deficiency of function in damaged proximal segments with which they were in series (Biber et al., 1969). Previous knowledge of function in pathological nephrons had been based on clearance studies. Smith (1951) had pointed out that from the combined information supplied by inulin and PAH clearance, Tm_{PAH} and PAH extraction, it should be possible to assess the extent of the inert or nonfunctional tissue in a diseased kidney, although he considered inulin clearance might be inaccurate under such conditions. Concepts of nephron function based on clearance studies in disease kidneys (Bricker et al., 1960, 1965) have led to the conclusion that only those nephrons with structural integrity continue to function. These results had been widely accepted and the concept of only undamaged nephrons remaining active was referred to as the "intact nephron hypothesis." The results of micropuncture studies are consistent with the hypothesis that nephrons exhibit a spectrum of functional activities dependent upon their individual structural characteristics. The "intact nephron hypothesis" is now not favorably regarded.

One technical development from micropuncture has been the so-called "split oil drop method" (Shipp et al., 1958). With this technique, the tubule is punctured, a small oil drop is introduced into the lumen. A second puncture is made alongside the first and a solution of known composition is introduced into the oil drop which splits into two droplets, each then acting as a quarantine barrier to prevent the introduced solution from becoming contaminated with tubular fluid or from leaking out of the tubule at the puncture site. After 10–20 minutes, the tubule is again punctured and the fluid between the oil droplets collected. As with the stop flow technique, change in inulin concentration is the basis for volume change calculations. Using a refinement of this technique in combination with photographic measurement to estimate rate of fluid absorption from the column enclosed by the droplets, Gertz et al. (1965) have shown the rate of reabsorption of salt and water in the proximal tubule is proportional to surface area. The dilation of the proximal tubule with increasing filtered loads would increase the surface area which in turn would increase reabsorption of salt and water, and vice versa. Thus, the circumference of the proximal tubule is possibly the prime determinant for the maintenance of glomerulotubular balance which is essential to the continuation of life.

Another development from micropuncture has been the measurement of transtubular short-circuit currents, performed in the frog by F. W. Eigler (1961) and subsequently by Windhagen and Giebisch (1961) in the rat. This development is remarkable for its superb sophistication. It has recently been reviewed by Windhagen and Giebisch (1965). In both the proximal and distal tubule, the cell is electrically negative as compared with the lumen and peritubular fluid. There is no potential difference (PD) between the lumen and peritubular fluid but the membrane of the proximal tubule cell at either boundary has a PD of -70 mV. In the distal tubule, the lumen is electrically negative to the peritubular fluid, the PD being -50 mV; the distal tubule cell has a PD of -20 mV at the luminal membrane and -70 mV at the peritubular membrane.

All renal studies are influenced by the effects of extrarenal factors. By experimental design, these are kept minimal, but a kidney preparation free of such complications would have an important role in renal studies. The first successful attempt at an isolated perfused kidney system was a heart–lung–kidney preparation used by Verney (1947). Totally isolated perfused kidney systems have been reported by A. W. Bauman *et al.* (1963). Studies of renal function by the combination of micropuncture and isolated perfused kidney techniques were first performed by Bahlmann *et al.* (1967) (using rats). Such studies eliminate the effects of volume expansion, feedback control mechanisms, and influences of other organs (so that intrarenal mechanisms can be elucidated). The understanding of intrarenal control mechanisms on transport within the nephron is the exciting challenge of the future.

IV. HOMEOSTASIS AND THE KIDNEY

The living cell requires a very special environment to maintain itself in dynamic equilibrium and to function according to its specialized characteristics. Water, along with particular inorganic ions in particular amounts, is absolutely necessary for cells to perform the complex interactions which constitute living matter. The kidney plays a major role in the maintenance of water and electrolyte homeostasis; of particular importance is control of extracellular fluid (ECF) volume and acid–base balance.

A. WATER AND SODIUM HOMEOSTASIS

Because sodium is the principal electrolyte of the ECF and therefore makes the greatest contribution to the osmolarity, sodium excretion is primarily regulated to maintain the volume of the ECF constant. Maintenance of sodium homeostasis is therefore particularly critical. (Unlike humans, sodium is in comparatively high concentration in the red blood cell in both dog and cat.)

Although changes in both volume, osmolarity and ECF occur simultaneously, the mechanisms for control are independent. Volume control is primarily dependent on the sodium regulation whereas the osmolarity of the ECF is controlled by ADH.

The control of sodium concentration in ECF is solely by renal mechanisms. Variations in urinary excretion of sodium are entirely dependent on tubular reabsorption and independent of glomerular filtration rate (McDonald and de Wardener, 1965). In the proximal tubule, approximately 80% of sodium filtered is reabsorbed; regulatory processes responsible are the glomerulotubule balance (Rector *et al.*, 1966) and volume changes in ECF. (Dirks, 1968). It has been widely regarded that the fine regulation of sodium excretion occurs in the distal tubule under the control of several hormones of which aldosterone appears to have a dominant role. Increased aldosterone secretion is in response to ECF volume depletion and occurs by means of the renin–angiotensin system (Sims and Solomon, 1963). It is becoming increasingly clear that aldosterone activity plays only a limited part in the sodium renal control mechanism because of the ease of escape from its sodium-retaining effect (Jones *et al.*, 1963) due to alteration in proximal tubular reabsorption (Dirks *et al.*, 1965).

Sodium reabsorption causes increase of ECF osmolarity which in turn stimulates the release of ADH. With excessive sodium reabsorption, both thirst and secretion of ADH are stimulated and the resulting increased water intake and water reabsorption help offset the increased osmolarity of ECF. Adlosterone release is in turn primarily responsive to change in blood volume. In the healthy animal both mechanisms are ultimately affected through the kidney by their influence on the reabsorption of sodium and water. In kidney diseases, however, a third factor becomes superimposed, and these two regulatory mechanisms must compensate for decreased GFR. Detailed discussion of the role of aldosterone and ADH in the control of water and electrolyte is beyond the scope of this chapter. Sims and Solomon (1963) have published a diagram of the factors and proposed mechanisms of the activation of these two regulatory systems which illustrates the complexity of the nature of the control.

Plasma osmolarity is monitored at the hypothalamus. An increase of 2% in plasma osmolarity initiates the secretion of ADH or an equivalent decrease leads to cessation of secretion (Verney, 1947). ADH has a very prompt action on the kidney and as well has a very short biological half-life. For this reason the level of plasma ADH is constantly fluctuating to adjust to the osmotic conditions. The urine can only become concentrated to any degree when ADH is present and cells of the distal tubules and collecting ducts are capable of responding to it. The concentration or dilution of urine is the renal control system to maintain osmolar homeostasis of the body fluids. Change in urine volume, however, is not just a simple matter of concentration or dilution.

Increased urine volume is associated with either increased water excretion (water diuresis) or with increased excretion, both water and solute (osmotic diuresis). Water diuresis is defined as an increase in the water excretion without a simultaneous increase in solute excretion and occurs as a result of water loading. In such circumstances, urine becomes hypotonic and osmolarity may fall as low as 40 mOsm/liter. The ability of young animals to excrete a water load shows species variation; the calf has a prompt water diuresis (Dalton, 1968), whereas the pup has a poor response (McCance and Widdowson, 1955). Osmotic diuresis occurs whenever an excessive amount of osmotically active solute is presented to the distal tubules collecting ducts. The increased rate of fluid flow in this area of the nephron limits the effective reabsorption of water due to ADH. As the fluid at the start of the distal tubule is always slightly hypotonic, urine produced during osmotic diuresis approaches istonicity. Excessive solute with accompanying water being delivered to the distal tubules can arise in three ways. Increased filtered quantities of glucose, as in diabetes mellitus, or urea result in inadequate reabsorption of these solutes by the proximal tubule. Second, intravenous infusion of mannitol which is frequently employed after surgery to minimize renal hemodynamic alterations, also produces osmotic diuresis because increased quantity of nonreabsorbable solute in the proximal tubule fluid interferes with the reabsorption of sodium and potassium (Rapoport and West, 1950). Third, when an increased sodium load is presented to the proximal tubule, and although functional adaptation occurs and the amount of sodium emerging from the proximal tubule is unchanged (Rector *et al.*, 1966)), the distal tubular sodium reabsorption ability becomes limited and osmotic or saline diuresis results (Stein *et al.*, 1964). Osmotic diuretic agents, e.g., furosemide and ethnacrynic acid, diminish sodium reabsorption in both the proximal and distal tubules (Suzuki *et al.*, 1964) and the ascending limb of the loop of Henle (Goldberg *et al.*, 1964; Hook and Williamson, 1965).

Animals can produce only a small volume of concentrated urine. When an increased amount of solute has to be excreted from whatever cause, the urine volume increases and the osmotic concentration of the urine falls toward that of the plasma. From the clinical standpoint the concentration or dilution of urine must be considered in relation to the amount of solute being excreted. In veterinary practice, rarely is the urine volume measured; the most satisfactory index of urine volume is creatinine concentration which, in the dog, varies between 50 and 100 mg/100 ml and in the cat, is of the order of 100 mg/100 ml. In many conditions, particularly in chronic renal failure, it is found that the osmolarity of the urine is normal but there is a substantial increase in the amount of solute excreted. Only by simultaneous comparison of osmolarity with the creatinine concentration can the increased solute excretion be detected. A concurrent low solute (mOsm/liter) and creatinine (mg/100 ml) excretion can only occur in the presence of decreased GFR. When renal involvement is suspected, the change in the solute and creatinine excretion will precede any change in the plasma urea concentration by 24 hours or maybe 48 hours.

In clinical medicine, abnormalities of the body fluids should be investigated from the viewpoint of both sodium and water excesses or deficits. The following is a summary of specific water and sodium changes. It must be appreciated that there are many shades of "gray" between the extremes.

B. Water Deficit

Water deficit states may result from either insufficient water intake alone or in combination with excessive water loss due to renal inability to concentrate urine. Loss of water leads to hypertonicity of the body fluids, both intra- and extracellular, which stimulates thirst and ADH secretion to correct the deficit. In the absence of water repletion, the extent of hypovolemia is reflected by elevation of plasma sodium, urea nitrogen, and protein concentrations, and hemoconcentration. Prolonged thirst reduces appetite with the resultant ketosis. The renal response is decreased urine volume of high osmolarity with sodium and chloride both present in low concentrations in the urine. Urinalysis shows proteinuria, ketonuria, and casts. The dog with diabetes insipidus which is also water deprived, very quickly goes into coma, in which case, urinary changes are minimal.

Heat stress in dogs is a particular example of a water deficit (Iampietro *et al.*, 1966). Affected dogs have either a long coat, are older dogs with chronic respiratory problems, obese dogs, or show signs of excitement. Dogs have very few sweat glands and when placed in a thermal stress environment without access to water, their evaporative heat loss due to respiration quickly depletes ECF volume. Dogs can probably remain in this environment for 6 to 8 hours without irreversible change occurring. However, the excitable dog which undergoes vasoconstriction and renal ischemia can only stand a short exposure to thermal stress, due possibly to the renal changes associated with elevated cerebrospinal fluid pressures (James and Wise, 1969).

C. WATER INTOXICATION

Water intoxication can occur in any domestic species but it is probably most common in sheep and cattle (Kirkbride and Frey, 1967). It is always preceded by a period of water deprivation of considerable duration, 7 to 14 days, followed by excessive drinking. Most animals, when relieving such water depletion, have prompt diuresis, but some individuals do not. The explanation for the failure of diuresis has not been satisfactorily elucidated. It is not due to the rate of water absorption from the gut but due to the failure of renal excretion. Water intoxication is therefore primary water excess with dilution of plasma electrolytes especially sodium and bicarbonate, total protein and hemoglobin concentrations. The osmotic gradient between the hypotonic ECF and the isotonic intracellular fluid causes water movement into the cells. As a result, there is no initial fall in packed cell volume. Although sheep red blood cells are similar to other species with regards to *in vitro* osmotic fragility testing, water intoxication in this species always leads of hemolysis, increased serum hemoglobin, decreased packed cell volume, and hemoglobinuria. Before hemoglobinuria occurs, adequate urine volume of low osmolarity and moderate sodium concentration is found. Sodium excretion is increased in this situation due to the inhibition of aldosterone secretion. Once hemoglobinuria occurs, renal shutdown follows. In the normal animal, free hemoglobin has no effect on the kidney, and the effect under these circumstances is possibly due to decreased renal perfusion. In handling such cases of prolonged water deprivation, it would be best if the animals were initially given saline to relieve their thirst. Although hypervolemia occurs, the deleterious effects of water intoxication are those of hypotonicity and, therefore, treatment with hypertonic saline is recommended.

D. SODIUM DEPLETION

In animals, sodium depletion occurs as a result of diarrhea. Because sodium is the principle electrolyte of the ECF, sodium depletion is synonymous with ECF hypovolemia. Initially the sodium loss is matched by water loss and therefore electrolyte concentration remains normal. If sodium loss continues, hypovolemia leads to the classical signs of dehydration. Plasma urea concentration increases and hemoconcentration occurs. Renal response is decreased urine volume of low osmolarity; if severe, anuria results. Heat stroke in horses illustrates simultaneous sodium and water loss, but in this example, water loss exceeds that of sodium and the plasma becomes hypertonic.

E. SODIUM EXCESS

Primary sodium excess is recognized as a clinical entity in veterinary medicine, being due to ingestion of high salt content rations and the coincident lack of drinking water. Provided there is plenty of water, the ingestion of excess salt is not harmful. It occurs most frequently in pigs and chickens but also occasionally in sheep and cattle. Primary sodium excess of renal origin is however, not recognized as a clinical entity; the incidence of hypertension is much lower in animals than in man. Edema is a special case of ECF expansion in which primary expansion occurs in the interstitial fluid phase. Edema in animals may be either hepatic, renal, or cardiac in origin. Whatever the origin, the renal response is the same, urine volume being normal and slightly hypertonic with high sodium concentration. Serum protein and plasma urea nitrogen concentrations are low. Hemoglobin concentrations are low. Hemoglobin concentration and packed cell volume are either normal or low.

Because of the intimate renal control on sodium excretion, it is clinically important to distinguish between edema formation of renal and extrarenal origin because edema of hepatic origin will respond to diuretics. The mechanism for failure of homeostasis in edema of renal origin is not fully understood.

F. Water and Sodium Homeostasis in Liver Disease

Water and electrolyte disorders are serious, even ominous complications of liver disease. Although specific interrelations between the liver and the kidney have not been experimentally demonstrated, there is considerable clinical evidence that renal failure is a frequent sequel to hepatic failure (Shear et al., 1965; Summerskill, 1966; Baldus and Summerskill, 1967). Indeed the relationship has been accepted (Coppage et al., 1962). The term, "hepatorenal syndrome," although discouraged for academic reasons, is a frequent cliche because most clinical investigators are confident such a relationship exists.

There is no obvious reason why aldosterone secretion should be stimulated in liver disease, although increased secretion (Coppage et al., 1962), failure of hepatic inactivation (Chart et al., 1956) and increased urinary excretion (Dyrenfurth et al., 1957) have been reported. Schedl and Bartter (1960) showed that ADH did not play a primary role in the retention of water in patients with cirrhosis. There is again no reason why ADH secretion should be increased. Also, there is no impaired metabolism of this hormone in liver disease (Nelson and Welt, 1952; White et al., 1953). Schedl and Bartter advanced the hypothesis that the proximal tubular sodium absorption was so great as to allow little sodium to pass to the distal site where free water is generated. The role of aldosterone in this condition is now generally considered insignificant. The reduction of glomerular filtration and renal blood flow which occurs in many patients with cirrhosis (Rivera et al., 1961; Leslie et al., 1951; Ralli et al., 1945; Lancestremere et al., 1962; Tyler et al., 1962) could explain the increased proximal tubular reabsorption. However, changes in GFR are not demonstrable in all patients (Schedl and Bartter, 1960); also the cause for the disordered renal hemodynamics is not apparent because cardiac output (Tyler et al., 1962; Shear et al., 1965) and mean arterial pressure (Lancestremere et al., 1962) are adequate in the cirrhotic patient. Jick et al. (1964) postulated increased medullary blood flow to explain their findings of the renal concentrating defect in cirrhotic patients. This concept has been supported in part because of decreased PAH extraction found in three patients (Shear et al., 1965) and disputed (Lancestremere et al., 1962). In his extensive review, Summerskill (1966) proposed two other hypotheses as possible explanations. He suggested that (1) a substance liberated or inadequately inactivated could result in an increase in the resistance offered by the renal vasculature and could account for the various functional abnormalities observed, or (2) an increased interrelationship between the renal and hepatic circulations, mediated through the autononic nervous system could exist. The summary of the present knowledge is that the mechanism of water and electrolyte disorders in cirrhosis is open to question but it is certainly reversible (Vaamonde et al., 1967).

G. Potassium Homeostasis

Renal responsibilities in potassium homeostasis are more apparent in animals because, as compared with man, potassium appears in the urine of all animals in sizeable quantities. Herbivorous diets in particular place high-potassium and low-sodium loads on the ruminant kidney. By adjusting the urinary losses of these elements according to variations in their intake, the kidneys play an important part in sodium potassium balance (Dalton, 1964). R. S. Anderson and Pickering (1961) have shown that the ruminant kidney is very efficient in handling a potassium load. The precise mechanism of how the ruminant kidney handles the potassium load has not been investigated. Chickens, another species with a very large potassium intake, has been shown to handle potassium in a manner similar to that of rat, man, and dog (Orloff and Davidson, 1959). In many sheep-raising areas of the world, the natural water has a high salt content (Potter, 1963); the kidney is unusually tolerant and extremely efficient at handling excess sodium chloride and does so without altering GFR and RPF flow.

H. Phosphate Homeostasis

Red blood cell and plasma phosphate concentrations in animals are quite variable and independent of each other. In an individual healthy animal, the plasma phosphate concentration is not maintained within precise limits, varying from 2 to 8 mg/100 ml. Plasma phosphate is entirely filtered at the glomerulus and normally 85–90% is reabsorbed. Small changes in the amount filtered are offset by corresponding changes in tubule reabsorption (Goldman and Bassett, 1954). The common example of failure of phosphate homeostasis in dogs is in chronic nephritis, in which hyperplasia of the parathyroid is induced by hypercalcemia which follows the retention of phosphate due to the fall in GFR. Because the renal effect of parathormone is small when GFR is impaired, bone changes soon become prominent.

I. Acid–Base Balance

The hydrogen ion concentration of the body is regulated within narrow limits (pH 7.2–7.7) by the combined control of the lungs, kidney, and buffering salts of the body fluid and cells. Animals tolerate a much wider pH range than man (Iampietro et al., 1966).

Four buffering systems are operant within the body; all act immediately and continuously. Quantitatively the most important is the bicarbonate–carbonic acid system when carbonic acid dissociates, carbon dioxide is removed via the lungs and water via the kidneys. The other systems are the phosphate buffering system of the red blood cells and renal tubule cells, plasma and tissue cell proteins, and hemoglobin.

Respiratory acid–base control depends exclusively on regulating the plasma concentration of carbon dioxide. If this were the sole mechanism, the body would be quickly deprived of bicarbonate and no further carbon dioxide could be formed. The kidneys are therefore very important acid–base regulators because they compensate for the defects in the action of the buffer salts or the respiratory system.

J. Acidosis

Acidosis has been defined as the increase in anion content of the body relative to cation content (Black, 1958). In man three forms of acidosis, dependent on origin, are recognized: metabolic, respiratory, and renal. Renal acidosis is often not recognized as a clinical entity in veterinary medicine. Whatever the cause, the effects of acidosis are lowering blood pH and plasma HCO_3^- and increased respiratory rate. The renal response to metabolic or respiratory acidosis is increased urinary hydrogen excretion (increased exchange of hydrogen for sodium), fall in bicarbonate excretion, increased ammonium excretion (Dorman et al., 1954), and renal tubular intracellular pH (Roberts et al., 1955).

K. Alkalosis

Alkalosis is the opposite of acidosis, increased blood pH and plasma bicarbonate concentration. Alkalosis may be of metabolic or respiratory origin. It is commonly observed in the uremic stages of chronic interstitial nephritis when vomiting is severe. With the recent popularity of sodium bicarbonate therapy for prevention of urethral blockage in cats and in the treatment of uremia in dogs, clinical alkalosis may be more frequently observed in these species. The renal response is an alkaline urine, with high bicarbonate and little ammonium ion excretion and, because of the excessive sodium and potassium loss, diuresis. Roberts (Roberts et al., 1955) has pointed out that should potassium depletion occur from excessive renal loss, this would lead to increased hydrogen excretion and an acid urine. The further sequel to hypokalemia is the excretion of the hypotonic urine which is resistant to ADH (Giebisch and Lazano, 1959), due probably to lack of solute accumulation in medulla (J. O. C. Eigler et al., 1962).

V. NITROGEN EXCRETION

In all species, approximately 90% of the nitrogen derived from dietary protein is excreted in the urine. Almost all of this nitrogen is excreted as nonprotein nitrogenous compounds of which urea, 70–95%, ammonia, 1–10%, and creatinine, 1–10%, constitute the large bulk (Scheer and Ramamurthi, 1968). Because of this balance between metabolic nitrogen production and renal excretion of nonprotein nitrogen, protein metabolism is usually discussed in terms of urea nitrogen alone. For this reason, estimation of plasma urea nitrogen is the most common renal function test in animals. The excretion of urea is perhaps the most important single function of the kidney (Bernstein, 1965). The kidneys, however, do not regulate nitrogen balance of the body. In mature animals, the quantity of protein in the body is reasonably constant and therefore the urinary nitrogen excretion closely approximates the dietary nitrogen intake. As nitrogen comprises 16% of the average dietary protein, the nitrogen content of the urine multiplied by the value 100/16, provides a close estimate of the protein metabolized in the body. A small amount of nitrogen is also lost in feces. It has been determined experimentally that the total protein intake is approximately 6.9 times the quantity of nitrogen in the urine.

Because urea absorption is by passive diffusion along a concentration gradient, the urea excretion is dependent on water reabsorption from the tubule and particularly the collecting duct, to create the necessary gradient. As much as 90% of the filtered urea may be reabsorbed at low urine flows, 40% during water diuresis, and as little as 10% during osmotic diuresis. Except in the conditions of water and osmotic diuresis, urea clearance is dependent on urine flow. Nitrogen (urea) balance of the body is dependent on the amount filtered. If only 20% is excreted at low urine flows, the amount reabsorbed returns to the urea pool and raises plasma concentration so that if GFR remains constant, the amount filtered will then increase with the result that ultimately plasma concentration will become steady. It should be appreciated that normal plasma urea concentrations are very much dependent on the degree of hydration as well as protein intake. High protein diets result in significantly elevated fasting plasma urea concentrations (Lane and Robinson, 1968). Plasma urea concentrations increases after feeding, remaining elevated for approximately 12 hours in dogs (Street *et al.*, 1968).

With hydration, urine flow and urea clearance increase. When urine flow becomes greater than 1.5% of GFR, urea clearance reaches a maximum; however urine flow may not reach maximal until 6–8% of the simultaneous GFR (maximum water diuresis). At all levels of urine flow, urea reabsorption in the proximal tubule is constant, representing approximately 20% of the amount filtered. At maximum urea clearance, urea reabsorption in the distal tubule and collecting ducts approximately equals that of the proximal tubule. Also, it is independent of urine flow because the concentration gradients that develop are so small that they limit the amount which can diffuse out from the tubular urine at the distal sites. A feature of urea excretion which is unique to sheep is that on a low-protein diet, urinary urea concentration is independent of urine flow (Schmidt-Nielsen and O'Dell, 1959) and remains approximately five times the plasma urea concentration (Schmidt-Nielsen *et al.*, 1958; Schmidt-Nielsen and Osaki, 1958). This is in sharp contrast to the sheep capable of concentrating urea in the urine 200 to 300 times plasma concentration when fed a normal protein diet.

Urea excretion in osmotic diuresis deserves special mention because of the observation of normal or near normal plasma urea concentrations in some dogs with chronic interstitial nephritis, but low GFR. If reasonable urine flow can be established in dogs with chronic interstitial nephritis, osmotic diuretic therapy (10% mannitol or glucose) can successfully reduce plasma urea concentration due to increased urea excretion. The increase in osmotically active solute in the proximal tubule lowers the concentration gradient at that site and less urea is reabsorbed with the result that the concentration gradient is much reduced throughout the distal nephron. Under conditions of osmotic diuresis, as much as 90% of the filtered urea can be excreted; in a medium size dog, plasma urea clearances from 10 to as high as 20 ml/min can be achieved this way. Animals on a low protein intake and with chronic interstitial nephritis may have a normal or near normal plasma urea concentration, because the remaining functional nephrons have an osmotic diuresis.

In man, the major end product of purine metabolism is uric acid. All domestic animals including the dog, cat, monkey, rabbit, sheep, cattle, horse, and pig are capable of converting uric acid to allantoin in the liver by the action of the enzyme uricase. As a result, mostly allantoin and only a small amount of uric acid is found in the urine. In all these species, the ratio of allantoin to uric acid is in the order of 10 to 1 (Van Pilsun, 1969), whereas in man the reverse ratio is 1 to 5 to 10. The one exception is the Dalmatian dog, in which uric acid excretion is similar to that occurring in man. The Dalmatian dog has adequate liver uricase concentration but only a small amount of allantoin is available for excretion because uric acid is secreted by the tubule in this breed.

VI. HORMONE PRODUCTION BY THE KIDNEY

A. ERYTHROPOIETIN

The rate of production of red blood cells is in response to the status of tissue oxygen concentrations. Conditions such as anemia, hemorrhage, or diminution in the oxygen content of the inspired air cause decreased oxygen transport to the tissues and stimulate erythropoietin release and in turn, red blood cell production (Gordon, 1959). Many tissues are capable of producing erythropoietin, the kidney being the major site of production of this hormone in the dog, but species differences exist. It is a common clinical observation that whenever the renal mass is substantially decreased, anemia always occurs. An example is in the terminal stages of chronic interstitial nephritis. The converse may also happen. An increase in the renal mass may induce polycythemia. Tissue anoxia stimulates increased red blood cell production through the action of erythropoietin on the stem cells of the bone marrow (Alpen and Kranmore, 1959; Lajtha, 1964). This system operates on the conventional feedback mechanism. It has frequently been suggested in the literature that urea may have a toxic effect on the bone marrow and this is the explanation for the anemia observed in uremic states. Neats (1964) has shown this not to be true, it is decrease in renal mass and its effect on erythropoietin which is responsible.

B. RENIN

The renin content of the kidneys of domestic animals has been reported by Schaffenburg et al. (1960). Renin is formed in the group of cells comprising the juxtaglomerular apparatus (Cook and Pickering, 1962; Edelman and Hartroft, 1961). There is a close correlation between the degree of granularity of the juxtaglomerular cells and the extractable renin content of the kidney. Renin mediates its physiological effects through angiotensin which stimulates aldosterone production by the adrenal cortex. There is no evidence to establish that renin has an independent effect other than via angiotensin. Renin secretion is intimately associated with salt and water homeostasis (Peart, 1965). As hypertension of renal origin is not recognized as a clinical problem in animals, renin metabolism will not be further discussed.

VII.   PROCEDURES FOR STUDYING RENAL CLEARANCE

A. GLOMERULAR FILTRATION RATE

There is no method of measuring GFR directly. It can only be measured from the rate of urinary excretion of a substance that is freely filtered and is neither secreted nor reabsorbed by the tubules. Inulin is an ideal substance for this purpose (Smith, 1951). Glomerular filtration rate can be calculated from the following formula:

$$\text{GFR (ml/min)} = {}^{U}\text{IN}^{V}/{}^{P}\text{IN} \tag{1}$$

where ${}^{U}\text{IN}$ = urinary concentration inulin (mg %); V = urine flow (ml/min); ${}^{P}\text{IN}$ = plasma* concentration inulin (mg %).

In the dog, endogenous creatinine clearance is a satisfactory measure of GFR for clinical purposes. For precise work, creatinine must be infused in amounts sufficient to raise the plasma concentration to 15 mg/100 ml or more. Analytical methods for inulin are not difficult, the method of Roe *et al.* (1949), being preferred by most workers.

B. RENAL BLOOD FLOW

Smith *et al.* (1945) established that at plasma concentrations of less than 5 mg/100 ml the clearance of PAH approximates the RPF.

$$\text{RPF or } C_{\text{PAH}} \text{ (ml/min)} = {}^{U}\text{PAH}^{V}/{}^{P}\text{PAH} \tag{2}$$

where ${}^{U}\text{PAH}$ = urinary concentration PAH (mg %) and ${}^{P}\text{PAH}$ = plasma concentration PAH (mg %). If PAH was completely cleared from the plasma in one circulation through the kidney, then C_{PAH} would exactly equal RPF. However, in man approximately 9% (Bradley, 1947; Warren *et al.*, 1944) and in the dog 15% (Phillips *et al.*, 1946) of the PAH delivered by the renal artery is returned via venous output. Therefore, C_{PAH} only approximates the RPF and it has been suggested (Smith, 1951) that the term effective RPF or cortical plasma flow should be used as synonymous with C_{PAH}. That not all PAH is cleared in one circulation is probably due to PAH in the medullary circulation not being secreted. Also, the extent of the blood flow through the renal capsule is not known; in the cat, with its massive capsular vessels, the PAH extraction rate may be much less than 85% of the total blood flow.

If the plasma concentrations in both the renal arterial and venous blood is known, RPF can be calculated from Eq. (3).

---

*Plasma samples should not be withdrawn from abdominal vena cava, as these will probably have lower concentration of a substance which is excreted by the kidney than the renal artery.

$$\text{Total RPF (ml/min)} = {}^{U}\text{PAH}^{V}/{}^{A}\text{PAH} \tag{3}$$

$$({}^{A}\text{PAH} - {}^{V}\text{PAH})/{}^{A}\text{PAH}$$

where ^{A}PAH $-{}^{V}$PAH $=$ renal arterial concentration and PAH $=$ renal venous concentration. Once this is known, the following information can be calculated:

$$\text{RBF (ml/min)} = \text{RPF}/(1 - \text{PCV}) \tag{4}$$

where PCV $=$ packed cell volume (%).

$$\text{"Medullary" blood flow (ml/min)} = \text{RBF} - \text{ERBF} \tag{5}$$

C. TUBULAR SECRETION

If the quantity of the substance appearing in the urine is greater than the simultaneous quantity filtered, that substance is said to be secreted. With a substance which is freely filtered and secreted, tubular secretion can be derived from the formula:

$$\text{Amount secreted (mg/min)} = U_x V - C_{IN} P_x \tag{6}$$

where $U_x P_x =$ urine and plasma concentration of substance x in mg % and $x =$ any substance. The above equation makes the assumption that all of the substance is freely filtered at the glomerulus. Many substances are protein-bound and therefore are only partially filtered at the glomerulus. If the percentage of protein-binding is known, correction can be made for this. Under these circumstances tubular secretion becomes:

$$\text{Amount secreted (mg/min)} = U_x V - (100 - \% \text{ bound})/100 \, (C_{IN} P_x) \tag{7}$$

For example, PAH under most physiological circumstances is approximately 17% albumin bound, the factor for percentage protein-binding therefore becomes 0.83.

The quantity of any substance that can be secreted is quantitatively limited, that is, a tubular maximum exists. To create this condition, the plasma concentration of the substance under investigation is increased until the transport capacity is fully saturated. The tubular maximum (mg/min) occurs whenever the product of $U_x V$ is maximal.

Some substances undergo both secretion and reabsorption. Potassium, for example, is completely reabsorbed in the proximal tubule and secreted in distal tubules, the quantity appearing in the unit in the urine may be less than the simultaneous quantity filtered. Under such circumstances, there is no simple procedure for determining the quantity secreted except to make the assumption that the quantity appearing in the urine represents that derived solely from secretion.

D. TUBULAR REABSORPTION

When the clearance of the substance is less than the simultaneously determined filtration rate it is likely that the substance is reabsorbed during its passage along the tubule. With substances such as potassium, uric acid, phosphate, and magnesium which undergo glomerular filtration, tubular reabsorption, and tubular secretion, reabsorption cannot be measured. For the substance that is filtered and solely reabsorbed, the formula for determining the quantity reabsorbed is:

$$\text{Amount reabsorbed (mg/min)} = C_{IN}P_x - U_xV \qquad (8)$$

The tubular maximum for the substance being reabsorbed is reached when the difference between the quantity filtered and the quantity excreted in the urine per minute is maximal.

E. Osmolar Clearance, Free Water Clearance, and Free Water Reabsorption

In the same way that glomerular filtration rate is determined by the clearance of inulin, the clearance of osmotically active solute can be determined from knowledge of the plasma and urinary osmolarity and urinary volume (Zak *et al.*, 1954).

$$\text{Osmolar clearance (mOsm/liter)} C_{Osm} = \frac{V_{Osm}U}{P_{Osm}}$$

where V_{Osm} = urine osmolarity (mOsm/liter) and P_{Osm} = plasma osmolarity (mOsm/liter).

Normally urine is hypertonic as compared with plasma; for this to occur, water must be reabsorbed in excess of solute. Water reabsorption is derived from the following formula:

$$\text{Water reabsorption (ml/min) } T^c H_2O = C_{Osm} - V \qquad (10)$$

When the urine is hypotonic as compared to plasma, the water in excess of that required to create conditions of isosmosis with the plasma is described as free water. The equation for free water clearance therefore becomes:

$$\text{Free water clearance (ml/min) } C_{H_2O} = V - C_{Osm} - V \qquad (11)$$

VIII. FUNCTIONAL ALTERATIONS IN NEPHROPATHIES

A. Alterations in Renal Hemodynamics

Routine determinations of GFR constitute the most important procedures in assessing renal function. Normal clearance values for adult domestic animals are shown in Table II. These determinations have the advantage that comparison with normal animals can be made and if several tests are performed on the same animal at convenient time intervals, a precise prognosis can be made based on accurate assessment of the hemodynamic alteration. Furthermore, from knowledge of the filtration fraction it is possible to differentiate glomerular from tubular, interstitial, or vascular changes (Reubi, 1963).

In veterinary medicine, it is uneconomical to develop intensive care hospitalization and, therefore, sophisticated diagnosis based on extensive investigation is probably not justified. The essentials of diagnosis require that it be decided if there is renal

TABLE II NORMAL VALUES FOR RENAL FUNCTION IN ADULT DOMESTIC ANIMALS

C_{cr}	C_{IN}	C_{urea}	C_{PAH}	C_{PSP}
C				
Cat[a]				
7.5 (7.05–7.95)			23.8 (23.7–23.9)	
Cattle				
0.4 (0.28–0.51)			1.7 (1.10–2.40)	
1.68 (1.32–2.23)	1.84 (1.30–2.20)	0.84 (0.56–1.00)	9.11 (5.82–12.60)	
Dog				8.0 (4.70–10.9)
				7.82
	3.77 (1.74–5.86)		12.9 (6.3–21.2)	
	2.50 (1.80–3.20)			15.0 (8.60–21.4)
	3.0 (2.70–4.13)	1.66 (1.00–2.34)		
	3.45 (2.00–4.90)			10.0 (5.66–14.0)
4.46 (2.73–5.06)			12.7 (8.33–16.67)	
4.3 (2.20–8.30)		4.63 (2.35–6.92)	13.5 (8.10–22.4)	
5.0 (3.25–6.40)				
4.35 (3.15–6.95)			14.3 (10.1–21.3)	
4.20 (3.20–4.90)			11.2 (7.80–15.5)	
5.78 (4.66–7.00)	4.19 (3.37–5.00)		14.6 (12.1–17.0)	
			16.3 (12.5–19.0)	
	5.10 (4.25–6.33)		25.2 (15.0–30.1)	
		3.05 (1.67–4.03)		
Goat				
2.2				
2.75 (2.30–3.58)	2.01 (1.50–1.95)			
Horse				
	1.16 (0.78–1.53)			
1.46 (1.02–1.90)	1.66 (1.00–2.32)	0.76 (0.56–0.96)		
	1.66			
	1.40			
Monkey				
5.25 (3.85–7.80)[b]	3.80 (3.10–5.20)		12.2 (10.6–15.1)	

T_{PAH}	C_{DIO}	$C_{uric\ acid}$	Urine vol. (ml/kg-day)	Reference
1.68				Eggleton and Habib, 1950
			10–20	Hammett, 1915
0.34 (0.24–0.57)				R. R. Anderson and Mixner, 1959
0.94 (0.67–1.33)				R. R. Anderson and Mixner, 1960
				Paulsen, 1957
				Sellers et al., 1958
			17–45	Dukes, 1947
1.21 (0.43–1.89)				Asheim et al., 1961
				Blatteis and Horvath, 1958
				Clapp, 1965
				Corcoran and Page, 1938
				Glauser and Selkurt, 1952
				Houck, 1948
				Jolliffe and Smith, 1931
				Kubicek et al., 1953
0.78 (0.54–1.03)				Low et al., 1956
				Ramsay and Coxon, 1967
				Stevens et al., 1956
				Summerville et al., 1932
			20–100	Dukes, 1947
				Dziemian et al., 1950
			10–40	Ladd et al., 1957
				Ketz et al., 1956
				Knudsen, 1959a
	6.91 (5.29–8.53)			Knudsen, 1959b
			3–18	Poulsen, 1957
				Gagnon and Clarke, 1957

TABLE II (*continued*)

C_{cr}	C_{IN}	C_{urea}	C_{PAH}	C_{PSP}
3.08 (1.73–5.22)[c]	1.96 (1.18–3.03)		8.06 (6.71–10.9)	
6.20 (4.50–7.92)[b]	5.15 (3.66–6.63)			
3.47 (2.86–4.08)[d]	3.01 (2.46–3.54)			
	3.10 (2.20–3.80)[c]			
1.10 (0.90–1.30)[c]				
Sheep				
	2.78			
	2.52			
	2.78 (2.35–3.48)[e]		16.0 (12.0–20.6)	
	1.22 (0.97–1.43)[f]		4.75 (4.25–5.56)	
1.75 (1.70–1.79)	1.80 (1.72–1.87)			10.0 (2.75–17.6)
	1.50	0.64		
	1.56 (1.28–1.84)		12.0 (10.3–14.3)	
0.78 (0.76–0.80)		1.48 (1.40–1.55)		
Swine				
4.15 (4.07–4.40)	5.06 (4.87–5.32)		19.5 (19.3–19.7)	
Chicken				
	1.8 (0.2–3.4)			
	2.5 (1.80–3.50)		30.7 (20.8–40.6)	
	1.84	1.50		
	2.04			25.0
3.90 (2.00–6.80)	1.84 (1.04–2.83)		18.0 (10.5–25.8)	

[a] Values are ml/kg-min; in reducing values to ml/kg the following bodyweights (in kilograms) were assumed unless a specific value was recorded in the literature: cat, 2.5; cattle, 500; dog, 12; goat, 50; horse, 630; monkey, 12; sheep, 40. Values in parenthesis are ranges.

[b] Chimpanzee

T_{PAH}	C_{DIO}	$C_{uric\ acid}$	Urine vol. (ml/kg-day)	References
				Pickering and Sussman, 1962
				Smith and Clarke, 1938
				Smith and Clarke, 1938
				Sweet et al., 1961
				Vander and Cafruny, 1962
			70–80	L. Bauman and Oviatt, 1915
				Gans, 1964a
				Gans, 1964b
				Gans and Mercer, 1962
				Gans and Mercer, 1962
				Manning et al., 1959
				Schmidt-Nielsen et al., 1958
				Shannon, 1937
				Stacy and Brook, 1964a
				Stacy and Brook, 1964b
			10–40	Dukes, 1947
3.11 (3.00–3.21)			5–30	Mundsick et al., 1958
				Berger et al., 1960
1.58 (1.08–1.93)				Dantzler, 1966
		11.3 (0–23.0)		Nechay and Nechay, 1959
		19.8 (8.70–30.0)		Pitts, 1938
				Pitts and Korr, 1938
				Sykes, 1960a
				Sykes, 1906b
		25.1 (15.6–35.1)	6.2–7	Dixon, 1958

[c] Macaque
[d] Baboon
[e] High protein diet.
[f] Low protein diet.

involvement and if so, to establish the degree or extent of it so that an accurate prognosis can be made. Hence, there is the question as to whether the expense is justified of deciding whether the pathological alteration is primarily glomerular. Many pathologists consider that following glomerular nephritis, there is progressive tissue involvement, leading ultimately to chronic interstitial nephritis. Although this is true as a general statement, if the glomerular involvement is treated promptly, a dog may have a long and useful life before chronic nephritis threatens health. Thus the differentiation of glomerular lesions is important, and procedures which are often regarded as too sophisticated speak only to the limitations of those who do not use them.

The object of any clearance test is to assess the degree of renal damage. As the diseased kidney may consist of normal nephrons, aglomerular tubules, impotent nephrons, and inert tissue (Smith, 1951) the clinical requirement is to make some assessment of the number of functioning nephrons. There is no test as yet which will give this information. Because the kidney's capacity to hypertrophy is very great, for example, the removal of one kidney produces little or no permanent change in overall function (de Wardener, 1967); it is theoretically possible for renal disease to destroy about one-half of the nephron population and yet produce little or no change in renal function. Lapides and Bobcitt (1958) have reported that based on their clinical experience with man, glomerular function of 45% or more of normal is adequate for maintaining homeostasis in the presence of the most stressing operative procedures. Uremia may not appear until GFR has been reduced to less than 25% of normal. When renal function is persistently reduced to half its normal value, it is almost certain that a great deal more than half of the original renal parenchyma must have been destroyed.

All clearance tests require accurate measurement of urine flow rates and for this, catheterization is essential. Most animals require neither anesthesia or tranquilization to be catheterized. The common anesthetics, barbiturates or halothane, have no effect on renal function. Accurate clearance measurements also require constant plasma concentrations while urine flow is being determined. Constant intravenous infusions to maintain steady plasma concentrations are ideal. Although subcutaneous injection of inulin and PAH gives lower clearance values as compared with infusion studies (Ramsay and Coxon, 1967), for reasons of convenience, however, the former is probably the best clinical procedure.

Blood samples for plasma chemical determinations should be taken at the mid-point of urine periods. A less rigid sample collection procedure has been given by King and Wooton (1960) for human subjects. This sampling scheme is applicable where catheterization is impossible, e.g., in male sheep.

The procedure used in my laboratory is to give a subcutaneous injection of inulin and PAH and then to catheterize the animal with an indwelling catheter. With most animals, the 30 ml inflatable cuff is only inflated to 10 ml to limit the dead space within the bladder and thereby increase the accuracy in collecting urine. Immediately prior to the start of the urine collection period, the bladder is washed out with 10 ml water twice and then flushed with air. Urine collection periods are of 10 minutes duration. At the end of each period, the bladder is washed and flushed. All urine and washings are collected and the volume accurately measured. Normally only two clearance periods are made if the urine volume for the two periods are similar.

The importance of accurate measurement of urine volume in urine excretion tests cannot be overemphasized. There is no doubt that this is the most common source of error.

Inulin clearance is deliberately emphasized rather than creatinine clearance as a measure of GFR. Reproducibility of plasma and urine creatinine concentrations using the Jaffe reaction in most routine clinical laboratories is not as satisfactory as it should be. In attempting to follow the sequential alteration in GFR, however, the true alteration could be masked by analytical inaccuracies. The criticism of estimation of creatinine is largely overcome by the use of automated analysis. If this is available, creatinine clearance measurements are to be encouraged.

When glomerular involvement is suspected, measurement of GFR is warranted. It is progressively depressed in all forms of glomerular nephritis. Simultaneous determination of RBF and GFR provides information to assess whether a lesion is predominately glomerular or tabular. Decreased GFR with normal RBF is clear evidence a lesion is primarily glomerular. Under these circumstances the filtration fraction is much reduced. Decreased GFR and RBF with a disproportionate decrease in GFR is characteristic of chronic glomerular nephritis or predominately glomerular involvement in chronic interstitial nephritis. The hemodynamic alterations in chronic interstitial nephritis vary tremendously. For a considerable time after the pathological lesions would be apparent in histological examination of a renal biopsy, renal hemodynamics may be quite normal. Before any measured change in function would be recognized, greater than 50% of the nephrons would be involved. In terminal glomerular nephritis, RBF and GFR are decreased but the proportional decrease in each measurement throughout the course of the disease would vary.

Clearance studies are only meaningful if there is neither anuria or oliguria. Using conventional procedures, Bull et al. (1950) found essentially no renal blood flow in patients with acute oliguric failure. It has since been shown that the kidney in that state has approximately 50% of its normal RBF (J.G. Walker et al., 1963; Goldberg, 1962).

The obvious question is: why is there no production of urine? Onesti (1967) studied this problem using experiments in which partial constriction of the aorta was applied between two renal arteries. This produced in the left kidney: (1) a decrease in the mean arterial perfusion pressure of 15–20 mmHg, (2) minimal or no reduction in renal blood flow and glomerular filtration rate, (3) significant decrease in urine flow due to excessive tubular reabsorption of water. Intravenous infusion of heterologous hemoglobin to this preparation consistently produced acute renal shutdown of this kidney, whereas no changes were observed in the contralateral kidney perfused at normal arterial perfusion pressure. These experiments suggest that decreased RBF is not an important factor in producing acute renal failure, but that the excessive tubular reabsorption of water characteristic of "the low perfusion pressure kidney" results first in tubular stasis and subsequently in complete block. This sequence of events is typical of hemoglobinuric nephrosis which follows mismatched transfusions, water intoxication in calves, or copper poisoning in sheep (Kennedy, 1957). To explain the oliguria and anuria several other theories, back diffusion (Phillips and Hamilton, 1948), increased intrarenal pressure (Peters, 1945), and obstructive casts (Oliver et al., 1951), have been proposed but not convincingly demonstrated.

B. Fractional Clearance of Foreign Substances

Clearance studies are time consuming and for this reason, they cannot be classed as routine medical procedures. The rate at which the kidney removes chemical substances from plasma or the rate of appearance in urine are becoming common procedures for estimating the degree of kidney function in domestic animals. Rowntree and Geraghty (1910) first demonstrated the usefulness of assessing renal function by measuring excretion of phenol red (PSP) in urine. The classical papers showing fractional clearance of PSP as a measure of renal function in humans are those of Shaw (1925), Chapman and Halsted (1933), Goldring et al. (1936), and Lapides and Bobbitt (1958). The tests presently used in animals have been developed from this work. Fractional clearance of foreign chemical substances from plasma may become a routine clinical procedure in the near future.

With fractional clearance procedures based on rate of appearance in urine, a standard amount (6 mg in dogs, 3 mg in cats) of PSP is injected intravenously and urine collected at various intervals. Urinary catheterization is necessary for accurate volume collection. The ideal is to collect 10-minute urine samples, for 40–60 minutes after injection. Dogs and cats excrete approximately 60% of the injected dose in the first 30 minutes (Osbaldiston and Furhman, 1969). Unless collection conditions are well controlled, the test is not very sensitive (Bloom, 1937), with the result that most clinicians are hesitant to describe decreased renal function unless the 30 minutes excretion is below 25% of the injected dose. One major objection to the test is catheterization, especially in female dogs and cats. As most small animals will urinate in a few minutes following the administration of urecholine, this objection is largely overcome.

Recently, increased interest has been revived in the plasma disappearance of foreign substances, because of simplicity of the procedure, precision of measurement and the data being interpretable in kinetic terms, thus sequential, serial determinations can be performed so that renal function over long periods or the life history of an animal can be made. Such tests should be carried out on either minimally disturbed, unrestrained, conscious animals, or anesthetized animals. A blood sample is withdrawn prior to injection, and subsequently five or six blood samples are withdrawn at regular intervals during the next 30 minutes. A minimum of two samples is necessary. The principle of the test is identical to that of the bromosulfonphthalein clearance test used to estimate hepatic function, or the intravenous glucose tolerance test.

A number of substances have been investigated for this purpose. The ideal substance should be excreted exclusively by the kidney, should not be accumulated intracellularly, have a volume of distribution equal to that of plasma, and be easily determined. No substance has yet been found to meet all criteria, but three substances, inulin, PSP, and PAH approach the ideal in that they are principally excreted by the kidney.

Because vascular and extravascular ECF are in equilibrium, only those substances strongly protein-bound will have a distribution volume equal to plasma volume. PAH is poorly protein-bound, (10 to 20%); but because it is a comparatively large anion, it interchanges slowly between the compartments of the ECF, as compared with the smaller molecules like creatinine, so that its distribution volume should be primarily within the plasma. Phenol red is strongly protein-bound, 80–90% (Gault, 1966); its volume of distribution will be almost exclusively within plasma volume. All protein-bound substances may easily enter the lymphatic system; the extent to which this happens within the time period of the clearance study is probably very small. Inulin, because of its long equilibration time, and rapid urinary excretion, is distributed in significant amount in the extravascular compartment of the ECF (Schwartz et al., 1949).

PAH and PSP are not excreted exclusively by the kidneys. Depending upon the integrity of the liver cells, bile excretion may account for up to 20% of the total excretion of these substances (Kim and Hong, 1962). The mechanism of organic anion secretion in both bile and the proximal tubule has been suggested to be similar (Sperber, 1959). This is now considered unlikely because renal anion excretion is dependent on metabolic activity of the phosphorylase system, whereas hepatic excretory transport is dependent on different mechanisms (Gartner and Arias, 1969). There is evidence that inulin is slowly destroyed within the body, but in the time period of renal clearance studies, this would be negligible.

As inulin, PSP, and PAH are foreign substances, they are suited to plasma or urine clearance studies because no allowance need be made for an endogenous concentration. Inulin disappearance indicates glomerular function. PAH, because it is poorly protein-bound and at low concentrations is completely cleared from the kidney in one circulation, is the most sensitive index of overall kidney function. Its disappearance is influenced by both glomerular filtration and tubular excretion. Phenol red, on the other hand, is strongly protein-bound and its disappearance is essentially tubular excretion. Diminution of RBF usually parallels deterioration of renal function; PSP or PAH disappearance is a good indication of the extent of the disease process. Extrarenal factors do have a marked influence on RBF and falsely low values can occur. In veterinary medicine, the commonly encountered problems are fear, fever, and decreased cardiac output. Results of simultaneous estimation of inulin with PAH or phenol red disappearance, allow for the differentiation between glomerular and tubuler involvement in renal disease.

Figure 2 shows the relative plasma disappearance of PAH, PSP, inulin, and creatinine in normal sheep. All substances are cleared from the plasma at an exponential rate. The equations to derive the fractional clearance, the volume distribution, and the half-life of the substance have been previously discussed by Cornelius in Chapter 5, Volume I. The simplest terms for expressing results are $T_{1/2}$ (min) or the relative amount of substance cleared per minute (%/min).

As renal function deteriorates, the clearance of these substances from plasma becomes less so the slope of the exponential line is less steep and $T_{1/2}$ min increases while the relative clearance decreases. Because interpretation depends on the calculation of $T_{1/2}$ min, the test is not sensitive to minor alterations in renal hemodynamics. As standard deviation of normal clearance is small, the test is capable of accurately predicting a decrease in RBF of 25%.

In man (Gault et al., 1966), dog (Brobst et al., 1967), and cow (Mixner and Anderson, 1961) it has been demonstrated that, although clearance is probably constant, the plasma disappearance of PSP and PAH is biphasic rather than singly exponential. Gault et al. (1966) examined the effect of interstitial and intracellular movement, edema and ascites, biliary excretion, serum albumin binding, and metabolism of PSP on its fractional clearance. He concluded that the biphasic disappearance resulted from it being distributed in an open, multicompartment system with

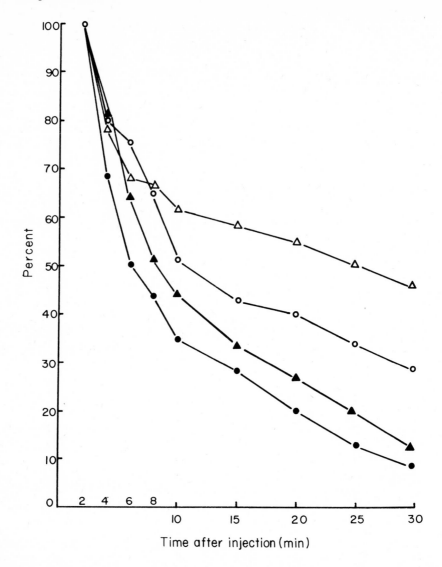

Fig. 2.   Fractional clearance of creatinine, inulin, PAH, and PSP from plasma of sheep. Plasma concentration 2 minutes after injection taken as 100%. (△) creatinine; (○) inulin; (▲) PSP; (●) PAH. (Osbaldiston and Fuhrman, 1969.)

constant clearance outflow from the smallest system. A similar explanation has been accepted by Brobst *et al.* (1967). The following evidence is not consistent with the multicompartment system. (1) PSP is strongly protein-bound and therefore its distribution is initially within the plasma volume. The plasma disappearance of phenol red is similar to that of the disappearance of inulin and PAH. As about 60% of the phenol red is excreted in 40 minutes, the amount of phenol red going into another compartment, for example, interstitial fluid, would be comparatively small. (2) PSP injected intravenously is not distributed to edematous or ascitic fluid. (3) There is no unequivocable demonstration that these compounds are absorbed into erythrocytes. The small percentage of PSP which cannot be accounted for in the plasma after centrifugation could be that which is trapped in plasma between erythrocytes. (4) The PSP is not stored in renal tubule cells (Puck *et al.*, 1952). (5) The disappearance in anuric animals is not exponential but linear.

Gault *et al.* (1966) have calculated that volume of distribution of PSP from the slower phase of the plasma PSP disappearance in humans, and found it to be similar to the estimated ECF volume. Calculating volume of distribution from both fast and slow phases of plasma disappearance after injection of 1, 3, or 5 mg/kg body weight PSP into 6 dogs (Brobst *et al.*, 1967) showed (1) volume of distribution of the slower phase was always greater than the volume calculated phase, (2) ratio of volume distribution for the two phases at any dose level were entirely unrelated, and (3) in all six instances, volumes of distribution were larger than plasma volume and smaller than ECF volume. This brief discussion illustrates that before this procedure can have wide application in clinical medicine, a much better understanding of the factors involved is required.

Osborne *et al.* (1967) have found that histological examination of renal biopsies has proved helpful in following structural alterations of advancing renal disease and that early stages of renal dysfunction can be diagnosed. At the present time, this is not a routine for the clinical laboratory, but chemical estimation of inulin, PAH, and phenol red is well within laboratory capability. For this reason the study of plasma clearance to establish simple procedures for the assessment of the kinetics of renal function is very important to the veterinary profession.

C. FUNCTIONAL ALTERATIONS AS MEASURED BY CLEARANCE STUDIES USING ISOTOPES

Clearance studies can be performed using radioactive-labeled compounds. The radiation effects of such procedures have recently been discussed by Mostofi (1966). Although pathological alteration has been described in experimental animals, it is unlikely that the accumulation of radioisotope by the kidney during infrequent clinical procedures would be harmful.

Estimation of GFR, RBF, and tubular maxima can be performed using radio labeled compounds (Oester *et al.*, 1968; Oester and Madsen, 1968). One major clinical application is the measurement of RBF in the anuric kidney (Brun *et al.*, 1955).

Renal disappearance of radioactivity following a single injection of a labeled compound has the dual advantages of demonstrating unilateral renal function and extent of functional nephron population (Winters and Myers, 1962). Studies on radioisotope renograms in dogs have been reported (Morgan and Gillette, 1963). Its application in veterinary medicine will be limited because of cost. However, the medical use of radioisotopes for screening selected populations for latent urinary tract dysfunction (Nordyke *et al.*, 1969) may have some limited application.

IX. URINALYSIS

Whenever an evaluation of renal function is needed, the first step should be a routine urinalysis. The methods for collecting and preserving urine, techniques, and interpretation have been set forth by Bloom (1960), Benjamin (1967), Coffin (1953), and others. We shall be concerned only with interpretation.

A. COLOR

The normal yellow color of the urine depends on the concentration of urochromes whose output is relatively constant. When urine volume is increased, the urochromes are diluted so that the urine is paler. Thus chronic interstitial nephritis, diabetes insipidus, diabetes mellitus, increased fluid load by ingestion or parenteral administration, and pyometra generally result in pale to colorless urine.

A dark urine due to concentration of urochromes occurs in cases where dehydration has resulted from fever, fluid losses in vomition, diarrhea, serous exudation, and reduced fluid intake. The early stage of acute renal insufficiency may have a concentrated, highly colored urine but the diuretic phase will be pale. In general, a rough approximation of specific gravity may be predicted from the color. Pale urines have low specific gravity; dark urines have high values.

Hemoglobin produces a urine of wine red color which in time may be changed to brown alkaline or acid hematin, depending on urinary pH. Pyrocatechins in horse urine change its yellow color to brown on standing. Horse urine will be brown on black from the excretion of myoglobin in azoturia. In cases of congenital porphyria, a faint pink from porphyrins may be seen in the urine and such urines will show an orange fluorescence under the Wood's light. A brownish orange to green color will be imparted by bilirubin which can be converted to green biliverdin by oxidation.

Drugs such as dizan and methylene blue give a greenish to blue color; phenothiazine (oxidized) and neoprontosil a red to orange color; phenol, salol, and creosote a brown to black color. Senna and acriflavine result in a yellow to green color.

B. CLARITY

Most of the time the urine is clear on being voided, but may become cloudy on standing. The more concentrated the urine, the more likely is precipitation to occur on standing. It is best that urine be examined as soon as possible after voiding.

When voided, horse urine is usually cloudy due to large amounts of calcium carbonate crystals which are suspended in a matrix of mucus.

Other materials causing turbidity are bacteria, epithelial cells, erythrocytes (in which case the urine may be pink to red), leukocytes sperm cells, casts, and Tamm and Horsfall mucoprotein (1950).

C. ODOR

The odor of urine is derived from volatile organic acids. The boar, tom cat, and billy goat have an especially strong odor to their urine. When urine is being broken down by bacteria or long retention has occurred, an odor of ammonia may be noted if urea is being converted to ammonia. The odor becomes more fetid when bacteria and pus cells are found because of the protein breakdown which accompanies their presence. Acetone may be detected in ruminant urine in pregnancy disease, ketosis, or displacement of the abomasum and other disease states.

D. Specific Gravity and Urinary Solute Concentration

The clinical interpretation to be made from specific gravity is the assessment of distal tubular function, that is, the ability of the kidney to maintain water and osmolar homeostasis. The precise knowledge required for this assessment, is the urinary solute concentration. Specific gravity is only an approximate measurement of the solute concentration because it is dependent on molecular size and weight as well as the number of molecules of solute. Equal numbers of molecules or urea, salt, albumin, globulin, fibrinogen, and glucose all make different relative contributions to the specific gravity because of their different molecular weights. Because the distal tubular function is dependent on the number and not the weight of solute, estimation of osmolarity is, therefore, to be preferred. For practical purposes a close correlation exists between specific gravity and osmolarity. If an animal is passing concentrated or dilute urine, the specific gravity is a satisfactory measure for clinical interpretation. The correlation between these two measurements is, however, not sufficiently precise for definitive clinical evaluation when the urine osmolarity approaches isotonicity. Bovee (1969) using a refractometer (TS meter, which is perhaps the most widely used instrument for specific gravity determination) has found that in dog's urine with the specific gravity 1.010, the predicted osmolarity is approximately 330 mOsm, with 95% confidence limits ranging from 160 to 540 mOsm. Likewise, at an osmolarity of 300 mOsm, the 95% confidence limits range from 1.003 to 1.016.

In chronic renal disease in which an extensive number of nephrons have been destroyed, the ability to concentrate and dilute the urine is limited. Because of the lack of precision in specific gravity estimation, the concept of a fixed specific gravity in isosthenuria has arisen. Fixed specific gravity has the clinical interpretation of failure to respond to either water loading or water deprivation. With more precise measurements using an osmometer, Bovee (1969) found that dogs with clinical isosthenuria had some concentrating ability and thus the concept of a fixed specific gravity is not physiologically sound. This does not embarass the conclusion that isosthenuria is associated with a very grave prognosis.

Because specific gravity or osmolality changes depending on the degree of hydration, random specific gravity determinations on urine have little clinical interpretation. Many textbooks present mean values and normal ranges for specific gravity determinations in various animals. These generally show an average specific gravity of 1.025 to 1.030, with a maximum specific gravity in the order of 1.045 for all species except the pig, which supposedly has a maximum specific gravity of 1.030. Average specific gravity is a meaningless concept clinically. What is important is the knowledge as to whether the animal has the capability to concentrate or dilute its urine. Repeated specific gravity determinations on random urine samples from dogs throughout the day showed variation from 1.006 to 1.025 under the conditions in my laboratory.

Maximum specific gravity is not so constant across the species as is suggested. Cattle and dogs have a maximum concentrating ability (specific gravity of 1.045) similar to that of man. Pigs and horses are capable of greater urinary concentration. With far greater concentration ability than the other species, are cats and sheep. Both of these species are capable of concentrating their urine to a specific gravity in the order of 1.070 and perhaps a maximum of 1.080.

E. FOAM

When urine is shaken after collection, foam will be produced. This foam will be abundant and slow to disappear when there is a high content of protein or bile salts and pigments. In the former instance there is no color and in the latter the color may be yellow, yellow-brown to green due to the bilirubin. When hemoglobin is present the foam is red to brown.

F. PROTEINURIA

For the most part, the normal glomerular membrane does not permit the passage of plasma proteins, and such protein which does pass the membrane is reabsorbed by the tubules so that the urine is free of protein when tested by the usual clinical methods. When the glomerular membrane is damaged, bleeding occurs anywhere along the urogenital tract from the kidney down to the orifice of the urethra or with pyelonephritis, protein may be detected in the urine. Ordinarily the glomerulus supplies the bulk of the protein which is seen in the urine. The first proteins to leak through the membrane are albumin and α-globulin so that the presence of albumin should be referred to strictly as albuminuria. However, the term has been used loosely to indicate any protein in the urine. When the damage is greater, β- and γ-globulins and fibrinogen may also appear. In cases of proteinuria, a portion of the protein will be reabsorbed by the tubules.

The presence of proteinuria is abnormal except at the time of estrus, during parturition, or in the first few days of life. Excessive ingestion of protein may give an albumin reaction in the human. After violent exercise or under great emotional stress, protein may give be found in the urine. Perhaps capillary dilation is responsible. Such exercise does not seem to produce any permanent damage but the proteinuria cannot be considered completely normal.

Abnormal proteinuria is brought about by a wide variety of conditions such as inflammation, trauma, neoplasia, parasitism, convulsions, exposure to cold, bleeding diatheses, renal poisons, and congenital conditions.

In acute renal failure, marked loss of protein in the urine occurs. Pyelonephritis produces varying degrees of proteinuria depending on the amount of tissue involvement and acuteness of the process. Cattle with pyelonephritis will generally have a strong protein reaction. Chronic inflammation of the kidney as in chronic interstitial nephritis usually leads to a trace reaction or a moderately positive reaction. Renal amyloidosis produces a strong protein reaction. The large volume of urine seen in chronic interstitial nephritis dilutes the protein so that the reaction is moderate, although the total amount of protein lost may be considerable.

Acute renal insufficiency, a frequent sequel to pancreatic necrosis, intestinal obstruction, trauma, adrenocortical insufficiency, or nephrotoxic poisons, is manifested by the presence of large quantities of urinary protein. The protein leakage is attributable to renal ischemia with damage to the capillary walls or is due to the direct effect or deleterious substances on the capillaries.

Viremia, endotoxin, and products of tissue destruction elsewhere in the body permit protein leakage from the glomerular capillaries. These capillaries are so susceptible to damage that pyrexia, passive congestion due to tumors, ascites, or heart disease can produce proteinuria. Infarction leads to proteinuria as does the presence of metastatic neoplasms such as lymphosarcoma. *Dioctophyma renale*, *Stephanurus denatus*, and *Dirofilaria immitis* infections may contribute protein to the urine. In the latter instance, passive congestion may be responsible for the proteinuria.

Although the kidney is most frequently the source of protein, ureteritis, cystitis, urethritis, vaginitis, prostatitis, metritis, pyometra, seminal vesiculitis, balanitis, calculosis, and *Capillaria plica* are incriminated in many instances. The contribution of protein from the genital tract may be avoided by catheterizing the bladder.

In summation, the glomerular membrane is extremely sensitive to toxic substances, ischemia, and inflammation. It is very difficult to determine the cause for a proteinuria on the basis of the amount. Proteinuria indicates urogenital tract pathology and is a sensitive index of the presence of such abnormality. Absence of proteinuria and the absence of other signs of renal or postrenal involvement tend to rule out disease in the urinary tract, but occasional exceptions may occur. Some localization of the lesion may be possible by palpation, radiography, and determination of the type of sediment.

G. Technique for Examination of Urine Sediment

For good results in examination of urine sediment, it is essential that the technique of collection and examination be performed with great care. If the urine is to be collected by catheter, gentle insertion and appropriate lubrication are important to avoid trauma. Examination should be made shortly after collection so degeneration and lysis of cellular elements will not occur and bacteria will not proliferate. Light centrifugal force should be applied to the urine so that casts are not broken up by marked packing with subsequent fragmentation on shaking up the sediment

The best procedure is to centrifuge 10–15 ml urine at 1000 rpm for 5 minutes. The resulting sediment should be examined for amount, color, and type of aggregation. Erythrocytes give a red button. Crystals are usually white. When bile pigments are present, the button is yellow. Lipids float in a centrifuged sample. Phosphate crystals may be suspended in a highly concentrated sample and produce a white cloudiness.

Heavy sediments should be diluted with the supernatant urine so it is easy to see the elements as a single layer without overlapping. It may be unnecessary to centrifuge samples with a heavy sediment. A drop of sediment is placed on a clean glass slide and a coverslip is then added. Reduction of light by appropriate use of a lowered condenser and closed diaphragm aid in microscopic examination. Low power examination at $100\times$ should precede high dry examination at $430\times$. Under low power the amount of sediment, the presence of casts, and staining with bile pigments become apparent. High power reveals the details of cell types and the presence of bacteria. The Gram stain will assist in identifying leukocytes and classifying bacteria. There is no need to stain the sediment for accurate recognition of components of the sediment. Some clinicians find one or two drops of New Methylene blue stain added to the urine before centrifugation helps identification. Wright's stain can confirm the presence of leukocytes and erythrocytes. A test of the sediment for hemoglobin will confirm that erythrocytes or ghost forms of red cells are present.

H. Classification of Urine Sediment

The sediment may be divided into organized and unorganized elements. Of greatest clinical value is the examination of the organized fraction which consists of epithelial cells, leukocytes, erythrocytes, casts, bacteria, protozoa, yeasts, fungi, metazoan parasites, and sperm. The unorganized elements are primarily crystals, pigments, and fat droplets.

I. Normal Sediment

The normal animal will show the presence of epithelial cells, an occasional erythrocyte, white blood cells, and a male dog, spermatazoa. It is often suggested that a recently mated bitch may have spermatazoa in urine specimen. Unless urine is voided within 30 minutes to 1 hour after mating, spermatozoa are not found in the urine. Normal urine is sterile in the bladder although the urethra may contain bacteria which get into the voided sample, but are not visible by microscopic examination. Dogs, cats, and other carnivores will usually show the presence of phosphate crystals. These same crystals may be seen in cattle or sheep, but in general the urine in these animals is more dilute and therefore show less precipitation. Typical horse urine is characterized by the presence of mucous threads and calcium carbonate crystals.

Many extraneous objects such as parasite eggs from fecal contamination, plant spores, and other organic matter may contaminate normal urine. If collection is made from a voided sample or in equipment which is not sterile or if the urine is not kept refrigerated, rapid growth of bacteria and yeast can occur.

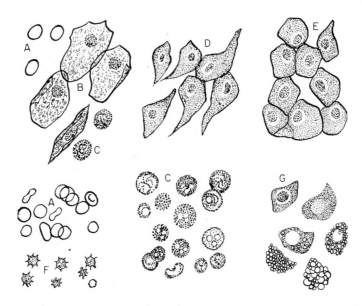

Fig. 3.   Organized sediments. (Sketch by J. S. Luick.) (*A*) Red blood cells. (*B*) Squamous epithelial cells. (*C*) Leukocytes or pus cells (*D*) Caudage epithelial cells from pelvis of kidney. (*E*) Transitional epithelial cells from bladder. (*F*) Crenated red blood cells. (*G*) Renal epithelial cells with and without lipid degeneration. (600 ×). (Courtesy C. E. Cornelius.)

J. White Blood Cells

Bloom (1960) states that more than 10 leukocytes in a high power field after centrifugation of 15 ml urine suggest that inflammation or necrosis of tissue must be present somewhere in the urogenital tract. When the animal is catheterized without permitting contamination from the vagina, prepuce, or penis any cells present must have come from the bladder, ureter, pelvis, or kidney. White blood cells may be difficult to identify because of degeneration of the nucleus or precipitation of crystals on their surface. Large numbers in an alkaline urine may decompose to give a mucilaginous quality to the urine.

K. Erythrocytes

Whereas white blood cells suggest inflammation or necrosis, erythrocytes appear in the urine not only because of necrosis or inflammation but also because of trauma, capillary damage in certain viral infections, infarction, chronic passive congestion, calculosis, hemorrhagic tendencies from clotting defects, parasites such as *Capillaria plica, Dioctophyma renale, Dirofilaria immitis* larvae, the administration or ingestion of poisons such as mercury, arsenic, or thallium, and capillary damage resulting from shock. Following catheterization, traumatic palpation of bladder or kidney, renal biopsy, or violent exercise, large numbers of erythrocytes may be found in the urine. Some localization of the bleeding can be inferred to be in the bladder if only the final act of micturition is contaminated with blood. When the blood is uniform by distribution throughout the sample, it is probable that bleeding is present in the kidney or ureter. Blood which appears only at the onset of urination is probably from a urethral lesion.

The appearance of the erythrocyte varies depending on the osmolarity of the urine of low specific gravity, the cell may be ballooned into a spherical shape or may lyse and become a ghost form which is then no longer slightly green in color, but similar to the hyaline cast in color. At specific gravities around 1.020, the cell is a biconcave disc which can sometimes be seen as it rolls over to reveal its thinner diameter. When viewed from above, it has an appearance of concentric rings. At high specific gravities, the erythrocytes become crenated so that cells bear "prickles" over the surface or are distorted and crumpled in outline.

L. Epithelial Cells

Epithelial cells are normally seen in the urine, but are increased in instances where there is a cystitis or any inflammation present. However, quantitative data are not available as to the normal limits of epithelial cells in centrifuged sediment of animal urine. Distribution of types of epithelial cells along the urinary tract is specific for any one species. In general, the epithelial cells of the collecting ducts and hilus of the kidney are cubodial, epithelial cells of the bladder are predominantly transitional, and epithelial cells of the lower urethra, vagina, and prepuce are squamous. Increased exfoliation of cells from any area of the tract will show itself as an increased proportion of these particular cells on cytological examination of the sediment. Perhaps one reason why cytological examination has been criticized in the past, is the very

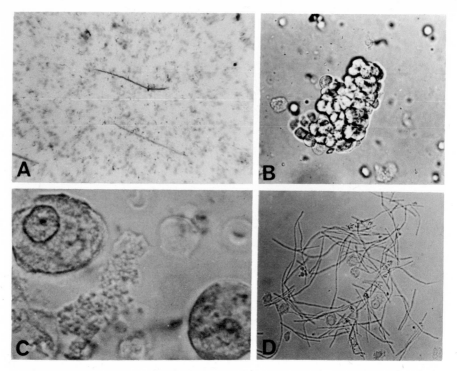

Fig. 4.   Cellular sediment from canine urine. (Courtesy C. E. Cornelius.) (*A*) Microfilaria (Wrights stain, 560 ×). (*B*) Aggregates of pus cells (leukocytes) in cystitis (560 ×). (*C*) Transitional epithelial cells (bladder cells) in cystitis (560 ×). (*D*) Terminal uremia: saprophytic bacteria and epithelial cells (140 ×).

poor preparations that have been made. Using proprietary cytological preparatory systems, excellent results can be obtained in the routine laboratory. Combined cytological and radiological examination is probably the best procedure for localizing areas of tissue destruction.

M. Casts

One of the most important findings in organized sediment is the cast which is formed from combination of protein and mucopolysaccharide. The protein is thought to be derived from glomerular leakage. As this dissolved protein passes down the tubule the filtrate becomes more and more acid. At the isoelectric point the protein tends to precipitate, so concentrated acidic urine will often show casts which are precipitates molded into a cylindrical form in the distal tubule. The mucopolysaccharide may be contributed by the tubule. The best characterized mucoprotein in urine is that isolated in 1950 by Tamm and Horsfall. This Tamm and Horsfall mucoprotein is a major constituent of urinary casts. The source of the protein has not been accurately determined and may be a result of degeneration of epithelial cells. Whatever happens to be in the tubule at the time of precipitation may be embedded in the cast. Epithelial cells will form epithelial casts, and as these cells degenerate, granules of the granular cast are formed. The final stage of degeneration

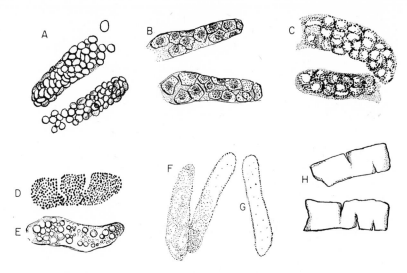

Fig. 5.   Organized sediments casts. (Sketch by J. S. Luick.) (*A*) Red blood cell casts. (*B*) Renal tubular epithelial cell casts. (*C*) Leukocyte or pus cell casts. (*D*) Coarsely granular tube cast. (*E*) Fatty cast. (*F*) Finely granular tube casts. (*G*) Hyaline cast. (*H*) Waxy tube casts (267 ×). (Courtesy C. E. Cornelius.)

is the refractile waxy cast. They are present in the urine most frequently in irreversible cases of renal failure. Erythrocytic or white blood cell casts are also formed. Crystals may be trapped to form crystalline casts. The absence of identifiable elements in the matrix results in a hyaline cast. Cylindroids differ from casts only in that the end is pointed; otherwise they have the same interpretation.

The presence of casts connotes that protein has been lost through the glomerulus or possibly from the tubular cells. Casts are seen in inflammatory or degenerative lesions of the kidney. Acute or chronic nephritis, renal poisons, and shock lead to the appearance of casts. Casts are seen fairly commonly in the concentrated acidic urine of the carnivore but are uncommon findings in the herbivore with its alkaline urine and larger volume output. Casts are rather uncommon in chronic nephritis because the urine is dilute. Whenever casts are seen, it indicates that the kidney is involved and it is therefore a localizing sign.

N. MUCIN

In inflammations of the lower urinary tract and in the normal horse, sinuous threads of mucus studded with crystals may be seen. Mucus threads may be differentiated from casts because of their serpentine form. They originate in the renal pelvis.

O. BACTERIURIA AND PARASITURIA

Freshly collected normal urine samples which have been obtained by catheter show no bacteria in the sediment when it is observed as a wet preparation or as a stained smear. When inflammation occurs, leukocytes and erythrocytes as well as bacteria

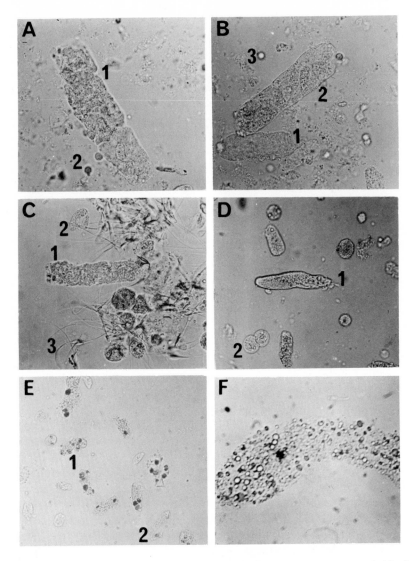

Fig. 6.   Casts in canine urine sediments. (Courtesy C. E. Cornelius.) (*A*) Acute nephritis: *1*, coarse granular and cellular cast; *2*, pus cells (560 ×). (*B*) Chronic interstial: *1*, fine granular cast; *2*, coarse granular cast; *3*, erythrocyte (560 ×). (*C*) Chronic interstitial nephritis: *1*, fine granular cast; *2*, transitional epithelial cell; *3*, spermatozoa (560 ×). (*D*) Cardiac failure: *1*, fine granular cast; *2*, unclassified epithelial cells (560 ×). (*E*) Chronic nephritis: *1*, granular cast containing erythrocytes and leukocytes; *2*, fine granular cast (140 ×). (*F*) Waxy cast; note various sized fat globules contained in cast (560 ×).

may be seen. Sometimes the bacteria are being phagocytized by leukocytes. The number of erythrocytes may be so great as to obscure the bacteria and leukocytes. This often occurs in pyelonephritis in cattle. The presence of yeasts is generally a result of contamination as is the presence of protozoa and parasite ova. The ova of *Capillaria plica, Dioctophyma renale*, and the larvae of *Dirofilaria immitis* can arise from the urinary tract.

P. Unorganized Sediment

For diagnostic purposes, unorganized sediment plays a minor role. Most normal urine samples (the horse is an exception) are clear on voiding and may become cloudy from cystalline precipitation as they cool. Calcium phosphate, magnesium ammonium phosphate, oxalates, and uric acid or urates are found in carnivore urine. The latter crystals are usually seen more abundantly in urine of the Dalmatian. Phosphates and oxalate crystals are frequently seen in cattle and sheep urine. Horse urine usually shows calcium carbonate or calcium oxalate crystals.

When calculi occur in the urine, the determination of the type of crystal in the sediment becomes important so that logical therapy may be instituted to prevent recurrence. The ingestion of ethylene glycol may result in the appearance of oxalates in the urine. Where sulfonamides have been administered, an oliguria, the presence in the sediment of erythrocytes and sulfa crystals all point to precipitation of these salts in the kidney.

Bloom (1960) states that leucine and tyrosine crystals are not normally seen except in severe liver disease due to poisoning from phosphorus, carbon tetrachloride, or chloroform. The excretion of cystine crystals may occur as a familial, inherited aberration in cystine transport in male dogs. The crystals are hexagonal plates. Fat

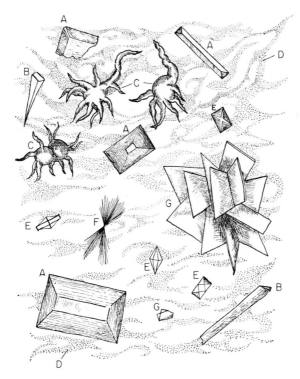

Fig. 7.   Unorganized sediments (sketch by J. S. Luick.) Alkaline urine: (*A*) triple phosphate crystals; (*B*) calcium phosphate crystals; (*C*) ammonium biurate crystals; (*D*) amorphous phosphates. Acid urines: (*E*) calcium oxalate crystals; (*F*) needles resembling tyrosine; (*G*) uric acid crystals, and (*D*) amorphous urates of acid urine (333 ×). (Courtesy C. E. Cornelius.)

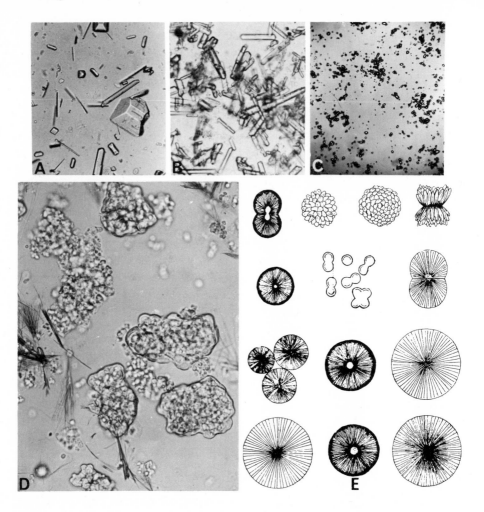

Fig. 8.   Crystalline (unorganized) urine sediments. (Courtesy C. E. Cornelius.) (*A*) Triple phosphates in canine urine pH 7.5 (280 ×). (*B*) Triple phosphates in ovine urine pH 8.6 (280 ×). (*C*) Calcium carbonate in equine urine (70 ×). (*D*) Aggregates of phosphatic "microcalculi" in urethers during experimental urolitheasis (280 ×). (*E*) Schematic diagram of calcium carbonate in horse urine (adapted after Fish, 1911).

droplets may be seen especially in cats. In severe cases of diabetes mellitus lipids may occur in the urine.

Observations of gross appearance, volume, specific gravity, protein, and sediment are essential in order to detect kidney damage. The remaining tests are often useful to elucidate systematic disease or other extrarenal lesions.

Q. Hydrogen Ion Concentration, pH

Cattle, horses, and sheep have a urinary pH of 7–8. The pig, which is an omnivore, may show either an acid or an alkaline reaction. Carnivores such as the dog and cat will generally give a reaction between pH 6 and 7. Nursing animals will show an acid urine even if in adult life they characteristically have an alkaline reaction on an herbivorous diet.

Low urinary pH may result from tissue catabolism as in fever, starvation, diabetes mellitus, and nephritis. The ingestion of large quantities of protein or acidifying salts such as ammonium chloride, ammonium mandelate, sodium acid phosphate, sodium chloride, and calcium chloride, produces an acid urine. Respiratory or metabolic acidosis tends to be reflected by an acid urine.

An alkaline reaction occurs when the urine is retained in the bladder due to an obstructive lesion or cystitis. Urea is broken down to ammonia simply by chemical decomposition or by bacteria which are "urea-splitters." The ingestion of salts such as sodium or potassium acetate, citrate, bicarbonate, lactate, and nitrate can give an alkaline reaction. Metabolic or respiratory alkalosis from vomiting or hyperventilation can be reflected in an alkaline urine.

R. GLUCOSURIA

Normal urine contains no glucose. Although the glucose is freely filtered at the glumerular membrane, reabsorption is complete in the proximal tubule if the load in the blood does not exceed 160–180 mg glucose/100 ml of blood. Above this value, glucose will occur in the urine.

A heavy meal of carbohydrates may elevate the blood sugar so that glycosuria is seen. Violent exercise, fear, excitement and shock stimulate the output of epinephrine and glucocorticoids which produce hyperglycemia. Hyperthyroidism may result in glycosuria from rapid intake of glucose from the gut. Occasionally a lesion of the brain in the region of the fourth ventricle may mediate glycosuria through its effect on the adrenal. General anesthesia or asphyxia results in more rapid release of glucose from liver glycogen. Convulsions, rabies, and the terminal stage of bacterial infections may act in the same way. Veterinarians may produce hyperglycemia by injecting glucocorticoids, epinephrine, or dextrose solutions.

Enterotoxemia will frequently produce glycosuria (Noyan, 1958) perhaps due to stimulation of the adrenal glands causing hyperglycemia or to specific inhibition of glucose reabsorption in the proximal tubule.

In diabetes mellitus, glucosuria varies from a trace to a heavy glucose content— the underlying mechanism is elevated blood glucose concentrations due to an absolute or relative lack of insulin which prevents glucose utilization by the cells. Diabetes mellitus follows acute pancreatic necrosis if the animal survives over 5 days. Large animals are rarely affected with diabetes mellitus so sugar reactions are much more uncommon. Overactivity of the anterior pituitary and adrenal cortex from neoplasia tends to have a diabetogenic effect. Chronic liver disease may be accompanied by glycosuria.

Certain other carbohydrates or reducing substances may give a false positive reaction when tested by a method which depends on the reduction of copper. These are chloral hydrate, formaldehyde, antibiotics (penicillin, streptomycin, auremycin, terramycin) lactose, matose, galactose, ascorbic acid, pentoses, salicylates, uric acid, glucuronic acid, and glucuronates. However, enzyme tests such as Tes Tape (Eli Lilly Co.) and Clinistix (Ames Corp.) which test for glucose alone, do not give false positives.

Lactosuria is not infrequent in lactating animals. Maltosuria or fructosuria follows ingestion of this sugar or accompanies severe liver damage and diabetes mellitus. Pentosuria is the result of ingesting large quantities of carbohydrates. In general, these other carbohydrates have little diagnostic importance.

S. KETONURIA

The passing of ketone bodies in the urine accompanies the accumulation of these substances in the blood. Ketone bodies consist of acetoacetic acid, β-hydroxybutyric acid, and acetone.

In small animals such as the dog and cat, the principal cause for ketosis is diabetes mellitus, although in young puppies or kittens high fever and starvation will result in ketonuria. Adult dogs and cats seldom show ketosis except from prolonged inanition produced by foreign bodies, neoplasms, or the like.

The situation in herbivorous animals is quite different. The cow, which because of its low glucose level of 40–60 mg/100 ml blood is in incipient hypoglycemia, develops ketosis readily from a large variety of conditions in which carbohydrate metabolism does not keep up with the carbohydrate needs of the body. Thus high-producing dairy cattle may show ketosis when improperly fed or anorexia develops from traumatic reticulitis, pneumonia, metritis, mastitis, pododermatitis, displaced abomasum, and other diseases. Cattle will also develop ketosis and thus ketonuria in the absence of a primary disease process where the carbohydrate intake is not adequate for the needs of the body.

In sheep, ketosis may be secondary to conditions as outline for cattle. Sheep develop an especially intense ketonuria in pregnancy disease, which accompanies the bearing of twin lambs.

T. BILIRUBINURIA

The old assumption that only direct and not indirect bilirubin can be excreted with urine seems to be logical, but no specific experimental evidence supports this contention. There is tremendous species variation in the degree of bilirubinuria, but unfortunately very little published work has been reported on the renal excretion of this substance. The horse is unique in the high plasma bilirubin concentration that it can contain. Beijers *et al.* (1950) and Osbaldiston and Fuhrman (1970) have both found no bilirubinuria in foals suffering from isoerythrolysis. The plasma threshold for bilirubinuria in dogs is particularly low, being 0.4 mg/100 ml (Rosenthal and Meier, 1921). This finding is in accord with Bloom's statement (1960) that normal dogs may show a mild bilirubinuria. A similar observation has been made with cattle (Kuhle, 1926). Bilirubinuria occurs in obstructive jaundice (Cameron *et al.*, 1963) and hepatic necrosis (Cornelius, 1963).

U. UROBILINOGENURIA

Urobilinogen is colorless when excreted in the urine, but on oxidation becomes converted to the greenish fluorescent pigment urobilin. Urobilinogen is formed in the intestinal tract by a bacterial reduction of conjugated bilirubin. Much of the urobilinogen is excreted in the feces as stercobilinogen or stercobilin. A portion of the urobilinogen is absorbed into the portal system. The liver excretes most of this urobilinogen, but a small amount is excreted in the urine. With (1968) has reviewed normal urobilinogen excretion in animals. Following a hemolytic crisis, increased urinary urobilinogen excretion occurs. If the hepatic cells are damaged, the removal of urobilinogen from the portal circulation may be depressed and higher levels can reach the kidney. Obstruction to the flow of bile into the intestinal tract cuts off the formation of urobilinogen as with certain antibiotics such as chloromycetin or aureomycin which interfere with the bacterial reduction of bilirubin.

V. Hemoglobinuria

Hemoglobinuria which results from the rapid hemolysis of erythrocytes, may be brought about by snake venons, intravascular poisons, phosphorus, acetanilide, potassium chlorate, lead poisoning, transfusion reactions, allergic reactions, *Hemobartonella*, piroplasmosis, babesiasis, infections due to *Clostridium*, *Streptococcus*, and extensive burns. Cattle will show an idiopathic hemoglobinuria after ingestion of a large volume of cold water.

Hematuria has been discussed under the section dealing with urine sediment. It should be realized that erythrocytes frequently rupture in dilute or alkaline urine to release hemoglobin and leave behind their stroma as ghost cells. Thus, not all hemoglobinuria may be the result of hemoglobin passing through the glomerular membrane.

W. Porphyria

Porphyrinuiria is produced by three different mechanisms. First, there may be an abnormality in the formation of the hemoglobin molecule so that porphyrinemia develops and porphyrins enter the urine as has been reported in cattle (Fourie, 1953). Second, liver damage, cirrhosis, hepatitis, or toxic damage from lead may impair the liver's ability to remove porphyrins from the circulation, and thus they enter the urine. Third, if the liver is damaged by certain toxic plants, the breakdown of chlorophyll to phylloerythrin will occur as usual, but when phylloerythrin is absorbed from the intestines it is not removed from the circulation and therefore passes the glomerular membrane.

X. Myoglobinuria

The rapid breakdown of muscle may cause myoglobin to occur in the urine. Crushing injuries, violent straining, tetanus, and azoturia may be associated with myoglobin in the urine.

Y. Indicanuria

Tryptophan is degraded in the intestine to indole, which after absorption is transformed to indoxyl which is ten coupled with sulfate to form potassium indoxyl sulfate in the liver. This is then excreted as indican in the urine. Increased breakdown of protein as in gastroenteritis or obstruction of the intestinal tract from constipation, foreign body, torsion, intussusception, volvulus, and stricture leads to elevated indican levels in the urine. Rapid breakdown of body tissue as in gangrene can elevate the indican in the urine. Thus, an increased indicanuria is usually associated with an intestinal lesion, but the reaction is nonspecific and does not localize the lesion.

REFERENCES

Ali, M. A., and Billing, B. H. (1968). *Am. J. Physiol.* **214**, 1340.
Allen, A. C. (1966). *In* "The Kidney" (F. K. Mostofi, ed.). Williams & Wilkins, Baltimore, Maryland.
Alpen, E. L., and Kranmore, D. (1959). *In* "Kinetics of Cellular Proliferation" (F. Stohlman, ed.), p. 53. Grune & Stratton, New York.
Anderson, R. R., and Mixner, J. P. (1959). *J. Diary Sci.* **42**, 545.
Anderson, R. R., and Mixner, J. P. (1960). *J. Dairy Sci.* **43**, 1476.
Anderson, R. S., and Pickering, E. C. (1961). *J. Physiol. (London)* **163**, 33.
Asheim, A., Persson, F., and Persson, S. (1961). *Acta Physiol. Scand.* **51**, 150.
Aukland, K. (1968). *Acta Physiol. Scand.* **74**, 173.
Bahlmann, J., Giebisch, G., Ochwadt, B., and Schoeppe, W. (1967). *Am. J. Physiol.* **212**, 77.
Baldus, W. P., and Summerskill, W. H. J. (1967). *Postgrad. Med.* **41**, 103.
Barac, G. (1951). *Rev. Med. Liege* **6**, 186.
Bard, P. (1961). "Medical Physiology." Mosby, St. Louis, Missouri.
Barraclough, M. A., and Mills, I. H. (1965). *Clin. Sci.* **28**, 69.
Bauman, A. W., Clarkson, T. W., and Miles, M. (1963). *J. Appl. Physiol.* **18**, 1239
Bauman, L., and Oviatt, E. (1915). *J. Biol. Chem.* **22**, 43.
Beijers, J. A., van Loghem, J. J., and van der Hart, M. (1950). *Tijdschr. Diergeneesk.* **75**, 955–970.
Benjamin, M. (1967). "An Outline of Veterinary Clinical Pathology." Iowa State Univ. Press, Ames, Iowa.
Berger, L., Yü, T. F., and Gutman, A. B. (1960). *Am. J. Physiol.* **198**, 573.
Berliner, R. W. (1960). *Harvey Lectures* **55**, 141.
Berliner, R. W. (1966). *In* "The Kidney" (F. K. Mostofi, ed.). Williams & Wilkins, Baltimore, Maryland.
Bernstein, L. N. (1965). "Renal Function and Renal Failure." Williams & Wilkins, Baltimore, Maryland.
Beyer, K. H. (1950). *Pharmacol. Rev.* **2**, 227.
Biber, T. V. L., Mylle, M., Baines, A. D., Gottschalk, C. W., Oliver, J. R., and MacDowell, M. C. (1969). *Am. J. Med.* **44**, 664.
Bing, R. J. (1943). *Am. J. Physiol.* **140**, 240.
Black, D. A. K. (1958). "Essentials of Fluid Balance." Blackwell, Oxford.
Blatteis, C. M., and Horvath, S. M. (1958). *Am. J. Physiol.* **192**, 353.
Bloom, F. (1937). *J. Am. Vet. Med. Assoc.* **91**, 679.
Bloom, F. (1960). "The Urine of the Dog and Cat." Gamma Publ., New York.
Bovee, K. C. (1969). *J. Am. Vet. Med. Assoc.* **155**, 30.
Bradley, S. E. (1947). "Factors Regulating Blood Pressure," Ist Conf. J. Macy, Jr. Found., New York.
Bricker, N. S., Morrin, P. A. F., and Kline, S. W. (1960). *Am. J. Med.* **28**, 77.
Bricker, N.S., Klahr, S., Lubowitz, H., and Rieselbach, R. E. (1965). *Medicine, (Baltimore)* **44**, 263.
Brobst, D. F., Carter, J. M., and Herron, M. (1967). *17th Gaines Vet. Symp. Univ. Minn.*, p. 15.
Brown, J. L., Samiy, A. H., and Pitts, R. F. (1961). *Am. J. Physiol.* **200**, 370.
Brun, C., and Munck, O. (1966). *In* "The Kidney" (F. K. Mostofi, ed.). Williams & Wilkins, Baltimore, Maryland.
Brun, C., Crone, C., Davidsen, H. G., Fabritius, J., Tybjaerg, Hansen, A., Lassen, N. A., and Munck, O. (1955). *Proc. Soc. Exptl. Biol. Med.* **89**, 687.
Bull, G. M., Joekes, A. M., and Lowe, K. G. (1950). *Clin. Sci.* **9**, 379.
Cameron, J. L., Stafford, E. S., Schnaufer, L., and Iber, F. L. (1963). *J. Surg. Res.* **3**, 39–42.
Chapman, E. M., and Halsted, J. A. (1933). *Fractional Phenolsulphonphthalein Test in Bright's Disease* **186**, 223.
Chart, J. J., Gordon, E. S., Helmer, P., and Lesher, M. (1956). *J. Clin. Invest.* **35**, 254.

Clapp, J. R. (1965). *Proc. Soc. Exptl. Biol. Med.* **120**, 521.

Clapp, J. R., Watson, J. F., and Berliner, R. W. (1963). *Am. J. Physiol.* **205**, 693.

Coffin, D. L. (1953). "Manual of Veterinary Clinical Pathology." Cornell Univ. Press, Ithaca, New York.

Cook, W. F., and Pickering G. W. (1962). *Biochem. Pharmacol.* **9**, 165.

Copp, D. H., McPherson, G. D., and McIntosh, H. W. (1960). *Metab., Clin. Exptl.* **9**, 680.

Coppage, W. S., Island, D. P., Cooner, A. E., and Liddle, G. W. (1962). *J. Clin. Invest.* **41**, 1672.

Corcoran, A. D., and Page, I. H. (1938). *Am. J. Physiol.* **126**, 254.

Cornelius, C. E. (1963). *In* "Clinical Biochemistry of Domestic Animals" (C. E. Cornelius and J. J. Kaneko, eds.), p. 225. Academic Press, New York.

Dalton, R. G. (1964). *Brit. Vet. J.* **120**, 69.

Dalton, R. G. (1968). *Brit. Vet. J.* **124**, 371.

Dantzler, W. H. (1966). *Am. J. Physiol.* **210**, 640.

Dent, C. E., and Harris, H. (1951). *Ann. Eugenics (London)* **16**, 60.

de Wardener, A. G. (1967). "The Kidney." Churchill, London.

Dirks, J. H. (1968). *J. Physiol. Pharmacol.* **46**, 315.

Dirks, J. H., Clapp, J. R., and Berliner, R. W. (1964). *J. Clin. Invest.* **43**, 916.

Dirks, J. H., Cirksena, W. J., and Berliner, R. W. (1965). *J. Clin. Invest.* **44**, 1160.

Dixon, J. M. (1958). *Poultry Sci.* **37**, 410.

Dorman, P. J. Sullivan, W. J., and Pitts, R. F. (1954). *J. Clin. Invest.* **33**, 82.

Dukes, H. H. (1947). "The Physiology of Domestic Animals," 6th ed. Cornell Univ. Press (Comstock), Ithaca, New York.

Dyrenfurth, I., Stacey, C. H., Beck, J. C., and Venning, E. H. (1957). *Metab., Clin. Exptl.* **6**, 544.

Dziemian, A. J., Wilson, P. P., and Meshane, W. P. (1950). *U.S. Army, Med. Center Chem. Corps., Res. Rept.* **29**, 1.

Eggleton, M. G., and Habib, Y. A. (1950). *J. Physiol. (London)* **110**, 458.

Eigler, F. W. (1961). *Am. J. Physiol.* **201**, 157.

Eigler, J.O.C., Salassa, R. N., Bahn, R. C., and Owen, C. A., Jr. (1962). *Am. J. Physiol.* **202**, 1115.

Eiler, J. J., Althausen, T. L., and Stockholm, M. (1944). *Am. J. Physiol.* **140**, 699.

Edelman, R. F., and Hartroft, F. B. (1961). *Circulation Res.* **9**, 1069.

Fourie, P. J. (1953). *Onderstepoort J. Vet. Res.* **26**, 231.

Fulop, M., and Brazeau, P. (1964). *J. Clin. Invest.* **43**, 1192.

Gagnon, J. A., and Clarke, R. W. (1957). *Am. J. Physiol.* **190**, 117.

Gans, J. H. (1964a). *Am. J. Vet. Res.* **25**, 914.

Gans, J. H. (1964b). *Am. J. Vet. Res.* **25**, 924.

Gans, J. H., and Mercer, P. F. (1962). *Am. J. Vet. Res.* **23**, 230.

Gartner, L. M., and Arias, I. M. (1969). *New Engl. J. Med.* **280**, 24.

Gault, M. H. (1966). *Can. Med. Assoc. J.* **94**, 61.

Gault, M. H., Kinsella, T. D., Gonda, A., and Ferguson, G. A. (1966). *Can. Med. Assoc. J.* **94**, 68.

Gertz, K. H., Mangos., J. A., Braun, G., and Pagel, H. D. (1965). *Arch. Ges. Physiol.* **285**, 360.

Gertz, K. H., Mangos, J. A., Braun, G., and Pagel, H. D. (1966). *Arch. Ges. Physiol.* **288**, 369.

Giebisch, G., and Lazano, R. (1959). *J. Clin. Invest.* **38**, 843.

Giebisch, G., Malnic, G., Klose, R. M., and Wrendhager, E. E. (1966). *Am. J. Physiol.* **211**, 560.

Gilman, A. (1958). *Ann. N. Y. Acad. Sci.* **71**, 355.

Glauser, K. F., and Selkurt, E. E. (1952). *Am. J. Physiol.* **168**, 469.

Goldberg, M. (1962). *J. Clin. Invest.* **41**, 2112.

Goldberg, M., McCurdy, D. K., Foltz, E. L., and Bulem, L. W. (1964). *J. Clin. Invest.* **43**, 201.

Goldman, R., and Bassett, S. H. (1954). *J. Clin. Invest.* **33**, 1623.

Goldring, W., Clarke, R. W., and Smith, H. W. (1936). *J. Clin. Invest.* **15**, 221.

Gordon, A. S. (1959). *Physiol. Rev.* **39**, 1.

Gottschalk, C. W., and Lassiter, W. E. (1967). *Proc. 3rd Intern. Congr. Nephrol., 1967* Vol. 1, p. 99.

Gottschalk, C. W., and Mylle, M. (1956). *Am. J. Physiol.* **185**, 430.

Gries, F. A., and Gries, G. (1957). *Klin. Wochschr.* **35**, 81.

Gutman, A. B., and Yü, T. F. (1957). *Am. J. Med.* **23**, 600.

Hammett, F. S. (1915). *J. Biol. Chem.* **22**, 551.

Harris, H., and Milne, M. D. (1964). "Biochemical Disorders in Human Diseases." Churchill, London.

Heinbecker, P., Rolf, D., and White, H. L. (1943). *Am. J. Physiol.* **139**, 543.

Hook, J. B., and Williamson, H. E. (1965). *Proc. Soc. Exptl. Biol. Med.* **118**, 372.

Houck, C. R. (1948). *Am. J. Physiol.* **153**, 169.

Iampietro, P. F., Fiorica, V., Higgins, E. A., Mager, M., and Goldman, R. F. (1966). *Intern. J. Bioclimatol. Biometeorol.* **10**, 2, 175–185.

James, I. M., and Wise, B. L. (1969). *Clin. Sci.* **36**, 99–108.

Jick, H., Snyder, J. G., Finkelstein, E. N., Cohen, J. L., Moore, E. W., and Morrison, R. S. (1963). *J. Clin. Invest.* **42**, 1561.

Jick, H., Kamm, D. E., Snyder, J. C., Morrison, R. S., and Chalmers, T. C. (1964). *J. Clin. Invest.* **43**, 258.

Jolliffe, N., and Smith, H. W. (1931). *Am. J. Physiol.* **98**, 572.

Jones, N. F., Barraclough, M. A., and Mills, I. H. (1963). *Clin. Sci.* **25**, 449.

Kean, E. L., Adams, P. H., Winters, R. W., and Davies, R. W. (1961). *Biochim. Biophys. Acta* **54**, 474.

Kennedy, P. C. (1957). *J. Am. Vet. Med. Assoc.* **130**, 15.

Kessler, R. H., Hierholzer, K., and Gurd, R. S. (1959). *Am. J. Physiol.* **197**, 601.

Ketz, H. A., Vogel, G., Lange, M., and Heym, E. (1956). *Monatsh. Veterinaermed.* **11**, 575.

Kim, J. H., and Hong, S. K. (1962). *Am. J. Physiol.* **202**, 174–178.

King, J., and Wooton, D. P. (1960). "Biochemistry for Medical Students." Churchill, London.

Kirkbride, C. A., and Frey, R. A. (1967). *J. Am. Vet. Med. Assoc.* **151**, 742.

Knudsen, A. (1959). *Acta Vet. Scand.* **1**, 52.

Knudsen, E. (1959). *Acta Vet. Scand.* **1**, 188.

Kramer, K., Thurau, K., and Dutzen, P. (1960). *Arch. Ges. Physiol.* **270**, 251.

Kubicek, W. G., Kottke, F. J., Laker, D. J., and Visscher, M. B. (1953). *Am. J. Physiol.* **174**, 397.

Kuhle, E. (1926). Inaugural Disertation, University of Berlin.

Ladd, M., Liddle, L., Gagnon, J. A., and Clarke, R. W. (1957). *J. Appl. Physiol.* **10**, 249.

Lajtha, L. G. (1964). *Mem. Soc. Endocrinol.* **13**, 239.

Laks, M. M., Pincus, I. J., and Goldberg, D. (1963). *Gastroenterology* **44**, 469.

Lancestremere, R. G., Davidson, P. L., Earley, L. E., O'Brien, F. J., and Papper, S. (1962). *J. Clin. Invest.* **41**, 1922.

Lane, D. R., and Robinson, R. (1968). *Brit. Vet. J.* **125**, 11.

Lapides, J., and Bobbitt, J. M. (1958). *J. Am. Med. Assoc.* **166**, 866.

Lathen, W. (1959). *J. Clin. Invest.* **38**, 652.

Lathen, W., Davis, B. B., Zweig, P. H., and Dew, R. (1960). *J. Clin. Invest.* **39**, 840.

Leslie, S. H., Johnston, B., and Ralli, E. P. (1951). *J. Clin. Invest.* **30**, 1200.

Lotspeich, W. F. (1959). "Metabolic Aspects of Renal Function." Thomas, Springfield, Illinois.

Low, D. G., Bergman, E. N., Hiatt, C. W., and Gleisen, C. A. (1956). *J. Infect. Diseases* **98**, 260.

McCance, L. A., and Widdowson, E. M. (1955). *J. Physiol.* (*London*) **129**, 628.

McDonald, S. J., and de Wardener, H. E. (1965). *Nephron* **2**, 1.

McQueen, E. G. (1962). *J. Clin. Pathol.* **15**, 367.

Malnic, G., Klose, R. M., and Giebisch, G. (1966). *Am. J. Physiol.* **211**, 529.

Malvin, R. L., Sullivan, L. P., and Wilde, W. S. (1957). *Physiologist*, **1**, 58.

Malvin, R. L., Wilde, W. S., and Sullivan, L. P. (1958). *Am. J. Physiol.* **194**, 135.

Manning, J. P., Reber, E. F., Malhstoa, P., Beamen, P. D., Boley, L. E., and Norton, H. W. (1959). *Am. J. Vet. Res.* **20**, 858.

Maxfield, M. (1961). *Biochim. Biophys. Acta* **49**, 548.

Mendel, D. (1959). *J. Physiol.* (*London*) **148**, 1.

Mills, I. H., Osbaldiston, G. W., Craig, G., and Wise, B. L. (1966). *J. Physiol.* (*London*) **186**, 113

Mixner, J. P., and Anderson, R. R. (1961). *J. Dairy Sci.* **41**, 306.

Morgan, J. P., and Gillette, E. L. (1963). *Am. J. Vet. Res.* **24**, 100.

Mostofi, F. K., ed. (1966). "The Kidney" Williams & Wilkins, Baltimore, Maryland.

Mudge, G. H., and Taggart, J. V. (1950a). *Am. J. Physiol.* **161**, 173.

Mudge, G. H., and Taggart, J. V. (1950b). *Am. J. Physiol.* **161**, 191.

Mundsick, R. A., Sawyer, W. H., and Van Dyke, H. V. (1958). *Endocrinology* **63**, 688.

Nechay, B. R., and Nechay, L. (1959). *J. Pharmacol. Exptl. Therap.* **126**, 291.

Nelson, W. P., and Welt, L. C. (1952). *J. Clin. Invest.* **31**, 392.
Nordyke, R. A., Gilbert, F. I., Jr., and Simmons, E. L. (1969). *J. Am. Med. Assoc.* **493**, 208.
Noyan, A. (1958). *Am. J. Vet. Res.* **19**, 840.
Oester, A., and Madsen, P. O. (1968). *Invest. Urol.* **6**, 322.
Oester, A., Olesen, S., and Madsen, P. O. (1968). *Invest. Urol.* **6**, 315.
Oliver, J., MacDowell, M. C., and Tracey, A. (1951). *J. Clin. Invest.* **30**, 1307.
Onesti, G. (1967). *In* "Renal Failure" A. N. Brest and J. H. Moyer, eds., p. 78. Lippincott, Philadelphia, Pennsylvania.
Orloff, J., and Davidson, D. G. (1959). *J. Clin. Invest.* **38**, 21.
Osbaldiston, G. W., and Fuhrman, W. (1969). Unpublished data.
Osbaldiston, G. W., and Fuhrman, W. (1970). *Can. J. Comp. Med. Vet. Sci.* (in press).
Osborne, C. A., Finco, D. R., Low, D. G., and Perman, V. (1967). *Minn. Vet.* **5**, 7.
Peart, W. S. (1965). *Pharmacol. Rev.* **17**, 143.
Peters, J. T. (1945). *Ann. Internal. Med.* [N.S.] **23**, 221.
Phillips, R. A., and Hamilton, P. B. (1948). *Am. J. Physiol.* **125**, 523.
Phillips, R. A., Dole, V. P., Hamilton, P. B., Emerson, K., Archibald, R. M., and Van Slyke, D. D. (1946). *Am. J. Physiol.* **145**, 314.
Pickering, D. E., and Sussman, H. H. (1962). *Am. J. Vet. Res.* **23**, 667.
Pitts, R. F. (1934). *Am. J. Physiol.* **109**, 532.
Pitts, R. F. (1938). *J. Cellular Comp. Physiol.* **11**, 99.
Pitts, R. F. (1959). "The Physiological Basis of Diuretic Therapy." Thomas, Springfield, Illinois.
Pitts, R. F. (1964). *Am. J. Med.* **36**, 720.
Pitts, R. F. (1968). "Physiology of the Kidney and Body Fluids," p. 86. Year Book Publ., Chicago, Illinois.
Pitts, R. F., and Alexander, R. S. (1944). *Am. J. Physiol.* **142**, 648.
Pitts, R. F., and Korr, I. M. (1938). *J. Cellular Comp. Physiol.* **11**, 117.
Potter, B. J. (1963). *Australian J. Agr. Res.* **14**, 518.
Poulsen, E. (1957). *Kgl. Vet.-log Land-Bohojskole, Ars.* p. 97.
Puck, T. T., Wasserman, K., and Fishman, A. (1952). *J. Cellular Comp. Physiol.* **40**, 73.
Ralli, E. P., Robson, J. S., Clarke, D., and Hoagland, C. L. (1945). *J. Clin. Invest.* **24**, 316.
Ramsay, D. J., and Coxon, R. V. (1967). *Quart. J. Exptl. Physiol.* **43**, 74.
Rapoport, S., and West, C. D. (1950). *Am. J. Physiol.* **163**, 175.
Rector, F. C., Brunner, F. P., and Seldin, D. W. (1966). *J. Clin. Invest.* **45**, 590.
Reubi, F. C. (1963). "Clearance Tests in Clinical Medicine." Thomas, Springfield, Illinois.
Rhodin, J. (1958). *Am. J. Med.* **24**, 661.
Rivera, A., Pena, J. C., Barcena, C., Rangel, S., and Dies, F. (1961). *Metab., Clin. Exptl.* **10**, 1.
Roberts, K. E., Randall, H. T., Sanders, H. L., and Hood, M. (1955). *J. Clin. Invest.* **34**, 666.
Robinson, J. R. (1967). "Renal Disease" p. 80. Blackwell, Oxford.
Roe, J. H., Epstein, J. H., and Goldstein, N. P. (1949). *J. Biol. Chem.* **178**, 839.
Rosenthal, R., and Meier, K. (1921). *Arch. Exptl. Pathol. Pharmacol.* **91**, 246.
Rowntree, L. G., and Geraghty, J. T. (1910). *J. Pharmacol. Exptl. Therap.* **1**, 579.
Schaffenburg, C. A., Hass, E., and Goldblatt, H. (1960). *Am. J. Physiol.* **199**, 788.
Schedl, H. P., and Bartter, F. (1960). *J. Lab. Clin. Med.* **42**, 116.
Scheer, B. T., and Ramamurthi, R. (1968). *Fed. Am. Soc. Exptl. Biol.*, Bethesda, Maryland.
Schmidt-Nielsen, B. (1958). *Physiol. Rev.* **38**, 139.
Schmidt-Nielsen, B., and O'Dell, R. (1959). *Am. J. Physiol.* **197**, 856.
Schmidt-Nielsen, B., and Osaki, H. (1958). *Am. J. Physiol.* **193**, 657.
Schmidt-Nielsen, B., Osaki, H., Murdaugh, H. V., Jr., and O'Dell, R. (1958). *Am. J. Physiol.* **194**, 221.
Schwartz, I. L., Schachter, D., and Freinkel, N. (1949). *J. Clin. Invest.* **28**, 1117.
Searcy, R. L. (1969). "Diagnostic Biochemistry." McGraw-Hill, New York.
Sellers, A. F., Prichard, W. F., Weber, A. F., and Sautter, J. A. (1958). *Am. J. Vet. Res.* **19**, 580.
Shannon, J. A. (1937). *Proc. Soc. Exptl. Biol. Med.* **37**, 379.
Shannon, J. A. (1939). *Physiol. Rev.* **19**, 63.
Shannon, J. A., Farber, S., and Troast, L. (1941). *Am. J. Physiol.* **133**, 752.
Shaw, E. C. (1925). *J. Urol.* **13**, 575.
Shear, L., Kleinerman, J., and Gabuzda, G. J. (1965). *Am. J. Med.* **39**, 185.

Shipp, J. C., Havenson, I. B., Windhager, E. E., Schatzmann, H. J., Whittembury, C., Yoshimura, H., and Soloman, A. K. (1958). *Am. J. Physiol.* **195**, 563.

Sims, E. A. H., and Solomon, S. (1963). "Clinical Metabolism of Body Water and Electrolytes." Saunders, Philadelphia, Pennsylvania.

Smith, H. W. (1951). "The Kidney." Oxford Univ. Press, London and New York.

Smith, H. W., and Clarke, R. W. (1938). *Am. J. Physiol.* **122**, 132.

Smith, H. W., Finkelstein, N., Aliminosa, L., Crawford, B., and Graber, M. (1945). *J. Clin. Invest.* **24**, 388.

Spargo, B. H. (1966). In "The Kidney" (F. K. Mostofi, ed.). Williams & Wilkins, Baltimore, Maryland.

Sperber, I. (1959). *Pharmacol. Rev.* **11**, 109.

Stacy, B. P., and Brook, A. H. (1964a). *Australian J. Agr. Res.* **15**, 289.

Stacy, B. P., and Brook, A. H. (1964b). *Quart. J. Exptl. Physiol.* **49**, 301.

Stein, R. M., Berchovitch, D. P., and Levitt, M. F. (1964). *Am. J. Physiol.* **207**, 826.

Stevens, C. E., Sellers, A. F., and Clark, J. J. (1956). *Am. J. Vet. Res.* **17**, 710.

Street, A. E., Chesterman, H., Smith, G. K. A., and Quinton, R. M. (1968). *J. Pharm. Pharmacol.* **20**, 325.

Summerskill, W. H. J. (1966). *Progr. Gastroenterol.* **51**, 94.

Summerville, W. W., Hanzal, R. F., and Goldblatt, H. B. (1932). *Am. J. Physiol.* **102**, 1.

Suzuki, A., Klutsch, K., and Heidland, A. (1964). *Klin. Wochschr.* **42**, 569.

Sweet, A. Y., Levitt, M. F., and Hodes, H. L. (1961). *Am. J. Physiol.* **201**, 975.

Sykes, A. H. (1960a). *Res. Vet. Sci.* **1**, 308.

Sykes, A. H. (1960b). *Res. Vet. Sci.* **1**, 315.

Tamm, I., and Horsfall, F. L. (1950). *Proc. Soc. Exptl. Biol. Med.* **74**, 108.

Terry, R., Watkins, D. R., Church, E. H., and Whiptle, G. H. (1948). *J. Exptl. Med.* **87**, 561.

Thorburn, G. C., Kopald, H. H., Herd, J. A., Hollenberg, M., O'Morchoe, C. C. C., and Barger, A. C. (1963). *Circulation Res.* **13**, 290.

Thurau, K. (1961). *Proc. Soc. Exptl. Biol. Med.* **106**, 714.

Thurau, K. (1964). *Am. J. Med.* **36**, 698.

Treacher, R. J. (1964). *Brit. Vet. J.* **120**, 178.

Trueta, J., Barclay, A. E., Daniel, P. M., Franklin, K. J., and Prichard, M. M. L. (1947). "Studies of Renal Circulation." Blackwell, Oxford.

Ullrich, K. J., Kramer, K., and Boylan, J. W. (1961). *Progr. Cardiovascular Diseases* **3**, 395.

Ullrich, K. J., Schmidt-Nielsen, B., O'Dell, R., Pehling, G., Gottschalk, C. W., Lassiter, W. E., and Mylle, M. (1963). *Am. J. Physiol.* **204**, 527.

Vaamonde, C. A., Vaamonde, L. S., Morosi, H. J., Klinger, E. L., and Papper, S. (1967). *J. Lab. Clin. Med.* **70**, 179.

Vander, A. J., and Cafruny, E. J. (1962). *Am. J. Physiol.* **202**, 1105.

Van Pilsun, J. F. (1969). "Metabolism." *Fed. Am. Soc. Exptl. Biol.*, Bethesda, Maryland.

Verney, E. B. (1947). *Proc. Roy. Soc.* **B135**, 25.

Walker, A. M., Bott, P. A., Oliver, J., and MacDowell, M. C. (1941). *Am. J. Physiol.* **134**, 580.

Walker, J. G., Wilver, H., Lawson, T. R., Ryder, J. A., and Sheldon, S. (1963). *Proc. Soc. Exptl. Biol. Med.* **112**, 932.

Warren, J. V., Brannon, E. S., and Merrill, A. J. (1944). *Science* **100**, 108.

Welsh, C. A., Rosenthal, A., Duncan, N. T., and Taylor, H. C. (1942). *Am. J. Physiol.* **137**, 338.

White, A. G., Rubin, G., and Leiter, L. (1953). *J. Clin. Invest.* **32**, 931.

Windhagen, E. E., and Giebisch, G. (1961). *Nature* **191**, 1205.

Windhagen, E. E., and Giebisch, G. (1965). *Physiol. Rev.* **45**, 214.

Winter, C. C., and Myers, W. G. (1962). *J. Urol.* **88**, 100.

With, T. K. (1968). "Bile Pigments: Chemical, Biological, and Clinical Aspects." Academic Press, New York.

Zak, G. A., Brun, C., and Smith, H. W. (1954). *J. Clin. Invest.* **33**, 1064.

2 _____ Fluids, Electrolytes, and Acid–Base
Balance

John B. Tasker

I. INTRODUCTION

There has been a remarkable increase in the clinical use of electrolyte solutions for therapy in the years since World War II. Although there may be universal agreement that this type of therapy is frequently indicated in veterinary medicine, there is often doubt about the scientific principles which are the foundation of this kind of treatment. It is not good enough to administer "fluid" to dehydrated patients; it is necessary to select the correct *kind* of fluid and to administer the optimal *volume* of fluid if the treatment is to be effective. These decisions should be made with an awareness of the anatomy and physiology of the body fluid and an appreciation of the potential derangements that can occur.

There are many characteristics of the body fluid that are important to students of differing disciplines. For example, the endocrinologist may be interested in glucose concentration and distribution in the various compartments of the body fluid; the nutritionist may be interested in trace elements in these fluids; the immunologist may be concerned with antibody distribution. When the clinician is concerned about fluid balance in his patients, however, he is concerned about only four general characteristics of the body fluids.

1. Is the volume of fluid in the body normal?
2. Is the osmotic pressure of the body fluid normal?
3. Is the acid–base balance of the body fluid normal?
4. Is the electrolyte composition of the body fluid normal?

When the preceding questions can be answered in the affirmative, one can conclude that the most fundamental requirements for cellular activity have been met. Conversely, when one or more of these important characteristics of the body fluid is abnormal, cellular metabolism cannot occur at the optimal rate and the normal function of the organism as a whole cannot occur.

For example, when an infectious agent causes enteritis, diarrhea usually occurs. This often results in severe abnormalities of the volume, osmotic pressure, acid–base balance and/or electrolyte composition of the body fluid. Elimination of the infectious agent with specific chemotherapy does not insure the recovery of the patient. The fluid derangements which have occurred may have modified normal cellular function to the extent that normal attitude, appetite, and activity do not return because of continuing abnormal function of the central nervous system; normal intestinal secretion, absorption, and motility do not return because of the effect of continuing abnormalities of the body fluid on cellular activity in the digestive tract. Normal function of the organism as a whole requires not only the elimination of the primary cause of disease but, in addition, the restoration and maintenance of normal conditions in the body fluids.

It is useful to recognize that normal function of the intact organism, health, is the result of normal function of its component parts (organs) and, in turn, individual cells. It could be said that "happy cells make a healthy body." Deviation from normal in volume, osmotic pressure, acid–base balance, and electrolyte composition of the body fluid interferes with normal cellular activity (the cells are not "happy") and the patient cannot return to health.

It is the task of the clinician to identify derangements of the body fluid which are present or imminent and institute rational therapy to correct these abnormalities.

II. BODY FLUID COMPARTMENTS

A. TOTAL BODY WATER

The "total body water" comprises from 45 to 70% of body weight. A horse weighing 450 kg (approx. 1000 lb) thus has approximately 270 kg (liters) of body water. The rather wide variation in total body water has been studied extensively in man. Infants have a very high body water content (70–83%) which gradually decreases during the first year of life. Marked differences in adults exist between the sexes. This has been shown to be related to the definite difference in fat between the two sexes. In advanced age there is also a decline in the total body water. Variations in the total body water of animals can be expected to be related to age and condition. Since the measurement of total body water includes the fluid of the gastrointestinal tract and fluid in the body cavities the degree of fluid accumulation in these areas may influence total body water measurements to a considerable degree.

Total body water is divided into two "compartments" in the body: the intracellular fluid and the extracellular fluid.

B. INTRACELLULAR FLUID

The intracellular fluid (ICF) comprises approximately 67–75% of the total body water or 35–45% of the body weight. It is apparent from these figures that the major fraction of the body water is intracellular.

Attempts have been made to determine the electrolyte composition of ICF (Graham, 1967). Since ICF cannot be examined directly, these determinations have, of necessity, been made on tissue specimens containing extracellular fluid as well as ICF. After making corrections for the extracellular fluid present, estimates of the intracellular electrolyte concentrations have been made. It is to be expected that

TABLE I   ELECTROLYTE CONCENTRATIONS IN THE BODY COMPARTMENTS (mEq/LITER)[a]

Electrolytes	Intracellular fluid	Interstitial fluid	Intravascular fluid
Cations			
Sodium	15	147	142
Potassium	150	4	5
Calcium	2	2.5	5
Magnesium	27	1	2
Anions			
Bicarbonate	10	30	27
Chloride	1	114	103
Phosphate	100	2	2
Sulfate	20	1	1
Organic acids	0	7.5	5
Protein	63	0	16

[a]Modified from Weisberg (1962).

the actual composition of the ICF will vary from species to species, from tissue to tissue, and probably even from one part of a single cell to another.

The electrolyte constituents of the body fluid compartments of man are shown in Table I.

It is of interest to note that the ICF has a very high potassium and phosphate concentration and a very low sodium and chloride concentration when compared with extracellular fluid.

The fallacy of applying these figures to all cells and to other species is made apparent by the observation that there is a marked interspecies difference in the electrolyte composition of the erythrocyte (Table II).

TABLE II   SODIUM AND POTASSIUM
            CONTENT OF MAMMALIAN
            ERYTHROCYTES (mEq/LITER
            CELLS)[a]

Species	Sodium	Potassium
Dog	107	9
Cat	104	6
Horse	—	88
Ox	79	22
Sheep[b]	16	64
Sheep	84	18
Swine	11	100

[a]From Prankerd (1961).
[b]There is a marked variation among sheep in the intracellular cation concentration.

C. Extracellular Fluid

The extracellular fluid (ECF) of man comprises about 25% of total body water or 15% of the body weight. Similar figures probably apply to most animals. This fluid compartment includes the intravascular fluid (plasma) and the interstitial fluid. Fluids in the digestive tract, urinary tract, ocular cavities, and other similar fluid spaces in the body are ECF also. However, they are not usually considered in a discussion of the properties of ECA since these fluids are present in small quantities and have very different characteristics. In most cases, the term ECF refers to plasma plus interstitial fluid.

It is this ECF which was first recognized by Claude Bernard as the *milieu interieur*— the internal environment which bathes the body cells and by its usual constancy of composition protects them from the drastic changes in the external environment.

The ECF is much more easily and more reliably described than the ICF because plasma, one of its component parts, can be sampled and studied directly. Inasmuch as water and the major electrolytes can diffuse freely across the vascular endothelium, the interstitial fluid is an ultrafiltrate of serum and has virtually the same electrolyte concentrations. The slight differences in composition of plasma and interstitial fluid that do exist result from the retention of plasma proteins within the vascular lumen. This results in a redistribution of the permeable ions in accordance with the Donnan equilibrium (Maxwell and Kleeman, 1962). It is apparent that sodium and chloride are the predominant cation and anion in the ECF (Table I).

III. PHYSIOLOGICAL CONSIDERATIONS

A. Osmotic Pressure

Cellular hydration depends upon the character of the ECF which surrounds each cell. It is believed that cell membranes are permeable to water and that the quantity of water within the cells is dependent upon the osmotic forces operative in the ICF and ECF. The intracellular solute exerts an osmotic pressure which tends to draw water into the cells. This is opposed by the opposite force created by the solute in the ECF.

The homeostatic forces of the body are directed toward maintenance of normal osmotic pressure in the ECF. This, in turn, results in normal osmotic pressure in the ICF. If the ECF is altered and has an increased osmotic pressure, water passes out of the cells until a new osmotic equilibrium is reached. It should be recognized that this extracellular movement of water has resulted in several changes in both the ICF and the ECF. (1) The cell has become dehydrated. (2) The intracellular osmotic pressure has increased. (3) The extracellular movement of water has decreased the hypertonicity of the ECF but not to the normal value. (4) A new equilibrium has been reached between ICF and ECF in which the effect of the initial change in osmotic pressure has been shared between both fluid compartments.

The osmotic pressure of a solution is related to the number of particles of solute in the solution. For practical purposes, the nature of the particle, its molecular weight, and its electrical change do not influence the osmotic pressure; it is the total number of particles in solution that determines the osmotic pressure of a solution. It is important to recognize that 1 gm of protein in 100 ml of water exerts a very small osmotic effect compared with a solution of 1 gm of sodium chloride in 100 ml of water. This is because the sodium chloride is completely ionized and 1 gm provides a very large number of individual, very small ions or particles. The protein solution, on the other hand, contains very large protein molecules. Being much greater in size, these particles are much fewer in number in the same weight of solute. Therefore the osmotic pressure created by them is smaller.

The osmotic effect of various substances is measured in terms of osmols (Osm) or milliosmols (mOsm). The gram-molecular weight (the molecular weight in grams) by definition contains 6.025×10^{23} (Avogadro's number) of molecules. This is equal to 1 Osm for an undissociated substance such as glucose. Since osmotic pressure depends on the number of particles in solution 1 Osm of an ionized substance is equal to the gram-molecular weight multiplied by the number of ions into which it dissociates. For example, the gram-molecular weight of glucose is 180. Thus, 180 gm of glucose equals 1 Osm. The gram-molecular weight of sodium chloride is 58.5. Since each molecule of NaCl dissociates in solution into two ions, 58.5 gm of NaCl equals 2 Osm.

The osmotic pressure of biological fluids is measured in terms of *milliosmols per kilogram of water* and this is called *osmolality*. A similar term *osmolarity* is used when the solution is described with respect to the osmol content *per liter of solution*. This is not as useful as osmolality since it does not make allowances for the volume occupied by proteins and lipoproteins and for the effect of temperature on volume. Osmolality values, on the other hand, allow comparison of the osmotic pressure of various body fluids, e.g., serum and urine (Hoffman, 1964). Thus, 180 gm of glucose dissolved in 1 kg of water has an osmolality of 1 Osm/kg of water or 1000 mOsm/kg of water. A solution containing 58.5 gm of NaCl/kg of water has an osmolality of 2000 mOsm/kg water. For comparison, the osmolality of plasma is about 310 mOsm/kg of plasma water.

The osmotic pressure of a solution can be determined by measurement of one of its other colligative properties (depression of vapor pressure, elevation of boiling point, depression of freezing point) since these are related to the number of particles in solution. The most common method of evaluating osmotic pressure is determination of the freezing point of the solution. Pure water freezes at $0°$ C. One osmol of solute per kilogram of water depresses the freezing point $1.86°$ C. Therefore, when the freezing point of a solution is $-1.86°$ C, it has an osmolality of 1 Osm/kg water or 1000 mOsm/kg of water.

In complex solutions, such as urine or serum, the osmotic pressure determined from the freezing-point depression does not usually correspond exactly to the theoretical value determined from chemical analysis of its constituents. This is because the degree of dissociation of ionizable constituents cannot be predicted with accuracy and certain other physical phenomena influence the behavior of the particles. For these reasons, the effective osmotic pressure of a solution can be determined more accurately from its freezing-point depression than from its chemical composition.

Instruments for determining osmolality of biological solutions by the measurement freezing-point depression are available commercially and are sometimes used in the evaluation of various disorders of fluid and electrolyte metabolism.

Since sodium and potassium are the most abundant ions in ECF and ICF, respectively, these ions are chiefly responsible for the osmotic pressure of the body fluids. The normal hydration of the body and its constituent cells depends not only upon the availability of water but to an equal degree on the maintenance of optimal concentrations of sodium and potassium in their respective locations. For this reason, among others, an understanding of the regulation of these major body electrolytes is essential.

B. Sodium

The most abundant ion in the ECF is sodium. Because of this, this ion is primarily responsible for the osmotic pressure of the ECF. In addition, the sodium ion is essential to the development of the membrane potential which is of fundamental importance in various specialized cell functions such as muscle contraction and nerve impulse transmission.

Since minerals such as sodium are not used up in the course of metabolism, the quantity of sodium in the body is controlled only by the intake and outgo of this substance.

1. Intake of Sodium

It has been observed for many years that among wild animals, it is only the herbivores that frequent salt licks. Although the diet of this group of animals contains enormous amounts of potassium, the sodium content of plants is very low. Carnivores in the wild do not need supplemental salt since their sodium requirements are satisfied by the ECF of the meat they consume.

In spite of these observations and the considerable research on nutrient requirements of man and animals over the last decades, the exact requirement of sodium is not known, even for man. One reason for the lack of useful information on this subject is that the dietary requirement is controlled by the losses of sodium from the body and these losses are extremely variable, being related to temperature, work, and other constituents of the diet, especially potassium. The usual goal in practical nutrition is to provide excess sodium in the diet and to rely on excretory mechanisms to control sodium balance.

Devlin and Roberts (1963) have studied dietary sodium requirements in lambs. The possible mechanism responsible for sodium appetite in sheep has been investigated by Beilharz and Kay (1963). Hamlin et al. (1964) reported on the effects on healthy dogs of a low sodium diet.

2. Excretion of Sodium

Sodium is lost from the body in the visible sweat which is seen during vigorous exercise or in a warm environment. Sodium is also present in the various secretions of the digestive tract. In carnivores and in some herbivores the sodium contained in these digestive secretions is almost completely resorbed in the lower alimentary canal and the sodium loss in feces is negligible. However, in herbivores with abundant feces of high water content, such as the ox and the horse there is an appreciable loss of sodium by this route.

The most important route of sodium excretion in all domestic animals is the kidney. The renal loss of sodium is very carefully controlled to maintain optimal sodium concentration in the ECF. More than 90% of the sodium filtered in the glomeruli is reabsorbed by the proximal tubules and the loops of Henle regardless of the sodium status of the body. The very small percentage of filtered sodium remaining can be reabsorbed or excreted depending upon the needs of the body.

The principal controlling factor which influences sodium reabsorption is the hormone aldosterone which is produced in the adrenal gland. In times of sodium excess, such as following the ingestion of large quantities of sodium chloride, aldosterone secretion is curtailed, the small percentage of sodium reabsorption controlled by this hormone does not occur, and sodium is lost in the urine. Conversely, when sodium intake is curtailed, aldosterone secretion increases markedly and sodium reabsorption in the kidney is essentially complete. Although the percentage of filtered sodium actually influenced is very small, the absolute quantity is very great since the quantity of sodium filtered by the kidney is enormous. It has been estimated in man that the 2–3% of filtered sodium which is under the influence of aldosterone is equal to 15–20 gm of sodium per day, one-tenth of the total sodium of the body (Guyton, 1966).

The mechanism controlling aldosterone secretion has been the subject of controversy for many years and a complete understanding of normal control over this hormone is still not available. It can be shown experimentally that reduced sodium concentration in the ECF causes an increased secretion of aldosterone as does a high extracellular concentration of potassium, reduced cardiac output, and physical stress. The question in dispute is how these various influences cause the change in adrenal hormone production. It has been suggested by some that these influences act directly on the adrenal cortex. Others have believed that these influences act on a diencephalic center, possibly the pineal body, causing the release of a hormonal substance to which the adrenal gland is responsive. Still others believe that the main factors known to influence aldosterone secretion act on the juxtaglomerlular cells of the kidney and cause the release of humoral substances which increase adrenal secretion of aldosterone. The net result, regardless of the intermediary mechanism, is that reduced sodium concentration in the ECF and reduced cardiac output (the two most important influences) cause increased secretion of aldosterone which, in turn, causes increased sodium readsorption in the kidney, i.e., reduced sodium loss from the body.

Pickering (1965) has investigated renal control of sodium in the ox.

3. Sodium Distribution in the Body

About half of the total body sodium is contained in the ECF where it exerts its greatest physiological effect. Most of the remainder is located in bone. Some bone sodium may be available to maintain ECF sodium during periods of sodium depletion but a large amount of sodium in the skeleton appears to be in the bone crystal and not available to the ECF.

Although most ICF of the body contains only very small amounts of sodium, the sodium content of the erythrocyte varies greatly among different species as shown in Table II. The sodium content of various fluids of the body is shown in Table I.

C. POTASSIUM

Potassium serves an important role in the maintenance of intracellular osmotic pressure. In addition, this element is essential to many physical and chemical processes in the body. Potassium concentration in the ECF influences the development of membrane potentials and in this way significantly influences nerve transmission and muscle function. Potassium is also important in carbohydrate metabolism and electron transport since a number of the enzymes in these metabolic pathways are potassium-dependent.

1. Intake of Potassium

Potassium is the most abundant cation in the ICF of both plants and animals. For this reason, this element is present in high concentration in almost all normal animal foods. The diet of the herbivores contains especially large quantities of potassium. For example, a high quality alfalfa–timothy hay mixture analyzed contained 393 mEq potassium/kg. Ten kilograms of this hay daily was adequate to maintain the body weight of several adult horses weighing approximately 450 kg (Tasker, 1967a). The daily potassium intake of these horses was equal to that in 283 gm of potassium chloride! By contrast the sodium contained in 10 kg of this hay was equal to that of less than 20 gm of sodium chloride.

Although the proportions of sodium and potassium in the diet of the carnivores are different from those in the diet of herbivores there is seldom, if ever, a deficiency of potassium in the normal diet of any animal.

2. Potassium Excretion

Because of the large quantities of potassium consumed by normal animals, large amounts must be excreted to prevent potassium intoxication of the organism. Most of the potassium is excreted in the urine but an additional quantity is lost in sweat and digestive tract fluids. As indicated in the discussion of sodium loss, animals with voluminous feces of high water content lose a significant quantity of electrolytes from the digestive tract, but in other animals the loss by this route is negligible.

The kidney is the principal organ for potassium excretion. It does this by glomerular filtration as well as by tubular secretion. Ordinarily, there is little need to conserve potassium in the body and the principal renal effect is to prevent the accumulation of toxic quantities. However, when potassium intake is interrupted, renal conservation of this element is necessary to prevent potassium depletion. The kidney is much less able to conserve potassium during these periods than sodium. Although sodium restriction is immediately followed by resorption of virtually all sodium from the urine, potassium restriction does not result in a similar response. Under these conditions, potassium excretion continues for several days in spite of body depletion.

The tubular resorption of potassium occurs continually as does that of sodium. However, when aldosterone causes increased resorption of sodium it does so by promoting the exchange of sodium in the tubular fluid for potassium in the renal tubular cell. Thus aldosterone promotes excretion of potassium. When sodium is scarce in the tubular fluid, potassium excretion by this mechanism is curtailed.

Renal control of potassium excretion has been studied in the dog by Lemieux *et al.* (1964) and in the ox by Pickering (1965).

3. Potassium Distribution in the Body

The potassium concentration in the ECF is very low, approximately one-thirtieth of the sodium concentration. On the other hand, the reverse is true of most cells of the body: the potassium concentration is many times greater than the sodium concentration. This is presumably the result of the active extrusion of sodium from the cell by the so-called sodium pump.

Several abnormal situations can influence the degree to which potassium is confined to the cell but in the normal individual more than 90% of the body potassium is in the ICF. Because of the preponderance of muscle tissue in the body, most of the body potassium is in muscle.

The concentration of potassium in the fluids of the body is shown in Table I. Ward (1966a) and Keynes and Harrison (1967) have reviewed potassium metabolism in ruminants.

D. OTHER CATIONS

The other important cations in the body fluids are calcium and magnesium. These are discussed in Chapter 9, Volume I.

E. ANIONS

1. Chloride

Chloride is the most abundant anion in the ECF. It is present in the ICF only in very small concentration. Although the clinical pathology literature of the past abounds with discussions of chloride measurement and its significance in clinical diagnosis, this is not because chloride is often of fundamental importance in fluid balance problems. Rather, it is because convenient methods for the measurement of chloride in biological fluids existed long before methods were available for measurement of the more important body cations, sodium and potassium. With the advent of a practical means for accurate measurement of these cations, the importance of chloride balance, per se, in clinical studies has decreased considerably.

Chloride occurs in the diet in association with the major cations and is in adequate supply when they are present in normal amounts. The absorption, distribution, and excretion of chloride is mostly passive since this ion usually accompanies sodium and is distributed passively according to electrical gradients established by the active transport of sodium. Active transport of chloride apparently does occur but this is not a process of major importance in the electrolyte balance of the body.

The normal concentrations of chloride in the body fluids are shown in Table I.

2. Bicarbonate

The bicarbonate ion is of fundamental importance in the control of acid–base balance in the body. It is largely of endogenous origin being produced by the hydration of carbon dioxide in the cells to carbonic acid and the subsequent dissociation of carbonic acid to bicarbonate and hydrogen ions. It is lost from the body in the secretions of the digestive tract and in the urine. The regulation of bicarbonate ion concentration in the body is discussed in the section on acid–base balance.

Bicarbonate ion concentration in the body fluids is shown in Table I.

3. Phosphate

This anion is discussed in Chapter 9, Volume I. Although it is desirable to express phosphate concentration in milliequivalents per liter of plasma in order to appreciate the contribution of this anion to total ECF cation–anion balance, this cannot be done with accuracy. Chemical methods for phosphorus determination in serum provide the amount of total inorganic phosphorus present. This exists in serum as variable proportions of phosphate (PO_4^{3-}), monohydrogen phosphate (HPO_4^{2-}), and dihydrogen phosphate ($H_2PO_4^{-}$). For practical purposes, the mEq/liter of phosphate can be estimated by multiplying the mg/100 ml by 0.58. However, the factor varies with the pH of the blood.

4. Plasma Protein

At the pH of plasma, plasma proteins exist as anions. An estimate of the contribution of plasma protein to cation–anion balance can be made by multiplying the total protein of plasma in gm/100 ml by 2.43 to obtain approximately mEq/liter.

5. Organic Acids

The remaining anions of plasma are organic acids, especially lactate and sulfate. In normal individuals these represent approximately 5 mEq/liter in the serum.

F. ACID–BASE BALANCE

Normal body chemistry is influenced greatly by intracellular enzymes. These enzymic reactions occur optimally only within a very narrow range of pH. For this reason, the regulation and maintenance of normal pH in the body fluid is of fundamental importance. Since water and electrolyte balance are closely linked with acid–base balance (Nuttall, 1965) and diseases that alter one of these often alter the others, acid–base balance is customarily included in discussions of body fluid balance.

1. Definition of pH

pH is a measure of acidity and is equal to the negative logarithm of the hydrogen ion concentration. It is thus inversely related to hydrogen ion concentration, $[H^+]$. In aqueous solution the product of $[H^+]$ and hydroxyl ion concentration, $[OH^-]$, is constant: 1×10^{-14} Eq/liter. When the two species are present in equal concentration (1×10^{-7}) the reaction is neutral and the pH is 7. When $[H^+]$ is greater than 1×10^{-7} the solution is acid and the pH is less than 7. When $[OH^-]$ is greater than 1×10^{-7}, $[H^+]$ is less than 1×10^{-7}, the solution is alkaline and the pH is greater than 7.

2. Buffers

The fluids of the body contain several buffer systems which tend to prevent sudden changes in pH as acids or bases enter the body from without or are produced as a result of normal physiological processes. An understanding of buffers is thus of importance in understanding acid–base control.

A buffer system is a mixture of a weakly dissociated acid and a salt of that acid. For example, a mixture of acetic acid and sodium acetate forms a buffer system. This mixture tends to prevent changes in the hydrogen ion concentration (pH) of a solution in the following manner. If a large amount of strong acid (H^+) were added to water the quantity of free hydrogen ion in the water would be large and the pH of the solution would fall sharply. However, if the acid were added to the buffer described above the following reaction would occur:

$$H^+ + C_2H_3O_2^- \rightleftharpoons HC_2H_3O_2$$

Because the added acid resulted in formation of acetic acid, much of which was undissociated, the amount of increase in free H^+ in the solution was decreased and the change in pH was therefore minimized.

Similarly, if a strong base (OH^-) were added to water the pH would rise sharply as the OH^- converted some of the hydrogen ions to water:

$$OH^- + H^+ \rightleftharpoons H_2O$$

However, if OH^- was added to the buffer solution described above the change in pH would be minimized by these reactions:

$$OH^- + H^+ \rightleftharpoons H_2O$$

$$HC_2H_3O_2 \rightleftharpoons H^+ + C_2H_3O_2^-$$

As the hydroxyl ion converts hydrogen ions to water, some acetic acid molecules dissociate to restore the hydrogen ion concentration.

The tendency of a weak acid to dissociate is indicated by its dissociation constant, K. The hydrogen ion concentration of a buffer solution such as that described above can be determined by the following formula:

$$[H^+] = K \frac{[acid]}{[salt]}$$

When this relationship is expressed in terms of pH it becomes

$$pH = pK + \log \frac{[salt]}{[acid]}$$

where

$\qquad$ pH = negative logarithm of $[H^+]$
$\qquad$ pK = negative logarithm of the dissociation constant, K
$\qquad$ [salt] = concentration of the ionized species
$\qquad$ [acid] = concentration of the undissociated acid

This equation is the Henderson-Hasselbalch equation which is basic to the chemistry of pH regulation in the body. It should be recognized in passing that the pH changes only when the *ratio* between the components of the buffer changes. Changes in the absolute concentrations of the buffer pair do not result in changes in pH if the ratio between them is not changed.

3. Blood Buffers

The blood is a complex liquid. It contains many buffer pairs which help to control blood pH. The total buffer capacity of the blood is the cumulative effect of these individual buffer pairs. The significant buffer pairs in the plasma are: bicarbonate–carbonic acid (HCO_3^-/H_2CO_3), monohydrogen phosphate–dihydrogen phosphate ($HPO_4^{2-}/H_2PO_4^-$), and proteinate–protein (Protein$^-$/H Protein). In the erythrocytes, organic phosphate and hemoglobin are important buffers in addition to bicarbonate and protein. It should be recognized that the addition of acid or base to a complex mixture of buffers such as plasma results in alterations in the equilibrium of all buffer pairs simultaneously. Thus these various buffers *share* the burden of preventing marked changes in blood pH.

In spite of the fact that the buffers function together in the plasma, the bicarbonate–carbonic acid buffer pair is the most important one to the clinician. This is because it is the most abundant buffer in the plasma, it is the easiest one to measure, and it is the buffer system over which the body has the most control. Since changes in pH affect all plasma buffers, evaluation of the bicarbonate–carbonic acid buffer pair makes possible inferences about the total plasma buffer.

The Henderson-Hasselbalch equation, applied to this important buffer pair becomes

$$pH = 6.1 + \log \frac{[HCO_3^-]}{H_2CO_3}$$

(6.1 = pK for the HCO_3^- – H_2CO_3 buffer pair).

The pH of the plasma is dependent upon the concentrations of bicarbonate and of carbonic acid, and, of more importance, on the *ratio* between these two constituents.

4.   The Genesis of Carbonic Acid and Bicarbonate

Carbon dioxide is generated by various decarboxylation reactions in the cells of the body. It diffuses out of the cells, across the interstitial fluid and into the plasma. Most of the carbon dioxide is in the molecular form; very little is hydrated to form carbonic acid. When the CO_2 enters the erythrocytes, hydration is catalyzed by the enzyme carbonic anhydrase and H_2CO_3 is formed very rapidly. A large proportion of the H_2CO_3 dissociates to hydrogen and bicarbonate ions since, at the pH of the blood, this satisfies the requirements of the Henderson-Hasselbalch equation.

5.   The Regulation of Carbonic Acid Concentration

An equilibrium exists between the partial pressure of CO_2 in alveolar air, partial pressure of gaseous CO_2 dissolved in the blood, and the carbonic acid of the blood. Because of this relationship, changes in the carbonic acid concentration in the blood are directly related to pulmonary function.

The conventional method of evaluating the carbonic acid or carbon dioxide in the blood is the determination of the partial pressure of carbon dioxide (pCO_2). The pCO_2 is expressed in millimeters of mercury. The carbonic acid concentration in milliequivalents per liter can be determined by multiplying pCO_2 by a factor of 0.03. Because of this constant relationship between pCO_2 and carbonic acid concentration these terms can be used interchangeably in discussing mechanisms in the body.

The respiratory center in the medulla oblongata is sensitive to changes in pCO_2 of the blood. When pCO_2 rises significantly above the normal value of approximately 40 mmHg the respiratory center is stimulated and respiration is increased. Increased respiration decreases the pCO_2 of the alveolar air and this in turn decreases the pCO_2 of the blood.

The respiratory center is also sensitive to changes in blood pH. If the blood pH falls significantly below the normal value of 7.4, respiration is stimulated (even when the pCO_2 is normal) and the pCO_2 is reduced.

The opposite stimuli, i.e., decreased pCO_2 and increased pH, cause decreased respiration and an increase in pCO_2 in the blood.

6. The Regulation of Bicarbonate Concentration

The principal organ regulating bicarbonate concentration is the kidney. At normal plasma bicarbonate concentrations the kidney tends to reabsorb most of the bicarbonate in the tubular fluid. When bicarbonate concentration rises, however, this ion is not usually reabsorbed but is excreted in the urine.

7. Excretion of Acid

Although the blood buffers can prevent a sudden change in pH of the body fluid when excess acid or alkali enter the ECF a mechanism is necessary for the excretion of hydrogen ions. This is accomplished in the kidney by the excretion of dihydrogen phosphate and ammonium ion. To the extent that these ions are excreted in the urine, hydrogen ion is removed from the body.

G. Water

The body is dependent upon optimal water for all metabolic processes. Cellular reactions occur in the aqueous ICF; the movement of nutrients from the digestive tract and of oxygen from the respiratory tract to the individual cells depends upon the adequacy of water in the blood and interstitial fluid; the removal of metabolic end products from the cells to the liver and kidney and of carbon dioxide from the cells to the lungs depends upon transport in the aqueous medium of interstitial fluid and plasma. When normal water content of the body is altered, the circulation of blood and perfusion of tissues is altered. Products of cellular reactions accumulate upsetting the chemical equilibria which are essential to health.

1. Intake of Water

The intake of water is apparently regulated by thirst centers in the hypothalamus. It has been shown experimentally that electrical stimulation of this area or instillation into it of hypertonic solutions, induces drinking. Destruction of these centers decreases drinking or totally stops drinking. It is likely that, in the intact animal, several factors serve as stimuli or inhibitors of the thirst centers. Of greatest physiological importance are the known stimulatory factors of extra- or intracellular dehydration and low cardiac output. Other alterations in volume and tonicity also induce thirst under experimental conditions but their practical significance is not fully understood. The studies of thirst reported by Andersson and McCann (1956) and Andersson and Larsson (1961) are especially interesting.

In evaluating quantitatively the daily intake of water it must be remembered that food consumed usually contains a large amount of water which becomes available to the body. Cured hay, for example, has a water content of approximately 10% by weight. Canned pet food often contains more than 70% water.

Another source of water for the body is that which arises in the oxidation of foodstuffs or body tissues. The oxidation of each gram of fat, carbohydrate, or protein results in the formation of approximately 1.07, 0.60, or 0.41 ml of water, respectively.

The total water available to the body is the sum of drinking water consumed, water in food consumed, and water arising from oxidative metabolism in the body.

2.   Water Losses from the Body

The principal route of water loss from the body is the urinary tract. This route is the most important because the water loss in urine is, in most animals, the largest water loss from the body and, of greater importance, because the kidney can increase water loss to prevent overhydration or decrease water loss to prevent dehydration.

Water regulation in the kidney results from the interrelationships between the kidney and antidiuretic hormone. In a normal kidney with adequate glomerular filtration and tubular function, sodium will be resorbed from the filtrate and concentrated in the medullary interstitium. This results in the formation of a very dilute urine in the ascending loop of Henle. If no further resorption of water occurs, water excretion will be maximal.

The extent to which water in reabsorbed in the distal tubule of the kidney is controlled by antidiuretic hormone (ADH). In the absence of this hormone the distal tubule and collecting duct are impermeable to water. When large quantities of ADH are present in the body fluids the cells of the distal tubule and collecting duct become permeable to water. Since this portion of the nephron passes through the renal medulla, water is drawn out of the tubule by the hypertonic medullary inter-stitium. Water removed from the nephron in this manner is retained in the body and expands the total body water.

Obviously, in the normal animal the presence or absence of ADH determines whether water will be conserved by the kidney or excreted maximally. ADH is found primarily in the supraoptic nuclei of the hypothalamus and accumulates in the neurohypophysis. Release of stored ADH is caused by nerve impulses from the hypothalamic nuclei. It is postulated that the neurons of the supraoptic nuclei function as osmoreceptors. According to this view, if the ECF is highly concentrated the neuron is reduced in size due to the egress of water from the cell by osmosis. This apparently causes excitation of the neuron, release of ADH, and reabsorption of water in the kidney. The reabsorbed water dilutes the ECF and thereby removes the stimulus of ADH secretion.

Conversely, when the ECF is hypotonic both production and release of ADH are inhibited, maximal water loss occurs in the kidney and the osmotic pressure of the ECF returns to normal.

The ADH mechanism makes possible the removal of excess water from the body in times of overhydration and causes the retention of water in the body in times of dehydration.

Water is lost in the feces to a very limited extent in those animals that produce a relatively dry stool of small volume, e.g., dog, cat, sheep. In animals producing voluminous feces of high water content the losses may be quite large, e.g., horse and cow. Water loss in feces of several mature horses (450 kg) was studied (Tasker, 1967a). In these normal individuals the average loss of water in feces was approximately 15 liters/day.

Water is also lost by diffusion through the skin and evaporation in the lungs. This insensible water loss may represent 50% of the water lost from the body. When visible sweating occurs, the cutaneous water loss is greatly increased. The water metabolism of tropical cattle has been studied by Siebert and McFarlane (1967). Responses of cattle to water loading were studied by Dalton (1964a).

H. BALANCE STUDIES

External balance studies of water and electrolytes have been made in the dog by R. C. Smith *et al.* (1964), in the cat by Hamlin and Tashjian (1964), in the sheep by English (1966a, 1967a,b), and in the horse by Tasker (1967a) and Fonnesbeck (1967). The water and electrolyte balance in man is summarized by Roberts (1962).

IV. EVALUATION OF THE CLINICAL PATIENT

The diagnosis of a fluid abnormality in a clinical patient depends upon obtaining an answer to these four important questions:
 1. Is there an abnormal volume of fluid in the body, i.e., does a fluid balance problem exist?
 2. Is the osmotic pressure of the ECF abnormal?
 3. Is there an abnormality in acid–base balance?
 4. Is there any other important abnormality in the composition of the ECF?

A. IS THERE AN ABNORMAL VOLUME OF FLUID IN THE BODY?

1. Measurement of Body Fluid Spaces

The most direct method of determining the volume of fluid in the body and its distribution is to measure the total body water, ECF volume, and plasma volume. From these results one can calculate the amount of ICF and the amount of interstitial fluid.

The measurement of the various fluid compartments of the body is done by the dilution technique. In this technique a substance is injected which has been shown to be uniformly distributed in the compartment to be measured. From the total amount of the substance injected and its concentration in the plasma after mixing is complete one can determine the total volume of fluid in which it has become distributed.

The substances used for total body water determination must be uniformly distributed in all fluid compartments including the intracellular space. Water labeled with one of the isotopes of hydrogen, either tritium or deuterium is the preferred substance for total body water determination. Where facilities for measurement of these isotopes are not available antipyrine has been used.

Extracellular water is measured by the dilution of a substance which passes through the capillary wall but does not enter the intracellular space. Inulin, sucrose, mannitol, thiocyanate, thiosulfate, sodium, and chloride have all been used for this purpose. The results obtained vary depending on the substance used. This is because each substance is distributed into a slightly different fluid space in the body. Differences between these tracer substances as well as certain theoretical considerations suggest that accurate measurement of the extracellular space may be impossible. However, the various substances used do provide an estimate of this compartment and also do permit a reliable measurement of *changes* in the volume of fluid in the specific space into which each is distributed.

Plasma volume is measured by determining the dilution of a substance which is distributed in the fluid in the intravascular space. Evans blue dye, T-1824, is frequently used for this purpose since it is bound to plasma albumin, most of which is confined to the vascular compartment. Where radioisotope counting equipment is available, plasma albumin labeled with ^{131}I is usually used. Since some escape of plasma protein outside the vascular space may occur, errors may be encountered in these measurements.

The ICF volume is determined by subtracting ECF from total body water. Similarly, the interstitial fluid volume is determined by substracting plasma volume from ECF volume.

It will be recognized by the reader that direct determination of the volume of the body fluid compartments is a procedure which requires the injection of foreign material into a patient and the withdrawal of several blood samples thereafter. Although it is sometimes done in human clinical patients in unusual circumstances, it is seldom done on clinic patients in the veterinary hospital.

2.   *Detection of Hemoconcentration and Hemodilution*

Changes in plasma water content and therefore, of extracellular water, can be inferred when sudden changes occur in the concentration of certain constituents of the blood. The most useful of these are the erythrocytes and the plasma proteins.

a. ERYTHROCYTES.   Except in instances of acute hemorrhage or hemolysis the red cell concentration in the blood is quite uniform from day to day. In the absence of red cell loss or destruction, sudden changes in the red cell concentration usually are due to loss or gain of plasma water. This can be recognized by changes in the total erythrocyte number per cubic millimeter, the packed red cell volume (hematocrit), or the hemoglobin concentration. Decreases in plasma water are reflected by increases in these erythrocyte values, whereas increases in plasma water cause a decrease.

Although this is the most popular method of detecting dehydration in clinical patients, misleading information can be obtained by this procedure. It is seldom possible to know the red cell concentration in the blood *before* the fluid balance problem occurred. The clinician must assume that this value is the mean for normal individuals of the same description. The assumption may be incorrect in many cases:

a patient with a red cell value which is in the high part of the normal range may be considered dehydrated when it has no fluid balance problem at all; a patient with a red cell value normally in the low part of the normal range may be dehydrated when this value reaches the mean for the group; most serious of all, a patient that is severely anemic and severely dehydrated may appear normal from inspection of the red cell values. In the latter case, both the anemia and the dehydration would be overlooked if the red cell value were the only criterion used to detect dehydration.

Another reason for the red cell values providing misleading information about changes in hydration, is the result of epinephrine causing circulation of erythrocytes previously sequestered in the spleen and small blood vessels. Large day-to-day variations in the red cell values, especially in the horse, can be attributed to apprehension, exertion, or excitement and an associated release of epinephrine. When the hemoglobin of a dehydrated horse rises 15–20% it may indicate serious dehydration; it may also indicate that the horse was alarmed when the sample was obtained.

b. PLASMA PROTEINS. The total protein content of plasma rises when water is lost from this compartment, and is decreased when water is returned to this compartment or when excess water is provided. Although subject to many of the same limitations as the red cell values, e.g., unavailability of baseline values, there is one distinct advantage of plasma protein determinations over the red cell values: the plasma proteins are not altered by epinephrine release.

The total protein determination can be made very quickly and quite reproducibly with a refractometer. By this means very slight changes in hydration can be detected from day to day in the course of an illness.

3. Clinical Signs

An experienced clinician can often evaluate the degree of dehydration better by physical signs than is possible from laboratory tests. The loss of normal skin turgor is the principal abnormality which can be detected. In man, mild, moderate, and severe clinical signs of dehydration have been correlated with fluid loss equal to 4, 6, and 8% of body weight, respectively.

These rules have been suggested for use in animals also. Since the ability to recognize mild abnormalities of skin turgor in animals may not be as great as in man, actual fluid loss may be greater in animals than suggested by this rule. For example, when horses had become dehydrated under experimental conditions, first changes in skin turgor were noted when body weight loss (presumably mostly fluid) was approximately 6%. Moderate abnormalities in skin turgor were evident when weight loss was 10–12% (Tasker, 1963).

Considerable experience in examining the turgor of the skin is necessary before accurate evaluation of dehydration is possible. The examination may vary considerably because of differences in species, thickness of hair coat, thickness of subcutaneous fat, and the part of the body examined.

Correlation between physical and laboratory findings may help to prevent misinterpretations such as are described for red cell values. Once the existence of dehydration is established, however, the laboratory tests, especially the total protein determination, provide a much more reliable, objective means of recognizing day-to-day changes in fluid volume than is possible by using clinical signs alone.

Overhydration is characterized by neurological signs and vomiting.

It is of considerable value, in evaluating day-to-day fluid balance changes, to know the daily changes in body weight. Marked changes in body weight over a short period of time usually reflect changes in total body water since weight changes due to increase or decrease in body tissue do not occur suddenly. Repeated determination of body weight is of special importance in anticipating or recognizing overhydration when large volumes of fluid are being administered to a patient with inadequate renal function.

B. Is the Osmotic Pressure of the Extracellular Fluid Abnormal?

This question is best answered by determination of the serum osmolality.

If equipment for determining serum osmolality is not available, the serum sodium can be used to estimate the osmolality quite reliably in most patients. This is because sodium and its associated anions represent approximately 95% of the osmotically active solute in the serum. It has been suggested that serum osmolality could be estimated by multiplying serum sodium concentration by 2.1. Leaf (1962) has discussed the clinical significance of serum sodium determinations.

The solutes which contribute the remaining 5% to serum osmolality are the other electrolytes (Ca^{2+}, Mg^{2+}, K^+, HPO_4^{2-}, SO_4^{2-}) and non-electrolytes (glucose, urea, amino acids, protein, lactate, and creatine) of serum. These substances do not ordinarily vary enough in concentration to influence the serum osmolality appreciably. However, in azotemia and hyperglycemia there may be a definite alteration in serum osmolality because of the increase in osmotically active solute. Each rise in serum glucose of 100 mg/100 ml contributes an additional 5.5 mOsm to the serum osmolality. A rise of 150 mg/100 ml in urea nitrogen adds 35 mOsm to the serum osmolality. In these situations a normal serum sodium does not indicate a normal osmotic pressure in the ECF. Of greater importance, it should be recognized that low sodium values in conjunction with hyperglycemia or azotemia may not be indicative of hypoosmolality of the ECF but may, instead, be the result of compensatory sodium reduction to preserve normal osmolality. It is apparent that the determination of both sodium and osmolality may provide information in occasional patients that cannot be recognized by either determination alone.

It has often been recommended that serum sodium concentration (and therefore serum osmolality) can be estimated by the sum of chloride concentration, bicarbonate concentration, and a factor of 12. This relationship between the major anions and sodium concentration was very useful when it was not possible to obtain accurate determination of sodium by flame photometry. Since it is now as easy to do a sodium determination as it is to do bicarbonate and chloride there is little justification for recommending this means of estimating sodium concentration. It is particularly apt to be erroneous in ketosis and uremia when severe retention of anions which are normally negligible (such as phosphate, ketones, and sulfates) causes alteration in the normal cation–anion balance.

One remaining application of this rule of thumb is in corroborating the accuracy of abnormal laboratory results. When the sodium, chloride, and bicarbonate have been determined they should be related as indicated by the rule. If the sum of major anions plus 12 is more than 10% greater than or less than the sodium concentration the possibility of ketosis or azotemia should be recognized. If these are not present, a laboratory error in one of the determinations should be considered.

C. Is There an Abnormality in Acid–Base Balance?

Although all of the buffers of the ECF share the function of regulating acid–base balance, the bicarbonate–carbonic acid buffer system is the one which is measured in the clinical evaluation of the patient. It was shown previously that the Henderson-Hasselbalch equation expresses the relationship between pH and the buffer:

$$pH = 6.1 + \log \frac{[HCO_3^-]}{[H_2CO_3]}$$

In clinical studies it is obviously important to know whether the pH is normal, above normal, or below normal. But in order to detect *incipient* abnormalities in pH it is important to know if each component of the buffer pair is normal or in which direction it has become abnormal. Evaluating the components of the buffer pair individually also provides information about the mechanism responsible for an acid–base disorder. Thus the desirable information for evaluating acid–base status in a patient includes all three of the unknown quantities in the Henderson-Hasselbalch equation: pH, $[HCO_3^-]$, and $[H_2CO_3]$.

It is obvious from inspection of this equation that one can determine any one of these values from the equation if the other two are known. Nomograms are available which simplify this procedure (Sigaard-Andersen, 1963; Henry, 1964). Convenient methods exist for determining each of the three components. Each laboratory chooses the two procedures which are most practicable in the individual circumstances. In most instances where the equipment is available, the blood pH is determined and either the bicarbonate or the carbonic acid is evaluated in addition.

It is desirable to use arterial rather than venous blood for complete description of the state of acid–base balance of a patient since oxygen saturation varies widely in venous blood and this introduces an additional factor in the calculation of pCO_2 by some techniques. Furthermore, the results obtained from venous specimens may be influenced by unpredictable variations in local venous pressure. Since arterial puncture is sometimes difficult, specimens for acid–base determinations in human patients have been obtained from "arterialized" blood in capillaries of hyperemic skin. Most routine studies, however, even in human patients, are performed on venous blood (Henry, 1964).

In animal patients, the difficulty of obtaining arterial or even "arterialized" capillary blood is even greater than it is in man. For this reason, almost all clinical studies of acid–base status in spontaneous disease as well as most studies of normal values have been based on venous blood specimens. It must be appreciated that stasis of blood in the vein prior to collection must be avoided if the results are to be meaningful.

1. Blood pH

Commercial pH meters are available from several manufacturers at the present time which have specially constructed electrodes for blood pH measurement. It is necessary that equipment for blood pH measurement be of sufficient quality to permit reproducible results within 0.01 pH units. It must also require a very small sample of blood to make measurements on small animals feasible. The pH electrodes used for blood pH measurement must be incubated to maintain the specimen at body temperature and be constructed in such a way that the specimen can be kept from exposure to air during the transfer from original container to the electrode and while the reading is being taken.

It is essential that the sample be kept anaerobic until after the pH measurement is made since equilibration of gaseous CO_2 between blood and air would alter the blood pH. Furthermore, the blood pH should be read as soon as possible after the sample is obtained since cellular metabolism in the blood will continue and this will alter the blood pH. If the reading cannot be made within 30 minutes the specimen should be refrigerated immediately or placed on ice until the reading can be done. Although the blood pH changes slightly even at 5°C, useful results can be obtained if the reading on refrigerated blood is made within 5 hours after the specimen is obtained (Henry, 1964). Heparinized whole blood is usually used for pH measurement but plasma obtained anaerobically is also satisfactory.

2. Determination of Carbonic Acid

There are no practical methods available for the direct measurement of carbonic acid in clinical patients. However, since the carbonic acid is always directly related to the pCO_2, which can be measured, this procedure is used to evaluate the acid concentration in the Henderson-Hasselbalch equation. The following relationship should be remembered.

$$H_2CO_3 \text{ concentration in mEq/liter} = 0.03 \times pCO_2 \text{ in mmHg}$$

3. pCO₂ Determination

Several commercial pCO_2 electrodes are available for clinical laboratory use. Most of these are of the type described by Severinghaus and Bradley (1958) in which the pCO_2 of the specimen is compared directly with that of gases of known concentration.

The pCO_2 can also be determined by the Astrup technique (Astrup, 1956) in which the specimen is equilibrated with gases of two known pCO_2 values and the pH then determined on the blood in which each known pCO_2 has been establish-ed. The resulting relationship between pH and pCO_2 can be represented graphically and from this information the actual pCO_2 of the specimen can be determined.

The precautions of specimen handling are the same as those described for pH determination. Adams et al. (1968) have discussed available methods and sources of error for both pH and pCO_2 analysis in blood.

4. Bicarbonate

The bicarbonate can be determined titrimetrically by the technique described originally by Van Slyke in 1919 (Henry, 1964). Several modifications of this technique have been published since that time (Henry, 1964). Plasma or serum is used for bicarbonate determinations. In obtaining specimens for bicarbonate determination it is important to remove the plasma from the cells as soon as possible and to keep the specimen anaerobic and refrigerated until this is done.

Bicarbonate can also be estimated from the total carbon dioxide content (TCO_2) of the specimen.

5. Total CO_2

This procedure consists of converting bicarbonate to carbonic acid by the addition of excess acid to the specimen and the extraction of gaseous CO_2 from the liquid by the application of vacuum. After determining the volume or pressure of the extracted gas and the use of appropriate factors the sum of bicarbonate, H_2CO_3, and CO_2 in the original specimen can be determined. This is usually expressed in milliequivalents of carbonic acid per liter and is called total CO_2 (TCO_2), CO_2 content, or merely "CO_2."

Since the bicarbonate of plasma is approximately 24 mEq/liter and the carbonic acid is approximately 1.2 mEq/liter, the TCO_2 is essentially a measurement of bicarbonate concentration. The bicarbonate concentration can be estimated quite satisfactorily by subtracting 1.2 mEq from the TCO_2 content.

It must be emphasized that this "CO_2" determination has quite a different significance from pCO_2 measurement. The former is a measurement of bicarbonate while the latter is a measure of carbonic acid. Unfortunately in casual usage, either one may be referred to as "CO_2."

D. Is There Any Other Important Abnormality in the Composition of the Extracellular Fluid?

In certain circumstances it is very important to determine the serum concentration of calcium, magnesium, or phosphorus (see Chapter 9, Volume I). Although most clinical laboratories are equipped to perform these tests routinely, they are not often used in the routine evaluation of a patient with a fluid balance problem. This is because disorders of these ions are not commonly of primary importance in dehydrated patients.

The other ions which are always of importance in studying dehydrated patients are potassium and chloride.

1. Potassium

Potassium is determined by flame photometry using serum or heparinized plasma. The mature erythrocytes of many species have a much higher potassium concentration than is present in the ECF. Even in those species that do not have a high-potassium fluid within the mature erythrocytes there seems to be a high-potassium fluid in immature erythrocytes. For this reason, it is essential that serum or plasma for potassium determinations be removed from the red cells before any leak of intracellular ions into the plasma has occurred. When hemolysis has occurred in collecting the blood sample an artifact in plasma potassium concentration is likely to be present. In addition, even when there is no grossly visible hemolysis plasma which has remained on the cells for several hours will have increased potassium values as the cells lose the ability to maintain concentration gradients and equilibration of intra- and extracellular potassium occurs. It has been shown experimentally that storage of whole human blood for 18 hours resulted in increases of serum potassium of 7.8 and 4.5 mEq/liter when storage was at 37° and 4°C, respectively (Henry, 1964).

It is important to remember that approximately 90% of the body potassium is in the ICF. A direct measurement of the intracellular content of potassium would be a much more valuable indicator of body potassium status than the serum potassium concentration. However, no practicable technique of evaluating intracellular potassium is available for routine use.

2. Chloride

Chloride ion concentration is determined in serum or plasma. A large number of chemical and physicochemical procedures have been recommended for chloride determination in biological fluids.

The chloride determination was of special importance in the past when it was used as a reflection of sodium changes when sodium could not be measured. It is not necessary for this purpose if sodium is measured directly. However, quantitation of this major anion of the ECF makes possible an appreciation of the relationship between the various anions and between the anions and the cations. This, in turn, provides insight into the mechanism responsible for certain electrolyte disturbances that would not have been possible otherwise.

E. Selection of Laboratory Tests for Clinical Patients

If laboratory tests are to be used to evaluate a clinical patient an effort should be made to evaluate each of the four areas of special concern: water, osmotic pressure, acid–base balance, and important electrolytes. This requires a battery of tests, the components of which will depend upon the capabilities of each laboratory. A good appreciation of the status of a patient can be obtained by using the packed cell volume and/or the total serum protein to evaluate water balance, the blood pH and pCO_2 to evaluate acid–base balance, serum sodium to evaluate osmolality, and serum potassium and chloride determination to evaluate these other important electrolytes.

Minimal laboratory evaluation of a dehydrated patient includes packed cell volume and serum sodium, potassium, and bicarbonate. With this small number of determinations useful information about the status of the patient can usually be obtained but occasionally false conclusions may be made, especially concerning acid–base abnormalities.

When no laboratory tests are used to evaluate the dehydrated patient one can only assume that the patient has abnormalities similar to those reported in other patients with the same disease. Any specific patient may differ quite markedly from the typical description. In those instances, such an indirect evaluation of the patient may be very misleading.

V. PATHOLOGICAL PHYSIOLOGY

Most clinical disturbances of fluid balance result in abnormalities in body water, body electrolytes, and acid–base balance. The clinical problem is, therefore, a complex one. Nevertheless, it will be useful, prior to a discussion of the important clinical problems, to consider the individual abnormalities that can occur and the causes and effects of these disturbances.

It can be stated quite simply that abnormalities in the body balance of water, electrolytes, and acids and bases is merely a question of intake and loss. Deficits theoretically will occur when intake is curtailed and/or losses are increased. Similarly, excesses can be expected whenever intake is excessive or losses are reduced. The mechanisms through which these changes occur, however, are often complex and deserve further consideration.

The papers on electrolyte abnormalities by Epstein (1962) and on acid–base derangements by Simmons (1962) are especially practical, clinically oriented discussions that are helpful in understanding clinical observations. The monograph by Deane (1966) provides more detailed information.

A. Sodium

It has been mentioned previously that regulation of the tonicity of the ECF is accomplished by regulation of both water and sodium. When either of these tends to be abnormal adjustments are made in the regulation of each in order to maintain isotonicity of the ECF. For example, when there is excessive intake of sodium, ADH is released and water is conserved in the kidney to prevent hypertonicity. The increased ECF volume which results suppresses the release of aldosterone and sodium excretion is enhanced. Thus both volume and tonicity of the ECF are maintained in the optimal range.

When abnormalities of sodium concentration occur, they are usually the result of conditions which interfere with the regulation of *both* water and sodium or are so extreme that the normal compensatory mechanisms are ineffective.

1. Hyponatremia

Abnormally low serum sodium concentration can result from too little sodium in the body or too much water. Each of these may result from abnormal intake or abnormal losses.

Inadequate intake of sodium is seldom a primary cause of hyponatremia. The renal conservation of sodium is so effective that depletion does not usually occur by this means alone.

Excessive loss of sodium occurs in many clinical conditions. When dietary sodium is abundant depletion may not occur even when sodium losses are increased. When losses are enormous or when dietary sodium is restricted, however, depletion will occur.

Renal losses of sodium are increased in disease of the kidney and the adrenal gland. In renal disease the active reabsorption of sodium may be impaired when there is damage to the tubules. Large quantities of sodium can thus be lost in the urine. Administration of certain diuretics can also result in accelerated renal loss of sodium. In diabetes mellitus there is often a large loss of sodium in the urine because of the osmotic diuresis which occurs. Adrenal insufficiency may lead to hyponatremia due to inadequate renal conservation of sodium in the absence of aldosterone.

Excessive sweating may result in a marked increase in sodium loss from the body. Exudation from burns or open wounds may also be associated with increased sodium loss.

The most common cause of sodium depletion is disease of the digestive tract in which large quantities of gastrointestinal secretions are lost by vomiting or diarrhea.

In many of these conditions in which increased loss of sodium occurs, the fluids lost have a lower concentration of sodium than is present in serum. Thus the losses of water are equal to or greater than those of sodium and hyponatremia should not result from these losses alone. However, it often occurs that the fluid lost is replaced by sodium-free water either consumed voluntarily by the patient or administered parenterally by the veterinarian (e.g., 5% dextrose). When sodium-containing fluid is lost and sodium-free fluid is replaced, hyponatremia may result.

Various factors which impair normal water excretion have been described as causes of hyponatremia in man. Similar conditions have not been identified in animals.

Hyponatremia is occasionally identified in association with hyperglycemia or lipemia. In hyperglycemia the large concentration of glucose tends to raise the osmolality of the ECF. Hypertonicity of this fluid is avoided by a compensatory reduction in sodium concentration. The hyponatremia is obviously desirable in this instance. If lipemia is severe, the lipid displaces a significant volume of the aqueous phase of the plasma. When a measured volume of plasma is obtained for sodium analysis, a smaller volume of the aqueous phase will be obtained and the sodium content will be less. However, if the sodium concentration is expressed in terms of plasma water rather than whole plasma it will probably be found to be normal.

The symptoms of hyponatremia have been described in man as excessive fatigue and a sense of exhaustion, muscle weakness and cramps, nausea, headache, faintness, and mental confusion. It can be anticipated that signs of similar abnormalities would be present in animals with hyponatremia. English (1967a) has investigated the effects of sodium depletion in sheep.

2. Hypernatremia

Abnormally high concentrations of sodium in the ECF are seldom seen. They may occur, however, when salt intake is excessive and water intake is restricted, or when water intake is restricted in spite of continuing losses from the body of fluid which contains sodium in a concentration less than that of plasma. Certain intracranial lesions have been associated with hypernatremia in man and experimental animals. Hypernatremia may be manifested by severe thirst, stupor, or coma.

B. Potassium

While sodium concentration in the plasma is a reliable index of the status of the body with respect to sodium, plasma potassium concentration is not always a meaningful indication of the status of the body with respect to potassium. This is because most of the potassium is intracellular and there is no consistently reliable relationship between intra- and extracellular potassium concentrations.

The normal cell, bathed by normal ECF maintains a disequilibrium between ECF potassium and intracellular potassium. This is the result of the active extrusion of sodium from the cell, the sodium pump, which is a process requiring energy. When intracellular carbohydrate metabolism is defective, as in diabetes mellitus, the sodium pump does not work optimally and intracellular potassium is lost in the ECF. Subsequently, after insulin administration, intracellular carbohydrate metabolism is accelerated and potassium is quickly redistributed from the ECF to the ICF. In neither of these conditions does the ECF potassium concentration reflect the nature of intracellular stores.

When cells of the body, especially muscle cells, become necrotic, large amounts of potassium move into the ECF. Once again the elevated ECF potassium does not reflect intracellular concentration.

The most common clinical problem in which serum potassium values are seriously misleading is acidosis. When the extracellular concentration of hydrogen ions is increased (acidosis) the cells tend to take up hydrogen ions and release potassium ions into the ECF. Thus, marked *elevation* of serum potassium may occur when the cells are *depleted.* In alkalosis, low serum potassium values may be found as hydrogen ions leave the cells and plasma potassium enters. Such findings do not always indicate potassium depletion.

1. Hypokalemia

Decreased concentration of potassium in the serum is called hypokalemia or hypopotassemia. This may be the result of decreased intake of potassium. It will be remembered that the kidney excretes the large quantities of potassium which are consumed daily but does not curtail potassium excretion promptly when intake ceases. Potassium depletion occurs even if the serum concentration is not recognizably altered. When anoretic animals continue to drink water or when they are kept hydrated by parenteral administration of potassium-free fluids for many days, frank hypokalemia may be recognized.

Potassium depletion and hypokalemia are also seen when the patient has lost large quantities of fluids by vomiting or diarrhea. This is especially apt to occur when fluid losses are replaced with potassium-free fluids.

Prolonged administration of adrenal steroids that have some mineralocorticoid activity may promote potassium excretion and result in hypokalemia. Hyperadrenocorticalism may also result in excessive renal excretion of potassium and hypokalemia.

Alkalosis, regardless of cause, results in increased exchange of potassium ions for hydrogen ions in the renal tubular fluid. This may cause marked hypokalemia.

Human patients with potassium deficiencies show neurological, muscular, and cardiac abnormalities. These do not usually appear until the serum potassium has dropped below 2.5 mEq/liter. The neurologic signs are drowsiness, irritability, mental confusion, and even coma. Severe muscular weakness is a common complaint.

Electrocardiographic abnormalities appear in hypokalemia. The characteristic changes are depression of the T waves and prolongation of the Q–T interval (Clark and McCrady, 1966). Electrocardiographic changes seen in potassium deficiency in swine have been described by Cox et al. (1966).

Necrosis of the myocardium has been reported in patients with chronic potassium depletion. Renal abnormalities also occur in potassium deficiency. Inability to concentrate the urine has resulted in a syndrome similar to diabetes insipidus. Characteristic histological lesions have been reported in the renal tubules of potassium-deficient patients (Epstein, 1962). Abbrecht (1969) studied the effect of potassium deficiency on renal function in the dog.

2. Hyperkalemia

Increased potassium within the cell is apparently not harmful, the toxic effects of excess potassium in the body are the direct result of increased levels in the ECF.

Hyperkalemia is most frequently the result of acidosis causing a redistribution of body potassium, i.e., the movement of intracellular potassium into the ECF. It may also occur in renal failure, although the significance of this in chronic renal failure is often overemphasized. Hyperkalemia resulting from renal failure is most likely to occur if renal failure is acute, if intake of potassium is continued in large amounts, if extensive cellular necrosis occurs simultaneously, or if serious acidosis exists.

The principal danger in hyperkalemia is cardiac arrest. Abnormalities may be observed when the serum potassium is 7 mEq/liter and are usually present (at least in man) when the serum potassium is greater than 8 mEq/liter. Death usually occurs when the serum potassium level is 10–12 mEq/liter. The characteristic electrocardiographic abnormalities are high, peaked, T waves, prolongation of the P–R interval, disappearance of P waves and prolongation of the QRS complex (Epstein, 1962; Goldberger, 1965; Clark and McCrady, 1966). Descriptions of electrocardiographic changes due to hyperkalemia have been made by Gentile and Venturoli (1960) in the horse and by Greenspan et al. (1965) in the dog. Ward (1966b) has reported the death of a cow following oral administration of potassium chloride.

C. Abnormalities in Acid–Base Balance

Disturbances in acid–base balance have been described as respiratory or non-respiratory (metabolic). The respiratory disturbances are the result of abnormalities in pulmonary gaseous exchange and are always characterized by alterations in the pCO_2 of the blood. The remaining disturbances in acid–base balance have many different causes, e.g., renal failure, vomiting, diarrhea, shock. These have been referred to collectively as metabolic disturbances. However, a more accurate and informative description would be nonrespiratory disturbances. These disturbances are always characterized by an alteration in the bicarbonate concentration in the blood.

There are four general classifications of acid–base disturbance: respiratory acidosis, respiratory alkalosis, nonrespiratory acidosis and nonrespiratory alkalosis. In each of these four types of disturbance the process may be uncompensated or it may be compensated. Compensation is the result of various homeostatic mechanisms in the body inducing a second acid–base disturbance which tends to correct the abnormality in hydrogen ion concentration caused by the primary disturbance. The compensatory mechanism will be opposite the primary disturbance in two respects. If the primary disturbance is respiratory, the compensatory mechanism will be nonrespiratory; if the primary disturbance is nonrespiratory, the compensatory mechanism will be respiratory. Furthermore, if the primary disturbance caused acidosis, the compensatory mechanism will be one that tends to cause alkalosis; if the primary disturbance caused alkalosis, the compensatory mechanism will be one that tends to cause acidosis. Thus the compensatory mechanism tends to neutralize the effects of the primary disturbance.

When a disturbance in acid–base balance has been recognized, it is important to try to classify the disturbance with respect to the primary mechanism responsible for it. This not only permits localization of the abnormality but is essential to the selection of rational therapy. In most cases of acid–base disturbance, identification of the abnormal mechanism involved is possible if the pH, pCO_2, and bicarbonate concentration are known. It should be remembered that direct measurement of two of these will permit evaluation of the third by use of the Henderson-Hasselbalch equation.

1.   Respiratory Acidosis

This condition is the result of hypoventilation. Carbon dioxide is not adequately eliminated and the $pCO_2(H_2CO_3)$ of blood rises. If there is no compensatory reaction the blood pH falls as the carbonic acid concentration increases.

Compensation for this disturbance occurs in the kidney. Increased quantities of H^+ are excreted and increased bicarbonate ion is reabsorbed. Chloride ion is excreted instead of bicarbonate.

It will be recalled that the Henderson-Hasselbalch equation shows the pH is not dependent upon the absolute concentration of carbonic acid or bicarbonate but on the *ratio* between them. The typical findings in a normal individual, a patient with uncompensated respiratory acidosis and one with compensated respiratory acidosis are shown in the tabulation below.

	pCO_2	H_2CO_3	HCO_3^-	$\dfrac{HCO_3^-}{H_2CO_3}$	pH
Normal	40	1.2	24	20:1	7.40
Uncompensated respiratory acidosis	90	2.7	24	8.8:1	7.20
Partially compensated respiratory acidosis	90	2.7	38	14:1	7.32

In the uncompensated patient the increase in pCO_2 (H_2CO_3) results in a decrease in the bicarbonate: carbonic acid ratio and the pH falls. As the bicarbonate increases due to renal compensation, the ratio is changed toward normal and the pH becomes less abnormal. Evaluation of pH, pCO_2, and bicarbonate indicates unequivocally that the problem is an acidosis, that it is of respiratory origin, and the degree to which compensation has occurred.

The most common clinical situation in which respiratory acidosis is recognized in veterinary medicine is in anesthesia with volatile anesthetics and a closed system apparatus. Under these conditions ventilation may be seriously reduced without hypoxia developing. The high oxygen content of the gas mixture supplied to the patient maintains high pO_2 in the blood and prevents an hypoxic stimulation of respiration. The well-oxygenated blood falsely indicates to the surgeon that ventilation is adequate. However, anesthesia of the respiratory center results in decreased respiratory movements and adequate CO_2 elimination does not occur. Although CO_2 accumulates (hypercarbia) the respiratory center does not respond by initiating increased respiration and serious respiratory acidosis may develop, *in spite of adequate oxygenation of the blood.*

Other causes of respiratory acidosis are widespread pulmonary disease, intrathoracic lesions that prevent normal ventilation, and lesions or drugs affecting the central nervous system which interfere with its regulation of normal respiration. In contrast to respiratory acidosis resulting from closed-system anesthesia, these other causes of hypoventilation are frequently accompanied by cyanosis because of coexisting hypoxia.

2. Respiratory Alkalosis

This condition is the result of hyperventilation and is characterized by decreased pCO_2 in the alveolar air and blood. If there is no compensatory reaction, the ratio of bicarbonate to carbonic acid rises and the pH is increased.

Compensation for this disturbance is by increased renal excretion of bicarbonate instead of chloride. This results in an increase in plasma chloride and a decrease in plasma bicarbonate. As plasma bicarbonate decreases, the bicarbonate–carbonic acid ratio decreases and the blood pH changes toward normal.

	pCO_2	H_2CO_3	HCO_3^-	$\dfrac{HCO_3^-}{H_2CO_3}$	pH
Normal	40	1.2	24	20:1	7.4
Uncompensated respiratory alkalosis	20	0.6	24	40:1	7.55
Partially compensated respiratory alkalosis	20	0.6	20	33.3:1	7.50

Respiratory alkalosis may be seen in animals in pain or psychological stress when increased respiration occurs. It may also occur in animals (especially dogs) which hyperventilate to prevent overheating when the ambient temperature is elevated. It is not of frequent occurrence in veterinary medicine.

3.   Nonrespiratory Acidosis

"Metabolic" acidosis is by far the most common type of acid–base disorder encountered in veterinary practice. It results from the loss of bicarbonate from the ECF. This reduces the bicarbonate–carbonic acid ratio and the pH.

Compensation for nonrespiratory acidosis occurs by hyperventilation. Thus a respiratory alkalosis is superimposed on the primary nonrespiratory acidosis and the disturbance in pH is ameliorated as the bicarbonate–carbonic acid ratio is returned toward normal.

	pCO_2	H_2CO_3	HCO_3^-	$\dfrac{HCO_3^-}{H_2CO_3}$	pH
Normal	40	1.2	24	20:1	7.40
Uncompensated metabolic acidosis	40	1.2	15	12.5:1	7.20
Partially compensated metabolic acidosis	32	0.96	15	15.6:1	7.30

The most common cause of metabolic acidosis in veterinary practice is diarrhea. The secretions of the intestinal tract are alkaline and contain a high concentration of bicarbonate. When the alimentary canal is functioning normally these secretions are largely reabsorbed in the lower digestive tract but in diarrhea the secretions are lost from the body. There is a serious depletion of bicarbonate as a result.

In certain other abnormalities of the digestive tract, e.g., obstruction, intestinal secretions may accumulate in the digestive tract and, being sequestered in that location, represent a significant loss of bicarbonate from the plasma and interstitial fluid. In certain acute intestinal disorders at least in the horse (salmonellosis, "colitis X"), there may be a large accumulation of fluid in the intestine before diarrhea is recognized. These animals may also have a serious metabolic acidosis.

The accumulation in the body of organic acids is another common cause of metabolic acidosis. In these instances the accumulating organic acids are buffered by bicarbonate and the bicarbonate concentration is decreased. This can be seen in the following equation where the organic anion is indicated by the symbol A:

$$HA + HCO_3^- \rightarrow H_2CO_3 + A^-$$
$$\hookrightarrow H_2O + CO_2$$

The hydrogen ions provided by the organic acid have been removed by the conversion of bicarbonate to carbonic acid but bicarbonate has been depleted in the process and has been replaced by the organic anion.

Since the ketone bodies are mostly organic acids, this may be seen in the clinical ketosis of cattle and sheep as well as in diabetes mellitus.

Shock and cellular hypoxia from other causes are characterized by a severe metabolic acidosis. This is because the failure of normal aerobic cellular metabolism results in the accumulation of lactic and pyruvic acids.

Renal failure also is characterized by metabolic acidosis. This may be due in part to the retention of phosphate, sulfate, and other acids by the failing kidneys but is probably also related to the inability of the kidney to excrete H^+ and to reabsorb bicarbonate.

4. Nonrespiratory Alkalosis

Metabolic alkalosis is characterized by the accumulation in the ECF of abnormally large amounts of bicarbonate ion. This decreases the bicarbonate–carbonic acid ratio and the pH.

Compensation for this abnormality is the result of hypoventilation. This increases the pCO_2 of the blood and tends to decrease the bicarbonate–carbonic acid ratio and the pH toward normal.

	pCO_2	H_2CO_3	HCO_3^-	$\frac{HCO_3^-}{H_2CO_3}$	pH
Normal	40	1.2	24	20:1	7.40
Uncompensated metabolic alkalosis	40	1.2	38	31.5:1	7.60
Partially compensated metabolic alkalosis	50	1.5	38	25.3:1	7.50

In compensating for metabolic alkalosis, the kidney may excrete increased quantities of bicarbonate as an additional compensatory measure. If the bicarbonate concentration were reduced while the pCO_2 were increasing, the change in bicarbonate–carbonic acid ratio would be greater and the compensation would be more complete.

Metabolic alkalosis is most commonly seen in digestive tract disorders in the ruminant. Any abnormality that results in the sequestration of abomasal juice in the abomasum or forestomachs may be a cause of metabolic alkalosis. This is seen in high intestinal obstruction and in atony, torsion, or displacement of the abomasum. The large amount of hydrochloric acid in the gastric juice is secreted by the mucosal cells by the following overall process (White et al., 1964):

$$NaCl + H_2CO_3 \rightarrow NaHCO_3 \text{ (plasma)} + HCl \text{ (secreted)}$$

The HCl which results is secreted in the gastric juice and the sodium bicarbonate moves into the plasma. If the gastric juice is subsequently reabsorbed in the lower digestive tract no acid–base disorder occurs. However, if abnormalities of the upper digestive tract prevent gastric juice from moving into the intestine for reabsorption serious metabolic alkalosis will occur as hydrogen ions are continuously removed and bicarbonate continuously contributed to the ECF.

Profuse vomiting in monogastric animals may cause metabolic alkalosis by the same mechanism although this is not as commonly encountered as might be expected.

Severe potassium depletion may be a cause of metabolic alkalosis since hydrogen ions tend to move into the cells to replace the lost potassium. This, by itself tends to cause alkalosis. In addition, however, there may be increased hydrogen ion secretion in the urine as a result of increased hydrogen ion concentration in the tubule cells. Whenever hydrogen ion is lost from the ECF alkalosis occurs which is characterized by increased bicarbonate as shown in the following equation:

$$H_2CO_3 \rightarrow H^+ + HCO_3^-$$

The removal of H^+ favors the dissociation of H_2CO_3 to restore the hydrogen ion concentration and produce abnormally high concentrations of bicarbonate.

5. Mixed Disturbances

Abnormalities in acid–base balance are usually the result of either a primary disturbance in respiratory control of carbon dioxide or nonrespiratory factors which alter bicarbonate. Each of these may be associated with an opposite, compensatory change. In some patients, however, a mixed disturbance exists which, at first inspection, may be confusing.

For example, if a patient had a pCO_2 of 80 and a plasma bicarbonate of 10 mEq/liter it would not be comparable with any of the simple disturbances, with or without compensation, described above. One would have to conclude that this patient had both a primary respiratory acidosis and a primary metabolic acidosis, a mixed disturbance. This type of abnormality could be seen in a patient with intestinal obstruction (metabolic acidosis) that has been anesthetized without adequate ventilation (respiratory acidosis).

6. Diagnosis of Acid–Base Disturbances

It should be apparent from the foregoing discussion how essential it is to know the three components of the Henderson-Hasselbalch equation if accurate evaluation of the acid–base status of the patient is to be made.

In the past, the common laboratory procedure for evaluating acid–base status has been the plasma bicarbonate determination or total CO_2, which is essentially the same measurement. Abnormally high results were interpreted as indicating alkalosis, abnormally low results suggested acidosis. This is valid if one is dealing with a primary nonrespiratory disturbance. However, in primary *respiratory* disturbances, the results may be normal or *exactly in the opposite direction from this rule of thumb*. That is, severe respiratory *acidosis* will be characterized by either a normal bicarbonate or, if compensation has occurred, by an elevated bicarbonate concentration.

Some have suggested that correlation of plasma bicarbonate with urine pH will make clear whether there is alkalosis or acidosis. However, there is a large number of clinical problems in which the urine pH is not reflective of blood pH and in these, false conclusions would result (Simmons, 1962).

Further discussions of acid–base disturbances can be found in the following references: Simmons (1962), Goldberger (1965), Weisberg (1962), Winters *et al.* (1967), and Nuttall (1965).

D. ABNORMALITIES OF BODY WATER

Normal water balance depends upon careful integration of many factors which involve most of the major body systems. The central nervous system is important in initiating drinking when water is needed and in producing and regulating the release of antidiuretic hormone; the kidneys are important in regulating water loss from the body; the digestive tract and the skin both function to prevent extraordinary losses of water in the normal animal; the endocrine glands, especially the pituitary and the adrenals produce hormones which, directly or indirectly, influence water balance; and the cardiovascular system is important in initiating humoral reactions which alter water balance. Abnormalities in water balance occur frequently, therefore, in association with a wide variety of diseases of these major body systems and, in addition, can be expected when the availability of water is restricted. In most instances, a single abnormality does not result in derangement of water balance because compensatory mechanisms are many and varied. When two or more abnormalities occur simultaneously, normal compensatory mechanisms may be vitiated and a serious derangement of water balance will result. For example, although diarrhea results in large, uncontrolled losses of water from the body, dehydration does not occur if normal kidneys cause maximal renal water conservation and a normal central thirst mechanism causes increased water intake. Diarrhea does result in dehydration, however, if the central nervous system is depressed so that the normal thirst mechanism is not responsive to the need for increased water intake or if adequate drinking water is not available.

1. Overhydration

Overhydration is not often considered as a potential fluid balance problem in veterinary medicine. It is apt to occur, however, when excessive volumes of fluid are administered intravenously at a very rapid rate. In addition, overhydration has been described in man in instances where there has been a sustained, unphysiological secretion of ADH and continued intake of water (Kleeman and Maxwell, 1962).

2. Dehydration

Water depletion occurs whenever the loss of water from the body exceeds the intake. This may occur when an animal fails to consume enough water to meet minimal losses, or when unusual losses have occurred without adequate compensatory increase in water intake.

a. DECREASED INTAKE. Inadequate intake of water may occur with accidental deprivation of drinking water; it may result from failure of the normal thirst mechanism because of central nervous system abnormalities; or it may be due to inability of the animal to drink or retain water because of paralysis, obstruction, or irritation of the upper digestive tract. The dehydration which ensues is of gradual onset because of the effects of at least three important compensatory factors: (1) There is immediate restriction of renal water loss as ADH is secreted in maximal quantities. (2) There is continued absorption of fluid from the digestive tract which tends to maintain ECF volume. (This is of considerable importance in the herbivores which have an especially capacious digestive tract.) (3) An appreciable quantity of water continues to be supplied to the body due to continuing oxidation of food or body tissues.

In spite of these mitigating influences, however, there is a continuing, minimal loss of water in the form of urine and water vapor from the skin and lungs. The minimal water loss for a normal adult man has been estimated to be 1500 ml daily. Although these losses are more related to body surface area ("metabolic size") than to body weight, this figure suggests the magnitude of continuing loss to be expected in animals.

b. INCREASED LOSS OF WATER.   By far the most common and serious cause of dehydration is that which results from sudden unusual increases in body water losses. Gradual increases in body water losses may not cause serious dehydration because gradual increases in water intake can usually compensate adequately. Moreover, the chronic diseases with which these losses are associated do not usually interfere with the mental processes involved in the thirst mechanism. In acute illnesses, however, there are often alterations in the sensorium which prevent compensatory increase in water intake and dehydration may develop rapidly.

The most common abnormality causing dehydration due to increased fluid loss in veterinary medicine is diarrhea. In all species acute, profuse diarrhea, especially that which is associated with systemic signs (e.g., altered sensorium) may be the cause of serious, life-threatening, dehydration. Vomiting and the sequestration of large quantities of fluid in the digestive tract or elsewhere may also cause severe dehydration. Fever results in increased loss of fluid by the insensible routes (skin and lungs). Visible sweating is a more obvious fluid loss, which, if not compensated by increased intake, will result in dehydration. Other routes of fluid loss which may be significant in the development of dehydration are exudation from burns or open wounds in the skin and loss of blood or other fluid during surgery.

Uncontrolled renal loss of water in polyuria regardless of the cause (diabetes mellitus, diabetes insipidus, nephritis, and nephrosis) will quickly lead to dehydration if adequate compensation by increased intake of water does not occur.

E. WATER–ELECTROLYTE RELATIONSHIPS

The laboratory findings in animals with fluid balance problems will reveal a broad spectrum of derangements. This is because of the possible combinations and permutations of water, electrolyte, and acid–base abnormalities which can occur, especially since many of these variables are independent of one another.

It is often useful, in designing a therapeutic regimen, to appreciate the significance of relative changes which have occurred, especially with respect to water and sodium losses. In many obviously dehydrated animals, the sodium concentration (and that of other electrolytes also) will be found normal. This can be referred to as "isotonic contraction" of the ECF. Instead of suggesting that body sodium is normal and can be ignored, this finding should be interpreted as indicating sodium losses of the same magnitude as the losses of extracellular water. A sodium deficit does exist, in spite of the finding of normal sodium *concentration* in the ECF.

Similarly, when sodium concentration in a dehydrated animal is higher than normal it does not mean there is a sodium excess. This "hypertonic contraction" merely indicates that water losses have been greater than sodium losses. If sodium concentration is abnormally low in a dehydrated animal, this "hypotonic contraction" indicates that the sodium deficit is relatively greater than the water deficit. Hypotonic contraction is most often the result of depletion of both water and sodium followed by replacement of water alone.

In Section VII of this chapter the abnormalities commonly encountered in clinical entities of veterinary importance will be discussed.

VI.   NORMAL VALUES FOR IMPORTANT LABORATORY DETERMINATIONS

The literature contains many references to studies that have been made in various species of the laboratory tests appropriate to the evaluation of fluid balance. These are usually in general agreement, one with another, but occasionally marked differences have been reported. While some of these differences may be attributable to different populations being studied, most of the differences are probably the result of inaccurate laboratory work, failure to recognize illness in the animals assumed to be normal, or artifacts such as prolonged stasis of blood in the vessel before collection, hemolysis, improper anticoagulants, or failure to handle the specimen properly for the specific test being done.

Tables III and IV contain suggested normal values for the tests of importance in

TABLE III   NORMAL VALUES FOR SERUM ELECTROLYTES (mEq/LITER)

Species	Determination	Range	References
Dog	Sodium	141.1–152.3	Robinson and Zeigler (1968)
	Potassium	4.37–5.65	Robinson and Zeigler (1968)
	Chloride	105.2–114.8	Michaelson et al. (1966)
Cat	Sodium	147–156	Albritton (1952)
	Potassium	4.0–4.5	Albritton (1952)
	Chloride	117–123	Spector (1956)
Ox	Sodium	132–152	McSherry and Grinyer (1954a)
	Potassium	3.9–5.8	McSherry and Grinyer (1954a)
	Chloride	97–111	McSherry and Grinyer (1954a)
Horse	Sodium	132–146	Tasker (1966b)
	Potassium	2.4–4.7	Tasker (1966b)
	Chloride	99–109	Tasker (1966b)
Sheep	Sodium	139–152	Pugh (1966)
	Potassium	3.9–5.4	Pugh (1966)
	Chloride	95–103	Pugh (1966)
Swine	Sodium	135–150	Bertho et al. (1964)
	Potassium	4.4–6.7	Bertho et al. (1964)
	Chloride	94–106	Bertho et al. (1964)
Man	Sodium	135–155	Henry (1964)
	Potassium	3.6–5.5	Henry (1964)
	Chloride	98–109	Henry (1964)

TABLE IV   NORMAL VALUES FOR ACID–BASE DETERMINATIONS

Species	Determination	Range	References
Dog	pH	7.31–7.42[a]	Spector (1956)
	pCO_2	38[b]	Spector (1956)
	TCO_2	17–24[c]	Spector (1956)
Cat	pH	7.24–7.40	Spector (1956)
	pCO_2	36	Spector (1956)
	TCO_2	17–24	Spector (1956)
Ox	pH	7.31–7.53	McSherry and Grinyer (1954a)
	pCO_2	34.7–44	Donawick and Baue (1968)
	TCO_2	25.6–33.4	McSherry and Grinyer (1954a)
Horse	pH	7.32–7.44	Tasker (1966b)
	pCO_2	38–46	Tasker (1966b)
	TCO_2	24–34	Tasker (1966b)
Sheep	pH	7.32–7.53	Spector (1956)
	pCO_2	38	Spector (1956)
	TCO_2	21–28	Spector (1956)
Swine	HCO_3	18–27	Aalund and Nielsen (1960)
Man	pH	7.31–7.45	Henry (1964)
	TCO_2	24–34	Henry (1964)
	HCO_3	22–30	Henry (1964)
	pCO_2	33–48	Henry (1964)

laboratory evaluation of fluid balance in the common domestic animals. The author has selected from the literature those reports which seem most representative of normal animals in his own experience. Additional sources of information are listed in Table V.

The balance and interrelationships of electrolytes can only be appreciated when concentrations are expressed in terms of milliequivalents per liter. Other terms have been used in the past and some persist today but fortunately one encounters them with decreased frequency at the present time. If other terms are used, the values can be converted to milliequivalents per liter by one of the factors in Table VI.

Some workers (Lane *et al.*, 1968) have reported on the concentration of electrolytes in whole blood. Since the intra- and extracellular concentration of electrolytes is quite different, results of determinations on whole blood vary greatly depending on the relative proportions of plasma and erythrocytes. Such values do not provide useful information about the fluid balance status of a patient. Plasma or serum should be used for electrolyte determinations.

Reports of the volume of the various fluid compartments of the body have been made by numerous investigators. Since the results obtained vary with the physiological status of the subjects, i.e., pregnancy, lactation, obesity, age, sex, it is of little value to present a table providing a single normal result for each species. For further information on this subject the reader is referred to the general discussions of Hansard (1964) and Reid *et al.* (1963) or to the specific reports concerning dogs (Becker and Joseph, 1955; Hannon and Durrer, 1963), cattle (Aschbacher *et al.*, 1965;

TABLE V   REFERENCES TO NORMAL VALUES FOR SERUM ELECTROLYTE AND ACID—BASE DETERMINATIONS
IN DOMESTIC ANIMALS

Subject	References
General	Spector (1956) Altman and Dittmer (1961) Albritton (1952)
Dogs	Van Stewart and Longwell (1969) Robinson and Ziegler (1968) Michaelson et al. (1966)
Horse	Tasker (1966b) Sreter (1959) Sova et al. (1965) Soliman and Nadim (1967) Simon (1964) Martinez (1963) El Amrousi and Soliman (1965) Bruning (1950)
Horses and cattle	Krapf (1938)
Cattle	Vrzgula (1963) Tashjian et al. (1968) Pozzi (1963) McSherry and Grinyer (1954a) Lebeda and Bus (1967) Kutas (1966) R. Gartner et al. (1966) Donawick and Baue (1968) Dalton (1967a) Bianca et al. (1962) Baucks (1967)
Cattle and swine	Forstner (1968)
Cattle and swine	Forstner (1968)
Swine	Wege (1967) Ullrey et al. (1967) Seidel (1964) Schroter et al. (1963)
Dog and swine	Bertho et al. (1964)
Sheep and swine	Birkeland (1968)
Sheep	Tumbleson et al. (1968) Pugh (1966) Long et al. (1965)

Dalton, 1964b; Hix et al. 1959; Howes et al., 1963; Payne et al., 1967), horses (Collery and Keating, 1958; Courtice, 1943; Cronin, 1954; Dalton and Fisher, 1963; Julian et al., 1956; Marcilese et al., 1964), sheep (Anand and Parker, 1966; English, 1966b) and swine (Ramirez et al., 1962; Tollerz, 1964). Additional information on several species can be found in Altman and Dittmer (1961).

TABLE VI   CONVERSION FACTORS

Sodium	mg/100 ml ÷ 2.3 = mEq/liter
Potassium	mg/100 ml ÷ 3.9 = mEq/liter
Calcium	mg/100 ml ÷ 2.0 = mEq/liter
Magnesium	mg/100 ml ÷ 1.2 = mEq/liter
TCO_2	vol % ÷ 2.2 = mEq/liter
Chloride	mg/100 ml ÷ 3.5 = mEq/liter
Chloride (expressed as NaCl)	mg/100 ml ÷ 5.8 = mEq/liter
Phosphorus	mg/100 ml ÷ 1.7 = mEq/liter
Sulfate	mg/100 ml ÷ 1.6 = mEq/liter
Protein	gm/100 ml ÷ 0.41 = mEq/liter

The value for serum potassium of swine cited in Table III is very high compared with other species. Other reports in the literature describe even higher values for normal swine. Since hemolysis occurs frequently in porcine blood specimens and since this results in false high potassium values, it is possible that these values are elevated for that reason. Some reports for serum potassium in cattle are also very high and a similar explanation is likely. It should be remembered that potassium is also falsely elevated if the serum (or plasma) remains in contact with the erythrocytes for several hours. Potassium values are only reliable when the specimen has been obtained without hemolysis and the serum or plasma has been removed promptly.

The normal value given in Table III for potassium concentration in horse serum is remarkable in that it is much lower than that reported for other species. Experience with clinical patients has shown that most normal horses have serum potassium greater than 3.0 mEq/liter. In several other surveys of groups of normal horses, however, individuals have been found in which the concentration has also been unusually low (Simon, 1964; Martinez, 1963).

Values in the literature for pH, pCO_2, and bicarbonate also tend to be variable. Technique in obtaining and handling the specimen is particularly important if reliable results are to be obtained in clinical patients or in surveys of normal animals.

The most reliable information on patients is obtained from laboratories that do a sufficient volume of these tests to have established an appreciation for normal results in each species when done by the routine procedure of that particular laboratory.

VII. CLINICAL DISORDERS OF WATER, ELECTROLYTE, AND ACID–BASE BALANCE

The most accurate evaluation of a clinical patient results from a careful physical examination of that patient and determination of blood pH and pCO_2 and plasma protein, urea nitrogen, sodium, potassium, and chloride. By this means an appraisal can be made of the patient's status with respect to the four important questions of water, ECF tonicity, acid–base balance, and specific ion abnormalities. This evaluation is indicated whenever there is obvious or possible dehydration, unusual losses of fluid from the body (vomiting, diarrhea, sweating, polyuria), respiratory abnormalities, fasting or thirsting, atony of the digestive tract, shock, abnormal intake of water or electrolytes (either inadequate or excessive), azotemia, diabetes mellitus, hyper- or hypoadrenocorticalism, or intensive therapy with water, electrolytes, or mineralocorticoid drugs.

In certain instances, a definite pattern of electrolyte and acid—base abnormalities can be anticipated with some degree of confidence in animals suffering from specific conditions. It is important to know these patterns since this knowledge will serve as a basis for the selection of fluid and other supportive therapy for these patients before the laboratory tests can be done on the patient at hand. In other instances, laboratory tests cannot be done at all. Here, it must be assumed that the disturbances in the patients are similar to those described in other comparable cases where the appropriate laboratory tests have been done. It must be remembered that individual variations are common and often marked. For this reason, the assumption that a given patient has the same type of fluid balance disturbance as another patient with the same disease is always subject to error.

In the paragraphs that follow a few of the more common patterns of fluid balance disturbance will be described.

A. DOGS

Hall (1967) has written a monograph on fluid balance problems in dogs. In it, he reviews fundamental principles, discusses diagnosis and treatment, and describes clinical cases. In the present author's experience, the following clinical problems have caused serious fluid balance problems in practice.

1. Fasting and Thirsting

Most dehydrated dogs have a fluid balance disturbance as a result of failure to eat and drink and have had no unusual losses of water and electrolytes. There is usually no abnormality in the concentration of serum electrolytes or in acid—base balance in these patients. This is probably due to renal adjustment of electrolyte losses to maintain normal concentrations in the ECF. The loss of electrolytes is therefore commensurate with the loss of water. Although the electrolyte determinations yield normal results, it must be appreciated that marked deficits of these ions are present.

2. Vomiting

When *continued* vomiting results in loss of a *large* volume of gastric juice, the patient becomes dehydrated due to this fluid loss and the failure to consume drinking water. The classical disturbance following prolonged vomiting with abundant loss of gastric juice is metabolic alkalosis manifested by elevated blood pH and plasma bicarbonate values, hypochloremia, and hypokalemia. It must be emphasized that this disturbance in fluid balance occurs only when vomiting has been severe and prolonged and there has been loss of a large volume of gastric juice. The majority of vomiting dogs do not have this disturbance because they have not lost a large volume of gastric juice. While these animals may be dehydrated, it is the result of inadequate intake of water rather than excessive loss of gastric juice and the classical electrolyte and acid–base disturbances of vomiting are not present.

3. Diarrhea

When fluid losses in diarrhea have been large and the patient has decreased food and fluid intake, dehydration develops. Since most of the secretions of the digestive tract below the stomach are alkaline due to high bicarbonate concentrations (especially bile and pancreatic juice) the unusual loss of this fluid may result in acidosis. This metabolic acidosis will be characterized by a low blood pH and low bicarbonate concentration in the plasma. It is difficult to predict changes in the other electrolytes. Sodium and chloride are often in the normal range. Serum potassium may be dangerously elevated due to movement of intracellular potassium into the ECF as a result of acidosis, but if potassium losses in the diarrheal feces have been large and intake of potassium has been decreased, normal or even decreased serum potassium values may be found.

It must be emphasized that most dogs with diarrhea do not have these abnormalities because the losses have not been great or because the patient has continued to eat and drink and thus has prevented depletion of water and electrolytes.

4. Chronic Renal Failure

Dogs with chronic renal failure are often dehydrated and a variety of electrolyte disturbances may be present. In dogs with severe signs of uremia there is usually metabolic acidosis due to the failure of the diseased kidneys to excrete hydrogen ions normally. This is usually characterized by an abnormally low blood pH and plasma bicarbonate concentration.

Serum sodium concentration is usually normal although marked depletion of body sodium may be present due to inability of the kidneys to conserve this ion (K. Gartner, 1962; Low, 1968).

There is considerable variation in the serum potassium concentration and no reliable assumptions about this electrolyte can be made. It has often been written that dogs with chronic interstitial nephritis have dangerously high serum potassium concentrations (Bloom, 1961; Wirth, 1962). This is true in some patients but in the majority of patients the serum value is normal and in occasional individuals there is hypokalemia. When the serum value is elevated it is probably due to the effect of severe acidosis causing extracellular shifts of potassium from the cells.

5. Diabetes mellitus

Serious fluid balance abnormalities are to be expected in dogs with diabetes mellitus whenever the patient is anoretic and depressed. Metabolic acidosis results from increasing quantities of ketone bodies in the body fluid. These organic acids are neutralized by buffers in the body fluids and plasma bicarbonate and blood pH decrease.

Severe glycosuria in diabetes causes an osmotic diuresis which results in abnormal losses of sodium, chloride, and water. This may result in hyponatremia if the patient continues to drink water to overcome the water deficit. Hyponatremia may also result from the osmotic effect of hyperglycemia causing movement of water from the cells to the interstitial fluid with dilution of extracellular sodium concentration.

Potassium depletion occurs in diabetes mellitus because of osmotic diuresis, lean-tissue breakdown, depletion of cellular glycogen, intracellular dehydration, and the effect of increased aldosterone secretion (Kleeman and Maxwell, 1962). In spite of these factors, serum potassium is often elevated in the terminal patient with diabetes because of the severe acidosis which is present. When insulin therapy is initiated, serum potassium may drop to very low levels as intracellular movement of potassium occurs due to improvement of cellular metabolism and correction of ketoacidosis.

6. Hyperadrenocorticalism

Since the hormones of the adrenal cortex, especially aldosterone tend to cause retention of sodium and excretion of potassium, it should be anticipated that hypernatremia and hypokalemia would be seen in hyperadrenocorticalism. These electrolyte changes are rarely seen in the dog. When they occur hypokalemia is the most significant change (Siegel, 1968).

7. Adrenocortical Insufficiency

Although serum cation abnormalities are rarely seen in hyperadrenocorticalism, changes are often seen in hypoadrenocorticalism. Inadequate production of mineralocorticoid hormones of the adrenal cortex permits excessive sodium loss in the urine and the development of hyponatremia and hypochloremia. Potassium retention occurs and hyperkalemia is present. Wilkinson (1969) has suggested that calculation of the ratio of serum sodium to serum potassium is a useful aid in diagnosis of this condition. He states that the normal Na:K is 27:1–34:1 and that dogs with hypoadrenocorticalism have ratios less than 23:1.

8. Congestive Heart Failure

It is believed by some that excessive aldosterone secretion occurs in congestive heart failure. This results in sodium and water retention and is important in the pathogenesis of edema. However, hypernatremia is not usually seen in this condition (Pensinger, 1969).

9. Shock

The subject of shock is a complex one which cannot be discussed in detail here. It should be emphasized, however, that metabolic acidosis is to be expected in shock. This is the result of cellular anoxia and the resulting accumulation of organic acids (lactic, pyruvic, keto acids) because of failure of aerobic metabolism (Simmons, 1962).

10. *Leptospirosis*

Finco and Low (1968) studied the water, electrolyte, and acid–base alterations in experimental canine leptospirosis. They found hyponatremia, hypochloremia, and hypokalemia in the early stages; in some animals they observed metabolic acidosis. Later, in the course of illness, hyperkalemia was noted.

B. CATS

The author has had very limited experience in studying fluid balance disorders in cats. It must be assumed that the general principles described for the dog are applicable to the cat until more clinical information can be obtained.

C. HORSES

1. *Salmonellosis*

A syndrome of acute febrile disease characterized by diarrhea and leukopenia is occasionally seen in horses, especially those subjected to unusual stresses such as shipping, fasting, anesthesia, or surgery. In some of these patients a diagnosis of salmonellosis can be substantiated by bacterial isolation and identification. In other horses with this syndrome the specific diagnosis cannot be confirmed.

These patients have a remarkably predictable fluid balance disturbance (Tasker, 1966a). There is hyponatremia, hypokalemia, hypochloremia, and metabolic acidosis. The hyponatremia and acidosis are especially predictable and often severe. One would anticipate that the severe acidosis would cause extracellular movement of potassium ions and hyperkalemia. This is rarely, if ever, seen. The serum potassium concentration may, however, be in the normal range until the acidosis is corrected, at which time hypokalemia becomes obvious. Low normal or subnormal potassium concentrations in severely acidotic patients suggest marked potassium depletion.

2. *Colitis X*

In the early 1960's a syndrome of unusually peracute illness with diarrhea and death was described as "colitis X." The laboratory findings in these patients, although usually more severe, were similar to those described in salmonellosis (Tasker, 1966a). It is to be anticipated in all cases that acute diarrhea in the horse, especially if associated with depression and anorexia, will be characterized by hyponatremia and acidosis.

3. *Intestinal Obstruction*

Severe dehydration and metabolic acidosis is often present in horses with severe clinical signs due to intestinal obstruction. Other fluid balance abnormalities are not predictable. The disturbances seen probably result from the accumulation in the digestive tract of large volumes of alkaline intestinal secretions, shock, and severe sweating.

4. General Anesthesia with Volatile Anesthetics in Closed Systems

Respiratory acidosis occurs frequently in horses which are maintained in surgical anesthesia for prolonged periods of time with closed system volatile anesthetic–oxygen apparatus. The development of this disorder has been discussed previously (Section V,C,1).

Since this abnormality jeopardizes the patients' welfare (Young et al., 1954), it must be appreciated and avoided whenever possible.

Experimental studies of this problem were reported by Tevik et al. (1968). Clinical patients have often been found, in the author's experience, to have even more severe abnormalities.

5. The Anhidrosis (Dry Coat) Syndrome

Veterinarians working with race horses in the tropics have reported a fluid and electrolyte abnormality called the anhidrosis syndrome (Gilyard, 1944; Correa and Calderin, 1966). This problem is seen primarily in Thoroughbred horses imported from temperate climates. It is characterized by fever, dyspnea, and the absence of sweating following exercise. Severe dehydration, hyponatremia, and hypochloremia have been reported. Although several theories have been advanced to explain this problem, complete elucidation of the mechanism has not been achieved.

6. Experimental Studies

The effect of fasting and thirsting and of diarrhea on electrolyte and acid–base balance in horses was described by Tasker (1967c).

D. CATTLE

1. Enteritis in Newborn Calves

Calves in the terminal stages of illness resulting from colibacillosis and related diseases are severely dehydrated and have predictable electrolyte and acid–base derangements. The most consistent finding is metabolic acidosis. This usually is associated with hyperkalemia. Death of these patients is probably the result of intolerably low pH of the body fluids or the direct effect of hyperkalemia on the heart. The work of McSherry and Grinyer (1954b), Fisher (1965), Fisher and McEwan (1967), Dalton et al. (1965), and Dalton (1967b) has been especially helpful in understanding these patients.

2. Disorders of the Abomasum and Upper Intestinal Tract

Cows with a wide variety of disorders of the cranial portion of the digestive tract have a similar electrolyte disturbance. This pattern may be seen in intestinal obstruction, in torsion and displacement of the abomasum, and in certain instances of abomasal impaction or atony. The abnormalities develop as a result of sequestration of a large volume of abomasal juice in the abomasum and forestomachs. The pathogenesis of this disturbance has been described previously (Section V,C,4).

An excellent discussion of this problem was based on studies of experimental intestinal obstruction in calves (Hammond *et al.*, 1964). This study provides a basis for understanding the disorders that develop in abomasal disorders in adult cattle as well. Laboratory findings in left displacement of the abomasum have been discussed by Robertson (1966) and by Poulsen (1967). Espersen and Simesen (1961) have studied the findings in dilation of the abomasum.

3. Postparturient Paresis in Dairy Cattle

Bovine practitioners have been concerned for many years by a syndrome in post-parturient cattle referred to as the "downer cow syndrome" or the "creeper cow syndrome." It has been suggested that this syndrome might be related to potassium depletion (Johnson, 1967), since potassium depletion is known to result in muscular weakness.

There is little evidence, however, to prove that hypokalemia or depletion of cellular potassium actually exists in these animals. The typical affected individual is alert, active, and eating. Since the diet of the herbivore is particularly high in potassium and since potassium depletion in man is characterized by drowziness and confusion, i.e., mental depression, these typical clinical findings are not suggestive of a state of potassium depletion.

4. Acute Impaction of the Rumen

The fluid, electrolyte, and acid–base abnormalities which develop in "toxic indigestion" or "rumen overload" have been studied by Dunlop (1961). Severe dehydration and metabolic acidosis develop as a result of the abnormalities in rumen digestion.

5. Water Intoxication in Calves

Calves which have had limited access to water occasionally develop acute nervous signs when permitted to drink unlimited quantities; hemoglobinuria is a much more common clinical sign (Kirkbride and Frey, 1967; Lawrence, 1965). Hyponatremia and hypochloremia were present in two patients in the author's experience although published reports have not described electrolyte changes.

E. OTHER SPECIES

1. Salt Poisoning in Pigs

D.L.T. Smith (1957) has induced salt poisoning in experimental swine and studied the pathogenesis of the disease. He found serum sodium levels up to 211 mEq/liter and serum chloride levels up to 147 mEq/liter in affected animals. The electrolyte concentrations in natural cases may vary considerably depending on the relative proportions and sequence of intake of water and salt by the animals.

2. Transmissible Gastroenteritis in Baby Pigs

The changes in fluid and electrolyte balance in baby pigs with transmissible gastroenteritis were reported by Cornelius et al. (1968). They reported a marked decrease in blood pH and plasma bicarbonate and, on the day of death, a marked rise in serum potassium. There were no consistent changes in plasma sodium values. Hemoconcentration was manifested by increased packed cell volume. The authors concluded that these changes were probably the result of the diarrhea that occurred in these pigs.

3. Ovine Pregnancy Ketosis

Katz and Bergman (1966) studied acid—base and electrolyte equilibrium in experimental ovine pregnancy ketosis. They reported a mild decrease in blood pH, plasma bicarbonate, and potassium in affected animals but the changes were not severe.

4. Acute Indigestion in Sheep

The acid—base status of sheep with acute indigestion has been studied by Huber et al. (1962) and by Blackburn and McCrea (1965).

VIII. FLUID THERAPY

As in all other aspects of medicine, sound therapy must be based on an accurate diagnosis. In reference to fluid therapy this means that rational therapy cannot be administered unless the needs of the patient have been determined with accuracy. This can best be accomplished by recording an adequate history, doing a careful physical examination, and making the appropriate laboratory tests. The information obtained in each of these ways must be interpreted with an adequate understanding of the physiological and pathological mechanisms which apply in each instance.

Of equal importance to accurate patient evaluation, in the design of sound fluid therapy, is knowledge of the composition of the fluids available for administration and the effect that each will have on the patient. Most products prepared for human use are clearly labeled with the electrolyte composition in milliequivalents per liter. These units are comparable to the units in which body fluid electrolyte composition is expressed. Therefore it can be determined easily from the label whether rehydration of a patient with a fluid having a certain electrolyte composition will tend to increase or decrease the concentration of each electrolyte in the ECF of the patient. For example, isotonic sodium chloride solution has a chloride concentration of 154 mEq/liter and normal plasma has a chloride concentration of approximately 105 mEq/liter. Administration of large volumes of this solution might tend to elevate the chloride concentration in the patient. If the patient were hypochloremic this would be desirable; if the patient were in need of bicarbonate rather than chloride, however, this fluid would be contraindicated.

Unfortunately, many fluid therapy products prepared for veterinary use are not labeled with useful information. These products are often labeled with the composition of the solution expressed as the milligrams of each constituent per 100 ml of solution. Isotonic sodium chloride would be labeled "each 100 ml of this solution contains 900 mg of sodium chloride." Unless the veterinarian converts this figure to milliequivalents per liter it will not be apparent to him that the chloride concentration is 150% of the normal serum value. When one is using complex formulations which contain several ingredients, the confusion is even greater. For example, one product available for use could be labeled "each 100 ml of this solution contains 516 mg sodium chloride, 89.4 mg potassium chloride, 27.8 mg calcium chloride, 14.2 mg of magnesium chloride, and 560 mg of sodium lactate." This information does not give the reader an appreciation of the effect the solution will have when added to the ECF of the patient. The same solution might also be labeled "this solution contains the following concentrations of electrolytes expressed in milliequivalents per liter: sodium 138, potassium 12, calcium 5, magnesium 3, chloride 108, and lactate 50." From this information it is readily apparent that this solution has a normal concentration of sodium, calcium, magnesium, and chloride ions and has an unusually high concentration of lactate and potassium.

Solutions containing bicarbonate cannot be sterilized by conventional procedures due to the heat instability of this ion. For this reason most solutions contain the organic anions lactate or acetate in place of bicarbonate. When these ions are metabolized, they are replaced, in the ECF, by an equivalent concentration of bicarbonate. Sterile solutions of bicarbonate are commercially available but are somewhat more expensive than those containing lactate or acetate.

Table VII contains the composition of some commonly used parenteral fluid therapy products. Several important observations should be made in this table.

1. Solutions of dextrose in water contain no electrolytes. Although they may be isotonic, they have the effect of an equal volume of pure water after the dextrose has been metabolized. When given in large quantities over a short period of time, this solution will tend to decrease the concentrations of electrolytes in the ECF.

2. Isotonic sodium chloride solution, although often called "physiological" is normal only in its osmolality and its sodium concentration. It is devoid of potassium and bicarbonate and has an unusually high concentration of chloride. Since the administration of this fluid would rehydrate a patient without replacing either potassium or bicarbonate, it would tend to aggravate hypokalemia or metabolic acidosis.

TABLE VII   PARENTERAL SOLUTIONS, ELECTROLYTE CONCENTRATIONS (mEq/LITER)

Solution	Na	K	Ca	Mg	Cl	Lactate	HCO_3
5% dextrose in water	0	0	0	0	0	0	0
0.9% sodium chloride	154	0	0	0	154	0	0
Ringer's solution	147	4	5	0	156	0	0
Lactated Ringer's solution	130	4	3	0	109	28	0
1/6 M sodium lactate	167	0	0	0	0	167	0
1.3% sodium bicarbonate	155	0	0	0	0		155

3. Lactated Ringer's solution is a balanced electrolyte solution which should permit rehydration of the patient without aggravating or inducing electrolyte disturbances. It must be recognized that Ringer's solution is quite different from *lactated* Ringer's solution. The former is seldom used for parenteral fluid therapy.

4. One-sixth molar sodium lactate solution or 1.3% sodium bicarbonate solution are strongly alkalinizing solutions which should have a favorable effect on the patient with metabolic acidosis. Because of their unphysiological composition they should only be given when indicated and always with caution.

A variety of commercial products is available which has been designed to meet the needs of patients with a variety of clinical entities in which peculiar electrolyte or acid—base disturbances are encountered.

The fundamental principle that is of most importance in designing rational fluid therapy is that the fluid(s) administered should have a composition which complements that of the ECF of the patient. Thus the patient with a metabolic alkalosis in which the bicarbonate concentration is abnormally high should be given a fluid devoid of this ion. Conversely, in metabolic acidosis, where the bicarbonate concentration is dangerously low, a high bicarbonate (or lactate or acetate) fluid is essential to the patient's improvement. Dextrose solutions in water are indicated in hypernatremia, contraindicated in hyponatremia.

When the status of the patient has been determined by the appropriate laboratory tests, fluid therapy can be designed with confidence and the fluids administered can be quite unusual in their composition. When the patient's needs can only be estimated from physical signs and experience with other similar patients previously, the fluid therapy cannot be as specific and it must be designed more conservatively.

Fluid therapy is supportive therapy; it does not eliminate the original cause of a patient's illness. When carefully designed, however, it corrects certain derangements which have resulted from the primary disease and thereby maintains the life of the patient while specific therapy or the patient's own protective mechanisms attempt to remove the cause of illness.

REFERENCES

Aalund, O., and Nielsen, D. (1960). *Nord. Veterinarmed.* **12**, 605–620.
Abbrecht, P. H. (1969). *J. Clin. Invest.* **48**, 432–442.
Adams, A. P., Morgan-Hughes, J. O., and Sykes, M.K. (1968). *Anesthesia* **23**, 47–64.
Albritton, E. C. (1952). "Standard Values in Blood." Saunders, Philadelphia, Pennsylvania.
Altman, P. L., and Dittmer, D. S. (1961). "Blood and Other Body Fluids." *Fed. Am. Soc. Exptl. Biol.,* Washington, D. C.
Anand, R. S., and Parker, H. R. (1966). *Am. J. Vet. Res.* **27**, 899–902
Andersson, B., and Larsson, S. (1961). *Pharmacol. Rev.* **13**, 1–16.
Andersson, B., and McCann, S. M. (1956). *Acta Physiol. Scand.* **35**, 312–320.
Aschbacher, P. W., Kamal, T. H., and Cragle, R. G. (1965). *J. Animal Sci.* **24**, 430–433.
Astrup, P. (1956). *Scand. J. Clin. & Lab. Invest.* **8**, 33.
Baucks, D. (1967). Inaugural Dissertation, Tieraerztliche Hochschule, Hannover.
Becker, E. L., and Joseph, B. J. (1955). *Am. J. Physiol.* **183**, 314–316.
Beilharz, S., and Kay, R. N. B. (1963). *J.Physiol. (London)* **165**, 468–483.
Bertho, E. M., Belanger, M., and Saint-Hilaire, B. (1964). *Laval Med.* **35**, 647–651.
Bianca, W., Findley, J. D., and Mabon, R. M. (1962). *Res. Vet. Sci.* **3**, 34.

Birkeland, R. (1968). *Nord. Veterinarmed.* **20**, 155–160.
Blackburn, P. W., and McCrea, C. T. (1965)*Vet. Record* **77**, 1250.
Bloom, F. (1961). *Vet. Scope* **6**, 2–9.
Bruning, P. (1950). Inaugural Dissertation, Tieraerztliche Hochschule, Hannover.
Clark, D. R., and McCrady, J. D. (1966). *Vet. Med./Small Animal Clinician* **61**, 751–760.
Collery, L. and Keating, J. (1958). *Vet. Record* **70**, 216–218.
Cornelius, L. M., Hooper, B. E., and Haeterman, E. O. (1968). *Am. J. Vet. Clin. Pathol.* **2**, 105–113.
Correa, J. E., and Calderin, G. G. (1966). *J. Am. Vet. Med. Assoc.* **149**, 1556–1560.
Courtice, F. C. (1943). *J. Physiol. (London)* **102**, 290.
Cox, J. L., Becker, D. E., and Jensen, A. H. (1966). *J. Animal Sci.* **25**, 203–206.
Cronin, M. T. I. (1954). *Vet. Record* **66**, 197–200.
Dalton, R. G. (1964a). *Brit. Vet. J.* **120**, 69–77.
Dalton, R. G. (1964). *Brit. Vet. J.* **120**, 378–384.
Dalton, R. G. (1967a). *Brit. Vet. J.* **123**, 48–52.
Dalton, R. G. (1967b). *Brit. Vet. J.* **123**, 237–246.
Dalton, R. G., and Fisher, E. W. (1963). *Brit. Vet. J.* **119**, 384–386.
Dalton, R. G., Fisher, E. W., and McIntyre, W. I. M. (1965). *Brit. Vet. J.* **121**, 34–41.
Deane, N. (1966). "Kidney and Electrolytes: Foundations of Clinical Diagnosis and Physiologic Therapy." Prentice-Hall, Englewood Cliffs, New Jersey.
Devlin, T. J., and Roberts, W. K. (1963). *J. Animal Sci.* **22**, 648–653.
Donawick, W. J., and Baue, A. E. (1968). *Am. J. Vet. Res.* **29**, 561–567.
Dunlop, R. H. (1961). Ph.D. Dissertation, Graduate School, University of Minnesota.
El Amrousi, S., and Soliman, M. K. (1965). *Can. Vet. J.* **6**, 253–256.
English, P. B. (1966a). *Res. Vet. Sci.* **7**, 233–257.
English, P. B. (1966b). *Res. Vet. Sci.* **7**, 258–275.
English, P. B. (1967a). *Brit. Vet. J.* **123**, 111–122.
English, P. B. (1967b). *Brit. Vet. J.* **123**, 123–132.
Epstein, F. H. (1962). *In* "Clinical Disorders of Fluid and Electrolyte Metabolism" (M. H. Maxwell and C. R. Kleeman, eds.), p. 38, McGraw-Hill, New York.
Espersen, G., and Simesen, M. G. (1961). *Nord. Veterinarmed.* **13**, 147–159.
Finco, D. R., and Low, D. G. (1968). *Am. J. Vet. Res.* **29**, 1799–1807.
Fisher, E. W. (1965). *Brit. Vet. J.* **121**, 132–138.
Fisher, E. W., and McEwan, A. D. (1967). *Brit. Vet. J.* **123**, 4–7.
Fonnesbeck, P. V. (1967). *J. Animal Sci.* **26**, 906.
Forstner, M. J. (1968). *Zentr. Veterinaermed.* **15**A, 76–80.
Gartner, K. (1962). *Berlin. Muench. Tieraerztl. Wochschr.* **75**, 109.
Gartner, R., Ryley, J., and Beattie, A. (1966). *Res. Vet. Sci.* **7**, 424–434.
Gentile, G., and Venturoli, M. (1960). *Nuova Vet.* [N. S.] **36**, 167–174.
Gilyard, R. T. (1944). *Cornell Vet.* **34**, 332–336.
Goldberger, E. (1965). "A Primer of Water, Electrolyte and Acid-Base Syndromes." Lea & Febiger, Philadelphia, Pennsylvania.
Graham, J. A., Lamb J. F., and Linton, A. L. (1967). *Lancet* **II**, 1172.
Greenspan, K., Wunsch, C., and Fisch. C. (1965). *Am. J. Physiol.* **208**, 954–958.
Guyton, A. C. (1966). "Textbook of Medical Physiology." Saunders, Philadelphia, Pennsylvania.
Hall, L. W. (1967). "Fluid Balance in Surgery." Baillière, London.
Hamlin, R. L., and Tashjian, R. J. (1964). *Vet. Med./Small Animal Clinician* **59**, 746–747.
Hamlin, R. L., Smith, R. C., Smith. C. R., and Powers T. E. (1964). *Vet. Med./Small Animal Clinician* **59**, 748–751.
Hammond, P. B., Dziuk, H. E., Usenik, E. A., and Stevens, C. E. (1964). *J. Comp. Pathol.* **74**, 210–222.
Hannon, J. P., and Durrer, J. L. (1963). *Am. J. Physiol.* **204**, 517–519.
Hansard, S. L. (1964). *Am. J. Physiol.* **206**, 1369–1372.
Henry, R. J. (1964). "Clinical Chemistry: Principles and Techniques." Harper, New York.
Hix, E. L., Underbjerg, G. K. L., and Hughes, J. S. (1959). *Am. J. Vet. Res.* **20**, 184–191.
Hoffman, W. S. (1964). "The Biochemistry of Clinical Medicine." Year Book Publ., Chicago, Illinois.
Howes, J. R., Hentges, J. F., Jr., and Feaster, J. P. (1963). *J. Animal Sci.* **22**, 183–187.
Huber, T. L., Mitchell, G. E., and Little, C. O. (1962). *J. Animal Sci.* **21**, 1025.

Johnson, B. L. (1967). *J. Am. Vet. Med. Assoc.* **151**, 1681–1687.
Julian, L. M., Lawrence, J. H., Berlin, N. I., and Hyde, G. M. (1956). *J. Appl. Physiol.* **8**, 651–653.
Katz, M. L., and Bergman, E. N. (1966). *Am. J. Vet. Res.* **27**, 1285–1292.
Keynes, R. D., and Harrison, F. A. (1967). *Vet. Record* **81**, 244–250.
Kirkbride, C. A., and Frey, R. A. (1967). *J. Am. Vet. Med. Assoc.* **151**, 742–746.
Kleeman, C. R., and Maxwell, M. H. (1962). *In* "Clinical Disorders of Fluid and Electrolyte Metabolism"
    (M. H. Maxwell and C. R. Kleeman, eds.), p. 145. McGraw-Hill, New York.
Krapf, W. (1938). *Jahresber. Veterinaermed.* **67**, 326.
Kutas, F. (1966). *Magy. Allatorv. Lapja* **21**, 112–115.
Lane, A. G., Campbell, J. R., and Krause, G. F. (1968). *J. Animal Sci.* **27**, 766–770.
Lawrence, J. A. (1965). *J. S. African Vet. Med. Assoc.* **36**, 277–278.
Leaf, A. (1962). *New Engl. J. Med.* **267**, 77–83.
Lebeda, M., and Bus, A. (1967). *Vet. Med. (Prague)* **12**, 573–576.
Lemieux, G., Warren. Y., and Gervais. M. (1964). *Am. J. Physiol.* **206**, 743–749.
Long, C. H., Ullrey. D. E., Miller, E. R., Vincent, B. H., and Zutant, C. L. (1965). *J. Animal Sci.* **24**,
    145–150.
Low, D. G. (1968). *In* "Current Veterinary Therapy III Small Animal Practice" (R. W. Kirk, ed.),
    p. 657. Saunders, Philadelphia, Pennsylvania.
McSherry, B. J., and Grinyer, I. (1954a). *Am. J. Vet. Res.* **15**, 509–510.
McSherry, B. J., and Grinyer, I. (1954b). *Am. J. Vet. Res.* **15**, 534–541.
Marcilese, N. A., Valsecchi, R. M., and Figueiras, H. D. (1964). *Am. J. Physiol.* **207**, 223–227.
Martinez, P. A. (1963). *Gac. Vet. (Buenos Aires)* **25**, 313–320.
Maxwell, M. H., and Kleeman, C. R., eds. (1962). "Clinical Disorders of Fluid and Electro-
    lyte Metabolism." McGraw-Hill, New York.
Michaelson, S. M., Scheer, K., and Gilt, S. (1966). *J. Am. Vet. Med. Assoc.* **148**, 532–534.
Nuttall, F. Q. (1965). *Arch. Internal Med.* **116**, 670–680.
Payne, E., Ryley, J. W., and Gartner, R. J. W. (1967). *Res. Vet. Sci.* **8**, 20–26.
Pensinger, R. R. (1969). *J. Am. Vet. Med. Assoc.* **154**, 413–424.
Pickering, E. C. (1965). *Proc. Nutr. Soc. (Engl. Scot.)* **24**, 73–80.
Poulsen, J. S. D. (1967). *Nord Veterinarmed.* **19**, 313–345.
Pozzi, L. (1963). *Atti Soc. Ital. Sci. Vet.* **17**, 363–368.
Prankerd, T. A. J. (1961). "The Red Cell." Thomas, Springfield, Illinois.
Pugh, D. M. (1966). *Irish Vet. J.* **20**, 142–147.
Ramirez, C. G., Miller, E. R., Ullrey, D. E., and Hoefer, J. A. (1962). *J. Animal Sci.* **21**, 1028–1029.
Reid, J. T., Bensadoun, A., and Paladines, O. L. (1963). *Ann. N. Y. Acad. Sci.* **110**, 327–342.
Roberts, K. E. (1962). *In* "Clinical Disorders of Fluid and Electrolyte Metabolism" (M. H. Maxwell
    and C. R. Kleeman, eds.), p. 215. McGraw-Hill, New York.
Robertson, J. M. (1966). *J. Am. Vet. Med. Assoc.* **149**, 1430–1434.
Robinson, F. R., and Ziegler, R. F. (1968). *Lab. Animal Care* **18**, 39–49.
Schroter, J., Seidel, H., Muller, I., and Kolb, E. (1963). *Arch. Exptl. Veterinaermed.* **17**, 827–857.
Seidel, H. (1964). *Arch. Exptl. Veterinaer med.* **18**, 669–675.
Severinghaus, J. W., and Bradley, A. F. (1958). *J. Appl. Phys.* **13**, 515.
Siebert, B. D., and McFarlane, W. V. (1967). *Australian J. Expt. Biol. Med. Sci.* **45**, 28.
Siegel, E. T. (1968). *In* "Current Veterinary Therapy III, Small Animal Practice" (R. W. Kirk, ed.),
    p. 552. Saunders, Philadelphia, Pennsylvania.
Siggaard-Andersen, O. (1963). *Scand. J. Clin., & Lab. Invest.* **15**, 211–217.
Simmons, D. H. (1962). *In* "Clinical Disorders of Fluid and Electrolyte Metabolism" (M. H. Maxwell
    and C. R. Kleeman, eds.) p. 71. McGraw-Hill, New York.
Simon, R. (1964). Inaugural Dissertation, Tieraerztliche Hochschule, Hannover.
Smith, D. L. T. (1957). *Am. J. Vet. Res.* **18**, 825.
Smith, R. C., Haschen, T., and Hamlin, R. L. (1964). *Vet. Med./Small Animal Clinician* **59**, 743–746.
Soliman, M. K., and Nadim, M. A. (1967). *Zentr. Veterinaemed*, **14A**, 53–56.
Sova, Z., Jicha, J., and Komarek. J. (1965). *Berlin. Muench. Tieraerztl. Wochschr.* **78**, 144–147.
Spector, W. S., ed. (1956). "Handbook of Biological Data" Saunders, Philadelphia, Pennsylvania.
Sreter, F. A. (1959). *Can. J. Biochem. Physiol.* **37**, 273–283.
Tashjian, R. J., Snyder, J. W., and Das, K. M. (1968). *Cornell Vet.* **58**, 8–11.

Tasker, J. B. (1963). Ph.D. Thesis, Cornell University, Ithaca, New York.

Tasker, J. B. (1966a). *Vet. Med./Small Animal Clinician* **61**, 765–776.

Tasker, J. B. (1966b). *Cornell Vet.* **56**, 67–76.

Tasker, J. B. (1967a). *Cornell Vet.* **57**, 649–657.

Tasker, J. B. (1967b). *Cornell Vet.* **57**, 658–667.

Tasker, J. B. (1967c). *Cornell Vet.* **57**, 668–677.

Tevik, A., Nelson, A. W., and Lumb, W. V. (1968). *Am. J. Vet. Res.* **29**, 1791–1798.

Tollerz, G. (1964). *Acta Vet. Scand.* **5**, 24–34.

Tumbleson, M. E., Littleton, C. A., Ticer, J. W., Komer E. G., and Bloomfield, R. A. (1968). *Am. J. Vet. Clin. Pathol.* **2**, 97–103.

Ullrey, D. E., Miller, E. R. Brent, B. E., Bradley, B. L., and Hoefer, J. A. (1967). *J. Animal Sci.* **26**, 1024–1029.

Van Stewart, E., and Longwell, B. B. (1969). *Am. J. Vet Res.* **30**, 907–916.

Vrzgula, L. (1963). *Folia Vet.* **7**, 223–232.

Ward, G. M. (1966a). *J. Dairy Sci.* **49**, 268–276.

Ward, G. M. (1966b). *J. Am. Vet. Med. Assoc.* **148**, 543–544.

Wege, V. (1967). Inaugural Dissertation, Tieraerztliche Hochschule, Hannover.

Weisberg, H. F. (1962). "Water, Electrolyte, and Acid-Base Balance." Williams & Wilkins, Baltimore, Maryland.

White, A., Handler, P., and Smith, E. L. (1964). "Principles of Biochemistry." McGraw-Hill, New York.

Wilkinson, J. S. (1969). *In* "A Textbook of Veterinary Clinical Pathology" (W. Medway *et. al.,* eds.), p. 190. Williams & Wilkins, Baltimore, Maryland.

Winters, R. W., Engel, K., and Dell, R. B. (1967) "Acid Base Physiology in Medicine." London Company, Cleveland, Ohio.

Wirth, W. (1962). *Deut. Tieraerztl. Wochschr.* **69**, 225–227.

Young, W. G., Sealy, W. C., and Harris, J. S. (1954). *Surgery* **36**, 636–649.

3   Gastrointestinal Function

B. C. Tennant and G. O. Ewing

I.   INTRODUCTION

The gastrointestinal system is composed of the alimentary canal, salivary glands, liver, and exocrine pancreas. Its principal functions are assimilation of nutrients and excretion of the waste products of digestion. Most nutrients are ingested in a form either too complex or insoluble for absorption. In the gastrointestinal tract, these substances are solubilized and degraded enzymically to simple molecules, sufficiently small in size and in a form which permits mucosal absorption. In the following chapter, we wish to describe the normal biochemical processes of intestinal secretion, digestion, and absorption. With these normal processes in perspective, we then will discuss the mechanisms involved in the pathogenesis of certain gastrointestinal diseases and the biochemical basis for their diagnosis and treatment.

II. GASTROINTESTINAL SECRETION

A. SALIVA

1. Mechanism of Secretion

Saliva is produced by three major pairs of salivary glands and by small glands distributed throughout the buccal mucosa and submucosa. Two types of secretory cells are found in the acinar portions of the salivary glands: (1) the *mucous cells* which contain droplets of mucus, and (2) the *serous cells* which contain multiple secretory granules. In those species which produce salivary amylase, the secretory granules are the zymogen precursors of this enzyme. A third cell type is found lining the striated ducts. The striations along the basal borders of these cells are caused by vertical infoldings of the cell membrane, seen in epithelial cells involved in rapid transfer of water and electrolytes. The primary secretion of the acinar cells is modified by active transport processes which occur in these ductal epithelial cells.

The distribution of the different types of secretory cells in the salivary glands varies among species. The parotid glands of most animals are serous glands which produce a secretion of low specific gravity and osmolarity, containing electrolytes and proteins including certain hydrolytic enzymes. The mandibular (submaxillary) and sublingual glands are mixed salivary glands containing both mucous and serous types of cells. They produce a viscous secretion containing large amounts of mucus (Dukes, 1955).

2. Composition

a. MUCUS.   Mucus is an aqueous mixture of protein–polysaccharide complexes and glycoproteins.* Both groups have relatively large amounts of carbohydrate bound to protein. Protein–polysaccharide complexes have long polysaccharide chains containing repeating units bound to a protein core. The glycoproteins contain numerous oligosaccharide residues distributed along the polypeptide chain.

One of the most completely studied glycoproteins is mucin from the submaxillary glands of ruminants. The carbohydrate portion is a disaccharide of N-acetylneuraminic acid and N-acetylgalactosamine. Approximately 800 such disaccharide molecules are present per molecule of mucin (Bhavanandan *et al.*, 1964; Bertolini and Pigman, 1967). An enzyme capable of linking protein with hexosamine was recently demonstrated in sheep submaxillary glands (McGuire and Roseman, 1967).

The physiological functions of mucin are closely related to its high viscosity. N-Acetylneuraminic acid is the component responsible for the formation of viscous aqueous solutions. At physiological pH, it causes expansion and stiffening of the mucin molecule (Gottschalk and Thomas, 1961). The resistance of mucin to enzymic breakdown is also due to the presence of disaccharide residues. Removal of the terminal N-Acetylneuraminic acid residues by neuranimidase significantly increases

*Classification of Gottschalk (1966).

the susceptibility of peptide bonds to trypsin (Gottschalk and Fazekas de St. Groth, 1960).

b. AMYLASE.   The saliva of most species contains the α-amylase, *ptyalin*. This enzyme is said to be absent, however, in the saliva of dogs, cats, and horses (Dukes, 1955). Salivary amylase splits the α-1,4 glucosidic bonds of various polysaccharides. The salivary enzyme is identical in all major respects to the α-amylase secreted by the pancreas. The pancreatic enzyme is discussed in detail below (Section II,D). Salivary amylase is responsible for initiation of digestion of starch and glycogen in the mouth. The optimum pH for amylase activity, however, is approximately 7 and activity terminates when the enzyme mixes with the acidic gastric contents.

3.   Functions of Saliva

Saliva bathes the oral cavity continuously serving to protect the surface epithelium. Ingested food is moistened and lubricated by saliva, facilitating mastication and swallowing. The teeth also are protected from decay by saliva which washes food particles from the surfaces of the teeth and, because of its buffering capacity, neutralizes the organic acids produced by bacteria normally present in the mouth.

Ruminants produce much greater quantities of saliva than simple-stomached animals and the saliva has a higher pH and bicarbonate ion concentration. In ruminants, saliva serves several unique functions. It is required for maintenance of the fluid composition of the rumen. The greater buffering capacity is necessary to neutralize the large quantities of short-chain fatty acids which are major end products of rumen fermentation. The saliva of ruminants contains significant amounts of urea which can be utilized by rumen bacteria for protein synthesis. Protein synthesized in the rumen eventually is used to meet protein requirements. In this way, urea nitrogen may be recycled through the amino acid pool of the body and in ruminants need not be considered an absolute end stage in protein catabolism. This ability to reutilize urea may be of particular benefit during periods of protein deficiency.

B. GASTRIC SECRETION

The stomach is divided into two main regions on the basis of secretory function (Grossman, 1958). The *oxyntic gland area* corresponds approximately to the body of the stomach in most species of domestic animals and also to the fundus in the dog and cat. The oxyntic glands contain *oxyntic or parietal cells* believed to be responsible for hydrochloric acid production, *peptic* (zymogenic, chief) *cells* which produce pepsinogen, and *mucous cells*. The *pyloric gland area* contains the pyloric glands which are composed primarily of mucous cells. The secretion of the pyloric glands is slightly alkaline and in addition to mucus, contains the polypeptide hormone gastrin.

1.   Control of Gastric Secretion

A variety of stimuli can initiate secretion of gastric juice. The sight or smell of food, or the presence of food within the mouth causes gastric secretion by reflex mechanism involving the vagus nerve. The presence of certain foods within the stomach or distention of the stomach alone can initiate both intrinsic and vagal reflexes which also cause secretion of gastric juice. In addition to these neural reflexes, such stimuli cause release of the polypeptide hormone *gastrin* from the pyloric gland area which enters the blood stream causing gastric secretion. The release of gastrin is inhibited by the presence of excess hydrogen ion and this negative feedback mechanism is believed to be of physiological importance in the control of hydrochloric acid production.

Gastrin has been isolated in pure form from the antral mucosa of swine (Gregory *et al.*, 1964; Gregory and Tracy, 1964; Tracy and Gregory, 1964). When administered intravenously, the purified hormone causes the secretion of hydrochloric acid and pepsin. It also stimulates gastrointestinal motility and causes pancreatic secretion.

Glu·Gly·Pro·Try·Met·Glu·Glu·Glu·Glu·Glu·Ala·Tyr·Gly·Try·Met·Asp·Phe·NH$_2$

Fig. 1.   Amino acid sequence of porcine gastrin I (Gregory, 1966). Gastrin II differs from gastrin I by the presence of a sulfate ester group on the single tyrosyl residue.

Two separate peptides have been obtained from porcine gastric mucosa and have been designated gastrin I and gastrin II. The structure of gastrin has been determined (Gregory *et al.*, 1964) and has been confirmed by synthesis (J. C. Anderson *et al.*, 1964). It is a heptadecapeptide amide, with a pyroglutamyl N-terminal residue and the amide of phenylalanine as the C-terminal residue (Fig. 1). In the center of the molecule is a sequence of five glutamyl residues which give the molecule its acidic properties. Gastrin II differs from gastrin I only in the presence of a sulfate ester group linked to the single tyrosyl residue. The C-terminal tetrapeptide amide, Try·Met·Asp·Phe·NH$_2$, is identical in all species so far studied (Gregory, 1967). The tetrapeptide has all of the activities of the natural hormone. It is not as potent as the parent molecule but activity can be increased by lengthening the peptide chain.

2.   Composition of Gastric Secretion

a. BASAL VERSUS STIMULATED SECRETION.   Gastric juice is composed of two components. One is secreted continuously by the surface epithelial cells and other mucus-producing cells. The other component is produced by the oxyntic glands in response to various stimuli. The basal component is neutral or slightly alkaline. The electrolyte composition is similar to an ultrafiltrate of plasma (Table I), and contains large amounts of mucus which protects the epithelium. The secretory component produced by the oxyntic glands in response to stimulation, contains free hydrochloric acid and pepsinogen, the principal substances involved in gastric digestion.

The composition of gastric juice depends on the relative amounts of the two secretory components present, which in turn, is a function of flow rate. In the dog, gastric juice is produced in the resting state at a rate of approximately 5 ml/hr (Gray and Bucher, 1941), and the composition is similar to that of the basal component, containing practically no peptic activity or hydrochloric acid. When the flow of gastric juice is stimulated maximally, the dog may produce 80 ml or more per hour

TABLE I   COMPOSITION OF PARIETAL AND NONPARIETAL
SECRETIONS OF CANINE GASTRIC MUCOSA

	Parietal secretion[a] (mEq/liter)	Nonparietal secretion[a] (mEq/liter)	Nonparietal secretion[c] (mEq/liter)
Na$^+$	—	155.0	138.0
H$^+$	159.0	—	—
K$^+$	7.4	7.4	4.0
Ca^{2+}	—	3.7	5.0
Cl$^-$	166.0	133.0	117.0
pH	< 1.0	7.54[b]	7.42

[a]Determined *in vivo* using dogs with gastric fistulae (Gray and Bucher, 1941).
[b]Calculated from bicarbonate concentration assuming CO_2 of 40 mmHg.
[c]Determined *in vitro* with isolated gastric mucosa (Altamirano, 1963).

(Gray and Bucher, 1941), and this secretion contains large amounts of peptic activity and hydrochloric acid. Sodium, which is the principal cation in the basal secretion is replaced to a large extent by hydrogen ion. The concentration of potassium is similar in both basal and stimulated secretions and therefore remains relatively constant at various rates of flow.

Hydrochloric acid and pepsinogen are secreted by separate mechanisms but these appear to be linked under physiological conditions. Stimulation of the vagus nerve (Bachrach, 1953; Hirschowitz and Sachs, 1965) or intravenous injection of gastrin (Hirshowitz, 1966) increases pepsinogen and hydrochloric acid levels together. Other stimuli may effect the two processes differently. In the dog, for example, histamine infusion stimulates hydrochloric acid production maximally, but inhibits pepsinogen secretion (Abrams and Brooks, 1960; Hirschowitz, 1966; Emas and Grossman, 1967).

b. PEPSIN.   Pepsinogen is the zymogen or inactive precursor of pepsin, the principal proteolytic enzyme of gastric juice. Pepsinogen was first crystallized from the gastric mucosa of swine (Herriott, 1938) and several separate pepsinogens now have been separated by Ryle (1965), Ryle and Porter (1959), and Ryle and Hamilton (1966). Porcine pepsinogen has a molecular weight of approximately 43,000 and is composed of the pepsin molecule and several smaller peptides (Fig. 2). One of these peptides has a molecular weight of 3200 and is an inhibitor of peptic activity (Herriott, 1962). The autocatalytic conversion of pepsinogen to the active pepsin begins below pH 6.0. At pH 5.4, the inhibitor peptide dissociates from the parent molecule and at pH 3.5–4.0 the inhibitor is completely digested by pepsin (Taylor, 1968).

Pepsin has a very acidic isoelectric point. It is stable in acid solution below pH 6.0 but is irreversibly denatured at pH 7.0 or above. In contrast, pepsinogen is stable in neutral or slightly alkaline solution. The optimum pH for peptic activity is generally between 1.6 and 2.5 but the effect of pH may vary with the substrate. Pepsin is capable of hydrolyzing peptide bonds of most proteins, mucin being one important

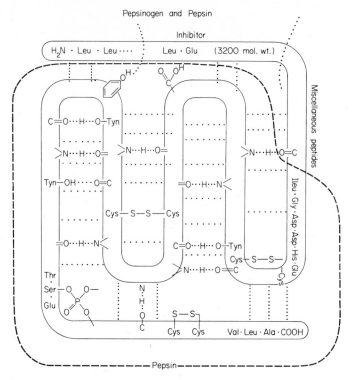

Fig. 2. Structure of pepsinogen–pepsin molecule showing position of inhibitor polypeptide, as proposed by Herriott (1962).

exception. Pepsin splits bonds involving phenylalanine, tyrosine, and leucine most readily but can hydrolyze almost all other peptide bonds.

c. RENNIN.   Rennin is another proteolytic enzyme produced by the gastric mucosa and has some characteristics which are similar to pepsin. It has been separated from pepsin in preparations from the stomachs of newborn calves. Rennin splits a mucopeptide from casein to form paracasein which then reacts with calcium ion to form an insoluble coagulum. The coagulated milk protein probably delays gastric emptying and increases the efficiency of protein digestion in young calves.

d. HYDROCHLORIC ACID.   Hydrochloric acid is produced by the oxyntic cells. When the normal mucosa is stimulated, both chloride and hydrogen ions are secreted together but current evidence suggests that H^+ and Cl^- are secreted by separate, closely coupled pump mechanisms. Small amounts of Cl^- are secreted continuously by the unstimulated oxyntic cells in the absence of H^+ secretion and this mechanism is responsible for the relative negative charge of the resting mucosal surface. H^+ and Cl^- secretory systems may also be differentiated *in vitro* by the demonstration of hydrogen ion secretion in the absence of Cl^-. A scheme for the secretion of hydrochloric acid is presented in Fig. 3. For every H^+ secreted, an electron is removed. The electron ultimately is accepted by oxygen to form OH^- which is neutralized within the cell by H^+ from carbonic acid. The bicarbonate ion produced enters the venous blood and explains why the pH of gastric venous blood frequently is

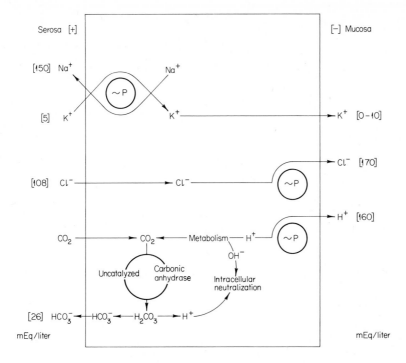

Fig. 3.   Movements of ions in the oxyntic cell during secretion of hydrochloric acid. [Modified from Davenport (1966) and based on the data of Harris and Edelman (1964).]

greater than that of arterial blood during hydrochloric acid secretion (Davenport, 1966).

The conversion of carbon dioxide and water to carbonic acid is catalyzed by carbonic anhydrase which is present in high concentration within the oxyntic cell. When the rate of acid secretion is high, this enzyme contributes to the secretory mechanism by maintaining the normal intracellular pH. Carbonic anhydrase inhibitors such as acetazolamide interfere with hydrochloric acid production in high concentrations and when the rate of acid secretion is high (Janowitz et al., 1952).

C. BILE

Bile is secreted continuously by the hepatocytes into the bile canaliculi and is transported through a system of ducts to the gall bladder where it is modified, concentrated, and stored. During digestion, bile is discharged into the lumen of the duodenum where it aids in emulsification, hydrolysis, and solubilization of dietary lipids. The digestive functions of bile are accomplished almost exclusively by the detergent action of its major components, the bile salts and phospholipids.

1.   Synthesis of Bile Acids

The primary bile acids are C-24 carboxylic acids synthesized by the liver from cholesterol. Bile acid formation represents the major pathway for cholesterol catabolism (Danielsson, 1963). Cholic acid ($3\alpha,7\alpha,12\alpha$-trihydroxy-5β-cholanoic acid) and chenodeoxycholic acid ($3\alpha,7\alpha$-dihydroxy-5β-cholanoic acid) are the primary bile acids formed by most species of domestic animals. In swine, chenodeoxycholic acid is hydroxylated at the 6α position by the liver to yield hyocholic acid which is a major primary bile acid in this species (Haslewood, 1964).

Bile acids are secreted as amino acid conjugates of either glycine or taurine. Taurine conjugates predominate in the dog, cat, and rat. In the rabbit, the conjugating enzyme system appears to be almost completely specific for glycine (Bremer, 1956). Both taurine and glycine conjugates are present in ruminants. In the new born lamb, 90% of the bile acids are conjugated with taurine. As the lamb matures, glycine conjugates increase, accounting for one-third of the total in mature sheep (Peric-Golia and Socic, 1968).

Under normal conditions, only conjugated bile acids are present in the bile and in the contents of the proximal small intestine. In the large intestine, the conjugated bile acids are hydrolyzed rapidly by bacterial enzymes so that in the contents of the large intestine and in the feces, free or unconjugated bile acids predominate. Several genera of intestinal bacteria including *Clostridium, Enterococcus, Bacteroides*, and *Lactobacillus* (Midtvedt and Norman, 1967) are capable of splitting the amide bonds of conjugated bile acids.

Intestinal bacteria also modify the basic structure of the bile acids. One such reaction is the removal of the α-hydroxyl group at the 7 position of cholic acid or chenodeoxycholic acid. These bacterial reactions yield the secondary bile acids, deoxycholic acid and lithocholic acid, respectively (Gustafsson *et al.*, 1957). Lithocholic acid is relatively insoluble and is not reabsorbed to any great extent (Gustafsson and Norman, 1962). Deoxycholic acid is reabsorbed from the large intestine in significant quantities and is either rehydroxylated by the liver to cholic acid and excreted (Lindstedt and Samuelsson, 1959) or is excreted as conjugated deoxycholic acid. The extent to which bacteria transform the primary bile acids depends on the nature of the diet, on the composition of the intestinal microflora, and the influences which these and other factors have on intestinal motility (Gustafsson *et al.*, 1966; Gustafsson and Norman, 1969a,b).

2. Detergent Properties of Bile

The carboxyl group of the bile acids is completely ionized at the pH of bile, and is neutralized by sodium ion forming *bile salts*. The bile salts are effective detergents. They are amphipathic molecules which have both hydrophobic and hydrophilic regions. In low concentrations, bile salts form molecular or ideal solutions but when their concentration increases above a certain critical level, they form polymolecular aggregates known as *micelles*. The concentration at which these molecules aggregate is called the *critical micellar concentration* (CMC).

Bile salt micelles are spherical in shape with a central nonpolar core and an external, polar region. Fatty acids, monoglycerides, and other lipids are solubilized when they enter the central core of the micelle and are covered by the outside polar coat. Solubilization occurs only when the CMC is reached. For the bile salt–monoglyceride–fatty acid–water system present during normal fat digestion, the CMC is approximately 2 mM which is ordinarily exceeded both in bile and in the contents of the upper small intestine (Hofmann, 1963). Phospholipids, principally lecithin, are also major components of bile. In the lumen of the small intestine, pancreatic phospholipase catalyzes the hydrolysis of lecithin forming free fatty acid and lyso-lecithin. The latter compound also is a potent detergent which acts with the bile salts to disperse and solubilize lipids in aqueous micellar phase.

3.   Enterohepatic Circulation of Bile Acids

The *enterohepatic circulation* begins as conjugated bile acids enter the duodenum and mix with the intestinal contents forming emulsions and micellar solutions. The bile acids are not absorbed in significant amounts from the lumen of the proximal small intestine. Absorption occurs primarily in the ileum (Lack and Weiner, 1961, 1966; Weiner and Lack, 1962) where an active transport process has been demonstrated (Dietschy *et al.*, 1966). The conjugated bile acids pass unaltered into the portal circulation (Playoust and Isselbacher, 1964) and return to the liver where the cycle begins again. This arrangement provides optimal concentrations of bile acids in the proximal small intestine where fat digestion and absorption occur and then efficient absorption after these functions have been accomplished. Absorption of unconjugated bile acids from the large intestine accounts for 3–15% of the total enterohepatic circulation (Weiner and Lack, 1968).

In dogs the total bile acid pool has been estimated to be 1.1–1.2 gm. The half-life of the bile acids in the pool ranged between 1.3–2.3 days and the rate of hepatic synthesis was 0.3–0.7 gm/day (Wollenweber *et al.*, 1965). The daily requirement for bile acids greatly exceeds the normal synthetic rate. This necessitates repeated reutilization of the bile acids which is accomplished by means of the enterohepatic circulation. Under steady-state conditions, the entire bile acid pool passes through the enterohepatic circulation approximately 10 times each day (Hofmann, 1966).

The size of the bile acid pool is dependent upon diet, the rate of hepatic synthesis, and the efficiency of the enterohepatic circulation. Surgical removal of the ileum in dogs interrupts the enterohepatic circulation causing an increase in bile acid turnover rate and in a reduction in the size of the bile acid pool (Playoust *et al.*, 1965). In diseases of the ileum, there may be defective bile salt absorption and bile salt deficiency. If severe, impaired utilization of dietary fat may occur resulting in steatorrhea and in impaired absorption of the fat-soluble vitamins.

D.   SECRETION OF THE EXOCRINE PANCREAS

The exocrine pancreas is an acinous gland with the same general structure as the salivary glands. The cytoplasm of the secretory cells contains numerous zymogen granules which vary in size and number depending on the activity of the gland. These granules contain the precursors of the hydrolytic enzymes responsible for digestion of the major dietary components. The cells of the terminal ducts probably secrete the bicarbonate ion responsible for neutralizing hydrochloric acid which enters the duodenum from the stomach.

1.   Composition

a. ELECTROLYTE COMPOSITION.   The cation content of pancreatic secretion is similar to that of plasma. Sodium is the predominant cation with smaller concentrations of potassium and calcium being present. A unique characteristic of pancreatic juice is its high bicarbonate ion concentration and alkaline pH. In the dog the pH ranges from 7.4 to 8.3 depending on HCO_3^- content. The volume of pancreatic juice is directly related to HCO_3^- concentration. As the rate of secretion increases, the HCO_3^- content and pH increase and the Cl^- concentration decreases. The sodium and potassium ion concentrations and osmolarity appear to be independent of secretory rate (Fig. 4).

b. α-AMYLASE. The amylase produced by the pancreas catalyzes the specific hydrolysis of α-1,4 glucosidic bonds which are present in starch and glycogen (α-1, 4-glucan-4-glucanohydrolase). Pancreatic amylase appears to be essentially identical to the amylase of saliva. It is a calcium-containing metaloenzyme (Vallee *et al.*, 1959). Removal of calcium by dialysis inactivates the enzyme and markedly reduces the stability of the apoenzyme. Pancreatic amylase has an optimal pH for activity of 6.7–7.2 and is activated by chloride ion.

Synthesis of pancreatic α-amylase occurs in the ribosomes. The enzyme is transferred from the endoplasmic reticulum to cytoplasmic zymogen granules for storage (Redman *et al.*, 1966). It is secreted in active form upon stimulation of the acinar cells. Newborn calves (Huber *et al.*, 1961) and pigs (Walker, 1959) secrete amylase at a significantly lower rate than mature animals. The rate of synthesis is also influenced by diet. Animals fed a high carbohydrate diet synthesize amylase at several times the rate of animals on a high protein diet (Ben Abdeljlil and Desnuelle, 1964).

Unbranched 1,4-α-glucosidic chains such as those found in amylose are hydrolyzed in two steps. The first is rapid resulting in formation of the disaccaride maltose and maltotriose. The second step is slower, involving hydrolysis of maltotriose with formation of glucose and maltose. Polysaccharides such as amylopectin and

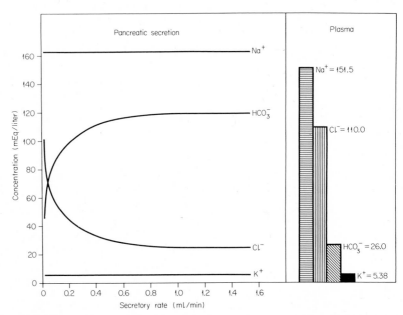

Fig. 4.   Influence of secretory rate on the electrolyte composition of canine pancreatic juice (From Bro-Rasmussen *et al.*, 1956.)

glycogen contain branched chains with both α-1,4 and α-1,6 glucosidic linkages. When α-amylase attacks these compounds, the principal products are maltose (α-1, 4 glucosidic bond) isomaltose (α-1,6 glucosidic bond) and small amounts of glucose. Final hydrolysis of the maltose and isomaltose occurs at the surface of the mucosal cell where the enzymes maltase and isomaltase are integral parts of the microvillous membrane.

c. PROTEOLYTIC ENZYMES. The proteolytic enzymes of the pancreas are responsible for the major portion of protein hydrolysis which occurs within the lumen of the gastrointestinal tract. Two types of peptidases are secreted by the pancreas. Trypsin, chymotrypsin, and elastase are *endopeptidases* which attack peptide bonds along the polypeptide chain producing smaller peptides. The *exopeptidases* attack either the carboxy-terminal or amino-terminal peptide bonds releasing single amino acids. The principal exopeptidases secreted by the pancreas are carboxypeptidases A and B. The endopeptidases and exopeptidases act in complementary fashion (Table II) producing free amino acids which are absorbed directly, or small peptides which are further hydrolyzed by the aminopeptidases of the intestinal mucosa (see Section III,C).

The pancreatic peptidases are secreted as inactive proenzymes or zymogens termed trypsinogen, chymotrypsinogen, and procarboxypeptidase A and B, respectively. Trypsinogen is converted to active trypsin in two ways. At alkaline pH, trypsinogen can be converted autocatalytically to trypsin, the activated enzyme converting more zymogen to active enzyme. Trypsinogen can also be activated by the enzyme *enterokinase* which is produced by the duodenal mucosa. This latter reaction appears to be highly specific in that enterokinase will not activate chymotrypsinogen. Chymotrypsinogen, proelastase, and the procarboxypeptidases A and B are converted to active enzymes by the action of trypsin.

The amino acid sequences and other structural characteristics of bovine trypsinogen and chymotrypsinogen now have been determined (Hartley *et al.*, 1965; Hartley and Kauffman, 1966; Brown and Hartley, 1966). The polypeptide chain of trypsinogen contains 229 amino acid residues. Activation of the proenzyme occurs with hydrolysis of a single peptide bond located in the 6 position between lysine and isoleucine. The C-terminal hexapeptide is released as enzyme activity appears. There is also substantial change in the helical structure of the parent molecule (Davie and Neurath, 1955; Neurath *et al.*, 1956). Chymotrypsinogen A is composed

TABLE II   RELATIONSHIP BETWEEN THE ACTIVITIES OF PANCREATIC ENDOPEPTIDASES
AND EXOPEPTIDASES

Enzyme	Type	Activity
Trypsin	Endopeptidase	Produces peptides with C-terminal basic amino acids
Carboxypeptidase B	Exopeptidase	Removes C-terminal basic amino acids
Chymotrypsin	Endopeptidase	Produces peptides with C-terminal aromatic amino acids
Elastase	Endopeptidase	Produces peptides with C-terminal nonpolar amino acids
Carboxypeptidase A	Exopeptidase	Removes C-terminal aromatic and nonpolar amino acids

of 245 amino acid residues and has numerous structural similarities to trypsinogen. Activation of the chymotrypsinogen also occurs with cleavage of a single peptide bond. For a complete discussion of this subject see the review by Keller (1968).

d. LIPASE.   The pancreas produces several lipolytic enzymes with different substrate specificities. The most important of these from a nutritional point of view is the lipase responsible for hydrolysis of dietary triglyceride. This enzyme has the unique property of requiring an oil–water interface for activity so that only emulsions can be effectively attacked (Sarda and Desnuelle, 1958). The principal products of lipolysis are glycerol, monoglycerides, and fatty acids. The monoglycerides and fatty acids accumulate at the oil–water interface and can inhibit enzyme activity. Their transfer from the interface to the aqueous phase is favored by the presence of sodium bicarbonate also secreted by the pancreas and by bile salts.

Mattson and Volpenhein (1966) have described two other carboxylic ester hydrolases in pancreatic juice. Both enzymes have an absolute requirement for bile salts in contrast to glycerol-ester hydrolase which is actually inhibited by bile salts at pH 8. One of these enzymes is a sterol-ester hydrolase responsible for hydrolysis of cholesterol esters. The other enzyme hydrolyses various water soluble esters. The two enzyme activities have been differentiated on the basis of stability and optimum pH.

The pancreas secretes a third lipolytic enzyme which hydrolyzes phospholids. Phospholipase A converts lecithin to lysolecithin, an effective detergent which aids in emulsification of dietary fat. Lecithin is present in significant quantities in the bile and contributes the precursor of lysolecithin in addition to the other important detergents.

2.   Control of Secretion

Pancreatic secretion is controlled and coordinated by neural and edocrine mechanisms. When ingesta or hydrochloric acid enters the duodenum, the hormone secretin is released into the circulation by the duodenal mucosa. Secretin increases the volume, pH, and HCO_3^- concentration of the pancreatic secretion.

Secretin is a polypeptide hormone which contains 27 amino acid residues. All 27 amino acids are required to maintain the helical structure of the molecule and its activity (Bodanszky et al., 1969). The C-terminal residue is the amide of valine. The presence of a C-terminal amide is a property of other polypeptide hormones such as gastrin and vasopressin which act on the flow of water in biological systems (Mutt and Jorpes, 1967). In addition to its effects on the pancreas, secretin increases the rate of bile formation (Wheeler and Mancusi-Ungaro, 1966).

The pancreatic juice which results from stimulation by secretin is large in volume with high bicarbonate concentration but is low in enzyme activity. Stimulation of the vagus nerve causes a significant rise in enzyme concentration. This type of response also is produced by pancreozymin, another polypeptide hormone secreted by the duodenal mucosa. Pancreozymin is now believed to be identical to cholecystokinin, an intestinal hormone which causes contraction of the gall bladder (J. C. Thompson, 1969). The C-terminal pentapeptide of pancreozymin-cholecystokinin is exactly the same as that of gastrin. This fascinating relationship suggests that gastrin and pancreozymin-cholecystokinin may participate in some unified but as yet poorly understood system of digestive control (J. C. Thompson, 1969).

III. DIGESTION AND ABSORPTION

A. WATER AND ELECTROLYTE ABSORPTION

1. *Mechanisms of Mucosal Transport*

The microvillous membrane of the intestinal mucosa, like other cell membranes, is a lipid structure which acts as a barrier to water and water-soluble substances. Water and polar solutes penetrate in one of two ways: (1) They may pass through *pores* in the membrane which are believed to be aqueous channels connecting the luminal surface of the cell with the apical cytoplasm. The "effective" diameter of jejunal pores has been estimated to be approximately 4 Å (Lindemann and Solomon, 1962). (2) The alternate route is to attach to *membrane carriers* which facilitate passage through the lipid phase of the membrane.

Transport of water and water-soluble compounds is influenced by the permeability characteristics of the limiting membrane and by the nature of the driving forces which provide energy for transport. Passive movement occurs either by simple diffusion or as a result of gradients in concentration (activity), pH, osmotic pressure, or electrical potential which may be present across the membrane. The passive movement of an ion in the direction of an electrochemical gradient is referred to as *single file* diffusion (Hladky, 1965). When a substance moves in a direction opposite that of an established electrochemical gradient, an *active transport* process is said to be responsible.

Most water-soluble compounds such as monosaccharides and amino acids cannot diffuse across the intestinal mucosal membrane at rates which are adequate to meet nutritional requirements. Transport of these substances is believed to be by means of membrane carriers. The nature of these carriers is not well understood but they are believed to be an integral part of the membrane and responsible for binding the transported substance in a rather specific way. Their existence is based primarily on kinetic evidence. Carrier mediated transport systems can be saturated and are competitively inhibited by related compounds.

Three types of carrier transport mechanisms are recognized (Curran and Schultz, 1968): (1) *Active transport*, as stated previously, involves movement of electrolytes against an electrochemical gradient. In the case of nonelectrolytes such as glucose, active transport is defined as movement against a concentration gradient. Active transport requires metabolic energy and is inhibited by various metabolic blocking agents or by low temperature. (2) *Facilitated diffusion* occurs when the passive movement of a substance is more rapid than can be accounted for by simple diffusion. Facilitated diffusion systems can increase the rate of movement across the membrane by 2 or 3 orders of magnitude. The carrier mechanism is similar to that involved in active transport in that it displays saturation kinetics, may be inhibited competitively, and is temperature-dependent. However, transport does not occur against concentration or electrochemical gradients and direct expenditure of energy is not required. (3) *Exchange diffusion* is a transfer mechanism similar to facilitated diffusion. It was postulated originally by Ussing (1947) to explain the rapid transfer of radioactive Na^+ across cell membranes. The mechanism does not give rise to net transport but contributes in a major way to unidirectional flux rates which are measured with isotopic tracers.

In the intestine, net water absorption is the result of bulk flow through pores in the membrane. Diffusion in the usual sense plays no important role in water movement (Section III,A,4). When bulk flow occurs, it is possible for solutes to move across the membrane in the direction of flow by a phenomenon called *solvent drag*. The effect of solvent drag on the transport of a given solute depends on the rate of volume flow and upon the *reflection coefficient* which is an expression of the relationship between the pore radius and the radius of the solute molecule being transported. A solute such as urea can be transported by the intestine against a concentration gradient by means of solvent drag (Hakim and Lifson, 1964).

2. Sodium Chloride Absorption

Studies with isotopic tracers have shown that transport of water and electrolytes by the intestinal mucosa is a dynamic process with rapid unidirectional fluxes of the substances occurring continuously in both directions. Net absorption occurs when the flow from lumen to plasma exceeds that in the opposite direction (Code *et al.*, 1960; Berger *et al.*, 1959; Hindle and Code, 1962).

Active transport of Na^+ can occur along the entire length of the intestine, but the rate of absorption is greatest in the ileum and colon where most net sodium and water absorption occurs. Sodium transport is believed to be accomplished by an energy requiring "sodium pump." The characteristics of this pump are not completely understood, but Skou (1965) has presented evidence which indicates that the pump is intimately related to the activity of a Na^+–K^+ dependent adenosine triphosphatase located within the cell membrane. This enzyme is inhibited by cardiac glycosides such as oubain which also are effective inhibitors of Na^+ transport, and it has been suggested that this enzyme system may actually be the pump. In the jejunum, net absorption of sodium occurs slowly unless nonelectrolytes such as glucose or amino acids are absorbed simultaneously. In *in vivo* studies by Fordtran *et al.* (1968), jejunal absorption of sodium appeared to be explained, in part, by solvent drag which was associated with active glucose transport. In the ileum, Na^+ absorption was independent of glucose absorption. Water absorption in the jejunum also appears to be almost entirely dependent upon the absorption of glucose while absorption from the ileum is unaffected by glucose (Barry *et al.*, 1961). The differential effect of glucose on absorption from the jejunum and ileum appears to be the result of fundamental metabolic differences between these two areas of the intestine (Curran, 1960; Gilman and Koelle, 1960).

As sodium is transported across the mucosal membrane, an equivalent amount of anion must be transported simultaneously to maintain electrical neutrality. A significant amount of chloride ion absorption can be accounted for on this basis. It is generally agreed that chloride transport in the intestine is a passive process (Clarkson *et al.*, 1961) although active secretion by the gastric mucosa seems well established. The intestinal mucosa can, under certain circumstances, absorb Cl^- independently of cation absorption and maintain electrical neutrality by exchange secretion of bicarbonate into the lumen (Ingraham and Visscher, 1936).

3. Potassium Absorption

Dietary potassium is absorbed almost entirely in the proximal small intestine. Absorption appears to be a passive process since movement across the mucosa occurs down a concentration gradient (high luminal concentration to a low concentration in plasma). The fluid which reaches the ileum from the jejunum has a potassium concentration and a sodium:potassium ratio which is similar to that of plasma. In the ileum and colon, the rate of sodium absorption is much greater than that of potassium so that, under normal conditions, the sodium:potassium ratio in the feces is much lower than that of plasma, approaching a ratio of 1.

4. Water Absorption

The absorption of water has been one of the most extensively studied aspects of intestinal transport. It is now generally agreed that water movement is the result of bulk flow through membranous pores and that simple diffusion plays only a minor role. The question of whether water is actively or passively transported has been the subject of considerable controversy and the controversy itself points to the fundamental difficulties which arise in trying to establish a definition of active transport. Hypertonic saline solutions can be absorbed from the canine intestine *in vivo* (Grim, 1962) and from canine (Hakim *et al.*, 1963) and rat (D. S. Parsons and Wingate, 1961) intestine *in vitro*. These observations indicate that water absorption can occur against an activity gradient and that the process is dependent upon metabolic energy. This would suggest that an active transport process is involved. Curran (1965), however, presents an alternate interpretation which is now generally accepted. This view is that water transport occurs secondarily to active solute transport and is the result of local gradients established within the mucosal membrane. Water transport is then coupled to the energy-dependent process responsible for solute transport but is one step removed from it.

In the dog and probably other carnivora the ileum is the main site of net sodium and water absorption. The colon accounts for no more than perhaps 20% of the total. In the case of herbivorous animals in which the large intestine is developed extensively, net secretion of water may occur in the ileum so that all net absorption of water must take place in the cecum and colon (Powell *et al.*, 1968).

B. Carbohydrate Digestion and Absorption

1. Polysaccharide Digestion

a. Starch and Glycogen.   Carbohydrate is present in the diet primarily in the form of polysaccharides of glucose. The most common polysaccharides are starch, glycogen, and cellulose. Starch and glycogen are composed of long chains of glucose molecules linked together by repeating α-1,4 glucosidic bonds. Branching chains are linked by α-1,6 glucosidic bonds. In those species which secrete salivary amylase, digestion of starch and glycogen begins in the mouth when this enzyme mixes with food. The action of salivary amylase is interrupted in the stomach, however, because of the low pH of the gastric secretion.

Starch digestion begins again in the proximal small intestine with the action of pancreatic amylase. This enzyme catalyzes a series of stepwise hydrolytic reactions resulting in formation of the principal end products of starch digestion, the disaccharides maltose and isomaltose, and small amounts of glucose. Glucose is absorbed directly by the intestinal mucosa and transported to the portal vein. The disaccharides are broken down further by hydrolytic enzymes of the brush border.

b. CELLULOSE. Cellulose, like starch, is a polysaccharide of glucose but differs from starch in that the glucose molecules are linked by β-1,4 glucosidic bonds. Starch can be utilized by all species, but cellulose is utilized as a source of energy only by animals which have extensive bacterial fermentation within the gastrointestinal tract. Ruminant species digest cellulose most efficiently but other animals, in which the large intestine is well developed, also can utilize cellulose to some degree.

In ruminants, hydrolysis of cellulose is accomplished by cellulytic bacteria which are part of the complex rumen microflora. The end products of cellulose fermentation are the short-chain fatty acids—acetic, propionic, and butyric acids. These are absorbed directly from the rumen and serve as the major source of energy for ruminants. Propionic acid is the major precursor for synthesis of carbohydrate.

2. Disaccharide Digestion

Maltose and isomaltose are the disaccharides (glucose–glucose) produced as end products of starch digestion. The diet also contains lactose (galactose–glucose) and sucrose (fructose–glucose). It once was believed that disaccharides were hydrolyzed within the lumen of the intestine by enzymes secreted by the mucosa. There is now general agreement, however, that disaccharide digestion is completed at the surface of the cell by disaccharidases which are components of the brush border (Table III). This is considered a form of intracellular digestion (Ugolev, 1965).

The disaccharidases have been solubilized from the brush border and partially purified. Two separate maltases have been isolated (Auricchio et al., 1965). Isomaltase and sucrase have been separated and purified together as a two-enzyme

TABLE III   ENZYMES OF THE MICROVILLOUS MEMBRANE

Enzyme	Reference
Lactase	Alpers (1969); Forstner et al. (1968)
Sucrase	Eichholz (1967); Forstner et al. (1968)
Maltase	Eichholz (1967); Forstner et al. (1968)
Isomaltase	Eichholz (1967); Forstner et al. (1968)
Trehalase	Eichholz (1967); Forstner et al. (1968)
Cellobiase	Forstner et al. (1968)
Leucylnapthylamidase	Rhodes et al. (1967); Eichholz (1968)
Leucylglycine hydrolase	Rhodes et al. (1967); Eichholz (1968)
Cholesterol ester hydrolase	Malathi (1967)
Retinyl ester hydrolase	Malathi (1967)
Alkaline phosphatase	Eichholz (1967); Forstner et al. (1968)
ATPase	Eichholz (1967); Forstner et al. (1968)

complex (Kolínská and Semenza, 1967). The mucosa also contains two enzymes with lactase activity. One of these is a nonspecific β-galactosidase which hydrolyzes synthetic β-galactosides effectively, but which hydrolyzes lactose at a slow rate. This enzyme has an optimum pH of 3 and is associated with the lysozomal fraction of the cell. The other lactase hydrolyzes lactose readily. It is associated with the brush border fraction of the cell and is the enzyme which is important in the digestive process (Alpers, 1969).

Maltase, isomaltase, and sucrase are almost completely absent from the intestine in newborn pigs (Hartman et al., 1961; Dahlqvist, 1961) and calves (Huber et al., 1961). Activity of these disaccharidases increases after birth and reaches adult levels during the first months of life. Lactase activity is highest at birth and decreases gradually during the neonatal period. The relatively high lactose activity seems to be an advantage to the newborn in utilizing the large quantities of lactose present in the diet. Recently Bywater and Penhale (1969) have demonstrated lactase deficiency following acute enteric infections and suggest that lactose utilization may be decreased in such cases.

3. Monosaccharide Transport

a. SPECIFICITY OF MONOSACCHARIDE TRANSPORT.   Regardless of whether monosaccharides originate in the lumen of the intestine or are formed at the surface of the mucosal cell, transport across the mucosa involves processes which have a high degree of chemical specificity. Glucose and galactose are absorbed from the intestine more rapidly than other monosaccharides. Fructose is absorbed at approximately one-half the rate of glucose, and mannose is absorbed at less than one-tenth the rate of glucose (Kohn et al., 1965). Glucose and galactose can be absorbed against concentration gradients and, by definition, are said to be actively transported. Active absorption requires metabolic energy and can be inhibited by a variety of substances which block oxidative phosphorylation.

The monosaccharides which are transported most efficiently against concentration gradients have certain common structural characteristics which were summarized by Wilson (1962). These include (1) the presence of a pyranose ring, (2) a carbon atom attached to C-5, and (3) a hydroxyl group at C-2 with the same stereoconfiguration as D-glucose. These features once were believed to be necessary for active monosaccharide transport, but recent observations suggest that they are not absolute requirements. Both D-xylose which has no substituted carbon atom at C-5, and D-mannose, which lacks the appropriate hydroxyl configuration at C-2, can be transported against concentration gradients under proper experimental conditions (Csáky and Lassen, 1964; Csáky and Ho, 1966; Alvarado, 1966b).

b. CHARACTERISTICS OF THE MEMBRANE CARRIER.   Most current concepts imply that during the initial phase of monosaccharide absorption, the monosaccharide molecule attaches to a mobile carrier located within the cell membrane (Crane, 1965). The evidence for such membrane carriers comes from kinetic studies of the overall transport process. The rate of glucose absorption is independent of luminal concentration over a rather wide range but a maximum rate of absorption can be demonstrated at very high concentrations. This limitation of transport is believed to be due to saturation of binding sites on the membrane carrier.

Glucose transport is competitively inhibited by galactose (Cori, 1925; R. B. Fisher and Parsons, 1953) and by a variety of substituted hexoses which compete with glucose for carrier-binding sites. The glucoside, phlorizin, is a very potent inhibitor of glucose transport (B. J. Parsons *et al.*, 1958; Alvarado and Crane, 1962). Phlorizin also competes for binding sites, but has a much higher affinity for these sites than glucose.

The absorptive surface of the mucosal cell is the microvillous membrane or brush border (Fig. 5a and b). It is through this part of the plasma membrane that glucose must pass during the initial phase of mucosal transport. Techniques have been developed recently for isolating highly purified preparations of microvillous membranes from mucosal homogenates (Eichholz and Crane, 1965; Forstner *et al.*, 1968). Faust *et al.* (1967) studied the binding of various sugars to these isolated membrane fractions. They found that D-glucose was bound by the membrane preferentially to L-glucose or to D-mannose and that glucose-binding was completely inhibited by 0.1 m*M* phlorizin. The specificity of their observations suggested that binding represented an initial step in glucose transport, namely attachment to a membrane carrier.

c. SODIUM REQUIREMENT.   The absorption of glucose and other monosaccharides is influenced significantly by sodium ion. When sodium is present in the solution bathing the intestinal mucosa, glucose is absorbed rapidly, but when sodium is removed and replaced by equimolar amounts of other cations, glucose absorption virtually stops (Riklis and Quastel, 1958; Csáky, 1961; Bihler and Crane, 1962; Bihler *et al.*, 1962). Glucose absorption is inhibited by oubain, digitalis, and other cardiac glycosides which also are inhibitors of Na–K dependent adenosine triphosphatase activity and of sodium transport (Csáky and Hara, 1965; Schultz and Zalusky, 1964). These observations suggest a close relationship between the transport of glucose and sodium. Based on their own observations, Crane and co-workers (1965) have suggested that sodium ion acts directly upon the membrane carrier to increase affinity of the carrier for glucose. Csáky (1963) interprets the apparent

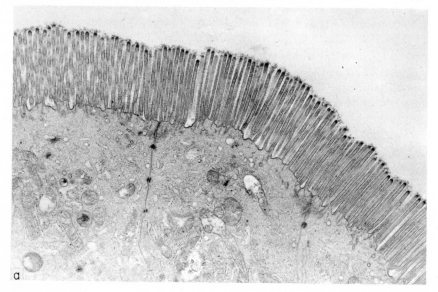

a

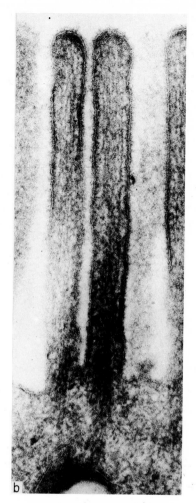

Fig. 5. (a) Absorptive surface of the mucosal epithelium showing the microvillous membrane and, below it, the apical cytoplasm. ($\times$ 8,500.)   (b) Electron photomicrograph of microvilli. ($\times$ 51,500.) (Electron photomicrographs courtesy of S. Lui and K. J. Isselbacher, Massachusetts General Hospital, Boston, Massachusetts.)

coupling of sodium transport to the transport of various nonelectrolytes as being due to the need to maintain a critical intracellular sodium concentration which, in turn, is essential for conversion of metabolic energy (ATP, etc.) to energy for transport.

C. Protein Digestion and Absorption

1. Enzymic Hydrolysis

The initial step in protein digestion is enzymic hydrolysis of peptide bonds with formation of smaller peptides and amino acids. The *endopeptidases* (proteinases) hydrolyze peptide bonds within the protein molecule and also hydrolyze certain model peptides. *Exopeptidases* hydrolyze either the carboxy-terminal (carboxy-peptidase) or the amino-terminal (aminopeptidase) amino acids of peptides and certain proteins.

Dietary proteins first come in contact with proteolytic enzymes in the stomach. The best known of the gastric proteinases are the pepsins (A–D) which attack most proteins with the exception of keratins, protamines, and mucins. Pepsins are relatively nonspecific endopeptidases and split peptide bonds involving many amino acids. The most readily hydrolyzed peptide bonds are those of leucine, phenylalanine, tyrosine, and glutamic acid (Ryle, 1965; Ryle and Hamilton, 1966).

The extent of proteolysis in the stomach depends on the nature of the dietary protein and upon the length of time spent in the stomach. The food bolus mixed with saliva has a neutral or slightly alkaline pH as it enters the stomach and a certain period of time is necessary for it to mix with gastric secretions and become acidified. Proteolytic digestion begins when the pH of the gastric contents approaches 4 and occurs optimally in two pH ranges, 1.6–2.4 and 3.3–4.0 (Taylor, 1959a,b). Because of the relative lack of specificity of the pepsins, some peptide bonds of almost all dietary proteins are split during passage through the stomach.

The partially digested protein passes from the stomach to the duodenum where the acidic contents are neutralized by sodium bicarbonate secreted in the bile and pancreatic juices. Peptic activity persists in the duodenum only during the period required to raise the pH above 4.0. The major peptidase activity in the lumen of the small intestine comes from the pancreatic enzymes trypsin, chymotrypsin, elastase, and carboxypeptidase A and B. The action of these enzymes is integrated so that the endopeptidases produce peptides with C-terminal amino acids which are appropriate substrates for the exopeptidases. Trypsin produces peptides with basic C-terminal amino acids which are particularly suited for the action of carboxypeptidase B. Chymotrypsin produces peptides with aromatic amino acids in the C-terminal position and elastase produces peptides with C-terminal amino acids which are nonpolar. Carboxypeptidase A hydrolyzes both types of C-terminal peptide bonds (Table II).

The intestinal mucosa contains a broad range of aminopeptidases which complete the process of protein digestion (Heizer and Laster, 1969). Approximately 90% of the aminopeptidase activity is found in the soluble fraction of the cell (Newey and Smyth, 1960). The remaining 10% is tightly bound to the microvillous membrane and may serve a digestive function at the cell surface similar to that described for the disaccharidases (Rhodes *et al.*, 1967). An endopeptidase from the intestinal mucosa has been studied recently by Hsu and Tappel (1965) using hemoglobin as substrate. Over 95% of the activity was located in the particulate fraction of the cell. Its association with other acid hydrolases suggests that it is a lysozomal enzyme. The relationship of this enzyme to the normal process of protein digestion is not known.

2. *Form in Which Products of Protein Hydrolysis Are Absorbed*

Despite the long interest and controversy regarding the subject of this section, we do not know the relative amounts of the various types of protein digestion products, i.e., peptides and amino acids, which are actually absorbed by intestinal mucosal cells during normal digestion. It is a difficult process to investigate from a kinetic point of view because the products of proteolysis are absorbed rapidly after they are formed. Studies of luminal contents, therefore, give only an estimate of the overall rate of protein digestion. In addition, dietary protein is continually mixed with endogenous protein in the form of digestive secretions and extruded mucosal cells. Endogenous protein is hydrolyzed and the amino acids absorbed in a manner similar to that of dietary protein and the two processes occur simultaneously. Endogenous protein accounts for a significant part of the amino acids of the intestinal contents (Nasset and Ju, 1961). Even when the dietary protein is labeled with a radioactive tracer, there is such rapid utilization that the tracer soon reenters the lumen in the form of endogenous protein secretion.

In adult mammals, protein is not absorbed from the intestine in quantities of nutritional significance without previous hydrolysis. Most neonatal animals absorb significant amounts of immunoglobulin and other colostral protein, but this capacity is lost soon after birth (see Section III, A, 4 below). The intestinal mucosa is not totally impermeable to large polypeptide molecules, however. The absorption of insulin (MW 5,700) (Laskowski et al., 1958; Danforth and Moore, 1959) and of ribonuclease (MW 13,700) (Alpers and Isselbacher, 1967) have been demonstrated. The intestine produces a part of the plasma β-globulin but this is believed to be the result of de novo synthesis of protein presumably from individual amino acid precursors.

During the digestion of protein, the amino acid content of the portal blood increases rapidly. Attempts to demonstrate parallel increases in the level of peptides in the portal blood have not been successful (Levenson et al., 1959). This has sometimes been taken as evidence that only amino acids can be absorbed by the intestinal mucosa and that the absorption of peptides does not occur. While it seems clear that a significant part of the dietary protein is absorbed in the form of free amino acids, peptides also may be taken up by the mucosal cell. Evidence of mucosal uptake of peptides has come largely from experiments with isolated loops of intestine (Wiggans and Johnston, 1959; Newey and Smyth, 1959). Various peptides were placed in solutions bathing the mucosa and analyses made subsequently of the serosal fluid. With the exception of small amounts of glycylglycine, peptides were never found on the serosal side but free amino acids were found in significant quantities. From these studies it appears probable that in the intact animal, peptides can be taken up in physiologically important quantities by intestinal mucosal cells and are hydrolyzed either at the cell surface or intracellularly to constituent amino acids. The individual amino acids then are transported to the apical part of the cell and finally enter the portal circulation.

3. Transport of Amino Acids

Amino acids, like glucose and certain other monosaccharides, are absorbed and transferred to the portal circulation by active transport processes. The same type of saturation kinetics observed in studies of monosaccharide absorption are observed with amino acids suggesting carrier transport mechanisms. Certain monosaccharides inhibit amino acid transport (Saunders and Isselbacher, 1965; Newey and Smyth, 1964). Inhibition generally has been of the noncompetitive type but Alvarado (1966a) has demonstrated competitive inhibition between galactose and cycloleucine suggesting that some form of common carrier may be involved.

Most amino acids are transported against concentration and electrochemical gradients and the overall transport process requires metabolic energy. The chemical specificity of these transport mechanisms is demonstrated by the observation that the natural *l*-forms of various amino acids are absorbed more rapidly than the corresponding *d*-forms and only the *l*-amino acids appear to be actively transported. Sodium ion is necessary for absorption of amino acids as it is for a variety of other nonelectrolyte substances.

Separate transport systems appear to exist for different groups of amino acids. Each member of a group inhibits the transport of other members competitively, suggesting that they share the same binding site. There is some overlap between groups indicating that in the overall transport process, certain steps may be common to all amino acids and other steps more specific (Saunders and Isselbacher, 1966; Matthews and Laster, 1965; Wiseman, 1968). These groups are:

1. Monoaminomonocarboxylic (neutral) amino acids including histidine. These amino acids show mutual competition for transport and have the greatest requirement for Na^+.

2. Monoaminodicarboxylic amino acids. Aspartic and glutamic acids are not transported against concentration gradients. Following uptake, they are transaminated and, under physiological conditions, almost all of the aspartic and glutamic acid enter the portal blood as alanine.

3. Dibasic amino acids. Cystine, lysine, arginine, and ornithine. These amino acids are apparently transported by the same transport system.

4. Proline and hydroxyproline, and the *N*-substituted glycine derivatives *N*-methyl glycine (sarcosine), *N*-dimethylglycine, and betaine. Proline and hydroxyproline can be transported by mechanism (1) but the affinity of both amino acids for this pathway is low.

4.   Neonatal Absorption of Immunoglobulin

At birth most domestic species, including the calf, foal, lamb, pig, kitten, and pup, absorb significant quantities of colostral protein from the small intestine (Brambell, 1958). γ-Globulin is either absent in the serum of these species at birth or is at a very low level. Within a few hours after ingestion of colostrum, the serum γ-globulin level rises (Fig. 6). This is the principal mechanism by which the young of the above-listed species acquire maternal immunity. Under normal environmental conditions, ingestion of colostrum is an absolute requirement for health of these species during the neonatal period.

Protein enters the absorptive cell by pinocytosis and passes across the cell to the lymphatics. The process is not selective because many proteins other than the immune globulins can be absorbed (Payne and Marsh, 1962a,b). The ability to absorb intact protein is lost by domestic species within 1 or 2 days following birth. In rodents, protein absorption normally continues for approximately 3 weeks. The mechanism of intestinal "closure" has been studied extensively by Lecce and co-workers (1964;

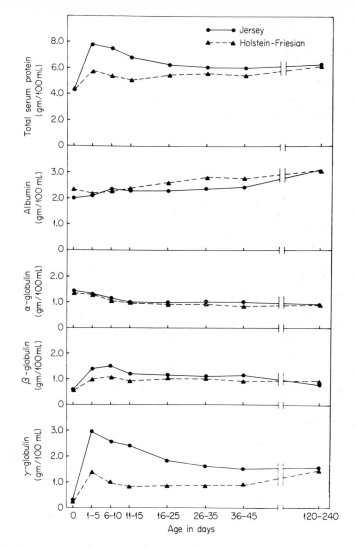

Fig. 6. Changes in serum globulin fractions and serum albumin which occur during the neonatal period in Jersey and Holstein-Friesian calves. Note significant differences between breeds in γ-globulin levels (Tennant *et al.*, 1969a).

Lecce, 1966; Lecce and Morgan, 1962). They have found that complete starvation of pigs lengthened the period of protein absorption to 4–5 days, whereas early feeding shortened the period. Feeding different fractions of colostrum including lactose and galactose resulted in loss of protein absorptive capacity. The route of feeding may not be the critical factor, however. Calves prevented from eating but which receive nutrients parenterally lose the ability to absorb protein at the same time as control calves (Deutsch and Smith, 1957).

D. Lipid Digestion and Absorption

1. Absorption of Fats

a. Luminal Phase.   The fat present in the diet is primarily in the form of triglycerides of long-chain fatty acids. The initial step in utilization of triglycerides
occurs in the lumen of the proximal small intestine where hydrolysis is catalyzed by
pancreatic lipase. This enzyme requires an oil–water interface for activity so that
only emulsions are attacked (Sarda and Desnuelle, 1958). Enzyme activity is directly
related to the surface area of the emulsion. The smaller the emulsion particle, the
greater the total surface area of a given quantity of triglyceride and the greater the
rate of hydrolysis (Benzonana and Desnuelle, 1965). Bile salts are not an absolute
requirement but they favor hydrolysis (1) by their detergent action which causes
formation of emulsions with small particle sizes, and (2) by stimulating lipase activity
within the physiological pH range of the duodenum (Borgström, 1954, 1964a).

Pancreatic lipase splits the ester bonds of triglycerides preferentially at the 1 and 3
positions (Sari *et al.*, 1966) so that the major end products of hydrolysis are 2-mono-
glycerides and nonesterified fatty acids (Mattson *et al.*, 1952; Mattson and Volpenhein,
1962, 1964). Both compounds are relatively insoluble in water but are brought rapidly
into micellar solution by the detergent action of bile salts. The mixed micelles so
formed have a diameter of approximately 20 Å (Borgström, 1964b; Laurent and
Persson, 1965) and are believed to be the form in which the products of fat digestion
are actually taken up by the mucosal cell (Hofmann and Small, 1967). The intraluminal events which occur in fat absorption are schematically summarized in Fig. 7.

b. Mucosal Phase.   The initial step in fat transport is the uptake of fatty acids
and monoglycerides by the mucosal cell from micellar solution. Just how this occurs

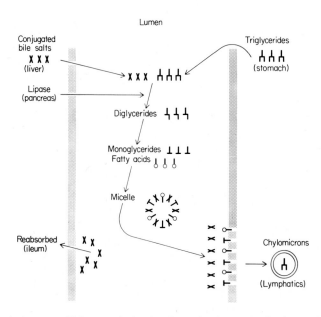

Fig. 7.   Intraluminal events which occur during fat absorption (From Isselbacher, 1967).

is not completely clear but present evidence suggests that the lipid contents of the micelle are somehow discharged at the cell surface so that they enter the cell in molecular rather than micellar form (Isselbacher, 1967). The net effect is the absorption of the end products of lipolysis with the exclusion of bile salts which are absorbed further down the intestine, primarily in the ileum (Lack and Weiner, 1963). Uptake of fatty acids appears to be a passive process having no requirement for metabolic energy (Johnston and Borgström, 1964; Strauss, 1966).

Within the mucosal cell, the fatty acids and monoglycerides are rapidly reesterified to triglyceride. The two biochemical pathways for triglyceride biosynthesis in the intestine are summarized in Fig. 8. Direct acylation of monoglyceride occurs in the intestine (Senior and Isselbacher, 1962) and probably is the major pathway for lipogenesis in the intestine during normal fat absorption (Kern and Borgström, 1965; Mattson and Volpenhein, 1964). The initial step in this series of reactions involves activation of fatty acids by acyl Co A synthetase, a reaction which requires Mg^{2+}, ATP, and Co A (Dawson and Isselbacher, 1960; Clark and Hübscher, 1960, 1961; Brindley and Hübscher, 1965) and which has a marked specificity for long-chain fatty acids (Dawson and Isselbacher, 1960; Brindley and Hübscher, 1965). This specificity appears to explain the observation by Bloom *et al.* (1951) that medium- and short-chain fatty acids are not incorporated into triglycerides during intestinal transport but enter the portal circulation as nonesterified fatty acids. The activated fatty acids then react sequentially with mono- and diglycerides to form triglycerides in steps catalyzed by mono- and diglyceride transacylases (Ailhaud *et al.*, 1964). The enzymes responsible for this series of reactions have been partially purified by Rao and Johnston (1966) from the microsomal fraction of the cell. They observed that purification of the separate enzyme activities occurred simultaneously, suggesting that these enzymes occur together in the endoplasmic reticulum as a "triglyceride synthetase" complex.

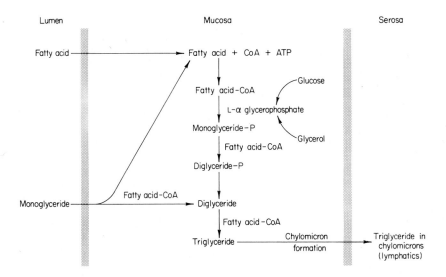

Fig. 8.   Biochemical reactions involved in intestinal transport of long chain fatty acids and mono-glycerides (From Isselbacher, 1966).

An alternate route which is available for fatty acid esterification involves L-α-glycerophosphate which may be derived from glucose or from dietary glycerol by the action of intestinal glycerokinase (Haessler and Isselbacher, 1963; Clark and Hübscher, 1962). Activated fatty acid Co A derivatives react with L-α-glycerophosphate to form lysophosphatidic acid (monoglyceride phosphate) which by a second acylation forms phosphatidic acid (diglyceride phosphate). Phosphatidic acid phosphatase then hydrolyses the phosphate ester bond forming diglyceride and by means of a transacylase step similar to that described in the previous paragraph, triglyceride can then be formed. Although this pathway appears to be one of minor importance for triglyceride synthesis in the intestine, Johnston (1968) has pointed out the importance of certain of the intermediates in this sequence of reactions in the synthesis of phospholipids which are necessary for stabilization of the chylomicron.

The next step in fat transport is formation of chylomicrons within the endoplasmic reticulum. The chylomicron is composed primarily of triglyceride and has an outer membranous coating of cholesterol, phospholipid, and protein (Zilversmit, 1965). The β-lipoprotein component of the chylomicron is synthesized by the intestinal mucosal cell (Isselbacher and Budz, 1963; Hatch et al., 1966; Windmueller and Levy, 1968). Inhibition of protein synthesis by puromycin or acetoxycycloheximide interferes with chylomicron formation and significantly reduces fat transport (Sabesin and Isselbacher, 1965).

The final step in fat absorption is extrusion of the chylomicron into the intercellular space opposite the basal lateral portion of the absorptive cell. This is accomplished by a process which is essentially the reverse of pinocytosis (Palay and Karlin, 1959). From the intercellular space, the chylomicron passes through the basement membrane and enters the lacteals through small pores. The chylomicron passes from the lacteal into lymph ducts and ultimately reaches the general circulation having bypassed the liver completely during the initial phase of absorption.

2. Absorption of Other Lipids

a. CHOLESTEROL. Dietary cholesterol is present in both free and esterified forms but only nonesterified cholesterol is absorbed (Vahouny and Treadwell, 1964). Cholesterol esters are hydrolyzed within the lumen of the intestine by sterol esterase secreted by the pancreas. Bile salts are required both for the action of this enzyme (Vahouny et al., 1965) and for the absorption of nonesterified cholesterol. In the mucosal cell, cholesterol is reesterified and transferred by way of the lymph to the general circulation. The type of triglyceride present in the diet significantly affects the absorption of cholesterol and its distribution in lymph lipids (Ockner et al., 1969).

b. VITAMIN A. The diet contains vitamin A activity in two principal forms: (1) as esters of preformed vitamin A alcohol (retinol) and fatty acids, and (2) as provitamin A primarily in the form of β-carotene. Vitamin A ester is hydrolyzed by a pancreatic esterase within the lumen (Murthy and Ganguly, 1962) and the free alcohol is absorbed in the upper small intestine by a process which apparently requires metabolic energy (Skála and Hrubá, 1964). Vitamin A alcohol is reesterified in the mucosa utilizing primarily palmitic acid (Mahadevan et al., 1963). The vitamin

An ester is absorbed by way of the lymph. After reaching the general circulation, it is rapidly cleared from the plasma and stored in the liver. In the postabsorptive state, vitamin A circulates as the free alcohol. This is also the form released from the liver as needed by the action of a specific hepatic retinyl palmitate esterase (Mahadevan et al., 1966). The blood level of vitamin A is independent of the liver reserve and as long as a small amount of vitamin A is present in the liver, the blood level remains normal (Dowling and Wald, 1958).

In diets which lack animal fat, the carotenes, mainly β-carotene, serve as the major vitamin A precursors. The intestinal mucosa plays the primary role in conversion of provitamin A to the active vitamin, although conversion can occur to a limited degree in other tissues (Bieri and Pollard, 1954; Zachman and Olson, 1963). The exact mechanism involved in the conversion of β-carotene to vitamin A is not completely established but studies by Olson (1961) suggest that there is central cleavage of β-carotene into two active vitamin A alcohol molecules which are subsequently esterified and transported by the lymphatics as with the preformed vitamin.

Bile salts are required for the mucosal uptake of β-carotene and for the conversion of β-carotene to vitamin A. Uptake of carotene and release of vitamin A ester into the lymph appear to be rate-limiting steps. Cattle also absorb substantial amounts of carotene without prior conversion to vitamin A and these pigments are responsible for much of the yellow color of the plasma. Most other species have no carotene in the plasma and it has been suggested that extraintestinal conversion may be more efficient in these species than in cattle (Ganguly and Murthy, 1967).

c. VITAMIN D.   Vitamin D, like cholesterol, is a sterol which is absorbed from the intestine by way of the lymph (Schachter et al., 1964). Intestinal absorption differs, however, in that vitamin D is transported to the lymph in nonesterified form (Bell, 1966). The uptake of vitamin D by the mucosal cell is favored by the presence of bile salts. Simultaneous absorption of fat from micellar solutions increases transport out of the cell into the lymph, a step which appears to be rate-limiting (G. R. Thompson et al., 1969).

One of the major actions of vitamin D is to enhance the intestinal absorption of calcium ion. The mechanism of action of vitamin D has been described recently by Wasserman and co-workers (1968; Wasserman and Taylor, 1966, 1968). They have shown that vitamin D causes synthesis of a calcium-binding protein present in the soluble fraction of the intestinal mucosal cell. They have accumulated a substantial amount of evidence which suggests that this protein plays a central role in the active transport of calcium.

IV.   DISTURBANCES IN GASTROINTESTINAL FUNCTION

A. VOMITING

Vomiting is a coordinated reflex act which results in rapid, forceful expulsion of gastric contents through the mouth. The reflex may be initiated by (1) local gastric irritation caused by a variety of toxic irritants or infectious agents, (2) foreign bodies, (3) gastric tumors, (4) obstruction of the pyloric canal or of the small intestine, or by (5) drugs such as apomorphine or other toxic substances which act centrally on the "vomiting center" located in the medulla.

Severe vomiting produces loss of large quantities of water and of H^+ and Cl^- ions. These losses cause *dehydration, metabolic alkalosis* with elevated plasma bicarbonate concentration, and *hypochloremia*. Chronic vomiting may also be associated with loss of tissue K^+ and hypokalemia. The K^+ deficit is caused primarily by increased urinary excretion which is the result of the existing alkalosis (Leaf and Santos, 1961). Gastric secretions contain significant quantities of K^+ (Section II,B) and losses in the vomitus also contribute to the K^+ deficiency. Potassium deficiency which develops initially because of alkalosis, ultimately may perpetuate the alkalotic state by interfering with the ability of the kidney to conserve H^+ (A. R. Koch *et al.*, 1956; Darrow, 1964). Both potassium deficiency and the hypovolemia caused by dehydration may result in renal tubular damage and ultimately in renal failure (Haden and Orr, 1923, 1924).

Vomiting occurs frequently in the dog, cat, and pig but is an unusual sign in the horse which has anatomical restrictions of the esophagus which interfere with expulsion of gastric contents. In cattle, sheep, and goats, the physiological process of rumination utilizes neuromuscular mechanisms similar to those involved in vomiting. Uncontrolled expulsion of ruminal contents is, however, an uncommon sign occurring most frequently after ingestion of toxic materials. The contents of the abomasum are not expelled directly even when the pyloric canal is obstructed. A syndrome does occur in cattle with pyloric obstruction, however, which is similar metabolically to that observed in nonruminants. The syndrome has been observed in right-sided displacement of the abomasum with torsion (Espersen, 1961; Boucher and Abt, 1968). We have also observed the syndrome in cows with functional pyloric obstruction (Hjerpe and Tennant, 1968), the result of reticuloperitonitis (a variety of "vagal indigestion"). When the pylorus is obstructed, abomasal contents are retained, causing distention of the abomasum which in turn stimulates further secretion and retention. Retained abomasal contents may be regurgitated into the large reservoir of the rumen and there are sequestered from other fluid compartments of the body. The net result is loss of H^+ and Cl^- ions and development of metabolic alkalosis, hypochloremia, and hypokalemia (Espersen and Simesen, 1961).

B. DIARRHEA

The term diarrhea is used loosely to describe the passage of abnormally fluid feces with increased frequency and/or with increased volume. The significance of diarrhea depends entirely upon the underlying cause and upon the secondary nutritional and metabolic disturbances which are caused by excessive fecal losses.

There are fundamentally three factors which act independently or in combination to produce diarrhea: (1) increased rate of intestinal transit, (2) decreased intestinal absorptive capacity, and (3) increased secretion into the intestinal lumen. An increase in the rate of intestinal transit is associated with various functional disorders of the gastrointestinal tract in which hypermotility is the primary cause. Increased intestinal motility also may be a secondary factor in the diarrhea of certain forms of intestinal parisitism or other inflammatory bowel diseases such as Johne's disease and canine ulcerative colitis.

Decreased intestinal assimilation of nutrients may result from either (1) decreased intraluminal hydrolysis of nutrients, e.g., *maldigestion* (Kalser, 1964) due to pancreatic exocrine insufficiency or to bile salt deficiency, or (2) defective mucosal transport of nutrients, *malabsorption*, which may be the result of various types of inflammatory bowel disease, intestinal lymphoma, or intrinsic biochemical defects in the mucosal cell which interfere with normal digestion and absorption. The role of increased intestinal secretion in the pathogenesis of various types of diarrhea is not completely clear, but it may be an important factor in certain types of acute enteric infections. Enteropathogenic strains of *E. coli* were shown recently to produce a powerful enterotoxin (Smith and Halls, 1967) which can cause diarrhea in intact animals (Kohler, 1968). The experiments of Smith and Halls (1967) suggest that this enterotoxin alters the bidirectional flux of fluid across the mucosa in a way which produces increased secretion.

Acute diarrhea is an important clinical problem in all species of domestic animals and represents the leading cause of morbidity and mortality in newborn calves and pigs. The pathogenesis of neonatal enteric disease is complex, often involving nutritional or environmental factors as well as infectious agents such as enteropathogenic strains of *Escherichia coli* or the virus of transmissible gastroenteritis (TGE). The severe clinical signs and frequently fatal outcome of acute diarrheal disease are often related directly to dehydration and to associated hydrogen ion and electrolyte disturbances (Dalton *et al.*, 1965; E. W. Fisher and McEwan, 1967; Tennant *et al.*, 1968).

In acute diarrhea with watery stools of large volume, the fecal fluid originates primarily in the small intestine. The electrolyte composition of the stool in such cases is similar to the fluid found normally in the lumen of the small intestine, which in turn is similar to an ultrafiltrate of the plasma. The rapid dehydration which accompanies acute enteritis in the newborn soon produces hemoconcentration and ultimately hypovolemic shock. Such cases are characterized by metabolic acidosis (Dalton *et al.*, 1965; Phillips and Knox, 1969) caused by decreased excretion of H^+ due to renal failure and by increased production of organic acids, the result of decreased tissue oxygenation which leads to excessive anaerobic glycolysis. Hyperkalemia also is observed characteristically in young, severely dehydrated animals. Hyperkalemia in such cases is the result of increased movement of cellular potassium into the extracellular fluid and to decreased renal excretion. Cardiac irregularities caused by hyperkalemia are demonstrable with the electrocardiogram and cardiac arrest related to the hyperkalemia is believed to be a direct cause of death in calves with acute diarrhea (E. W. Fisher, 1965; E. W. Fisher and McEwan, 1967). Marked hypoglycemia also has been observed occasionally prior to death in calves with acute enteric infections. Hypoglycemia is believed to be due to decreased gluconeogenesis and increased anaerobic glycolysis, the result of hypovolemic shock (Tennant *et al.*, 1968). The sequence of metabolic changes which occurs during acute neonatal diarrhea is summarized in Fig. 9.

In chronic forms of diarrheal disease, excessive fecal losses of electrolyte and

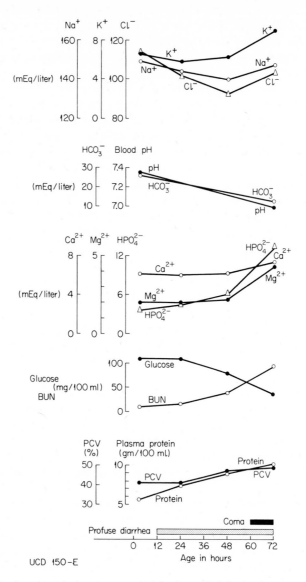

Fig. 9.   Metabolic alterations during the course of fatal enteric infection in a neonatal calf (Tennant *et al.*, 1970).

fluid may be compensated in part by renal conservation mechanisms and by oral ingestion. If water is consumed without adequate ingestion of electrolytes, hyponatremia and hypokalemia may develop (Tasker, 1967; Patterson *et al.*, 1968). In such cases, the osmolarity of the plasma is significantly decreased and *hypotonic* dehydration occurs. In long-standing cases of chronic diarrhea, the plasma K^+ may become dangerously low. It is imperative, in this situation, that intravenous fluids contain sufficient K^+ to prevent further reduction in the plasma level. Failure to do so may result in cardiac irregularities or in cardiac arrest.

C. Intestinal Malabsorption

Decreased assimilation of nutrients may occur as the result of either defective intraluminal digestion (maldigestion) (Kalser, 1964), or because of defects in mucosal transport. Intestinal malabsorption or the *malabsorption syndrome* is observed in several types of intestinal disease including chronic intestinal granulomatous diseases such as Johne's disease, intestinal parasitic infections, and lymphoma of the intestine. A primary or idiopathic form of intestinal malabsorption also has been reported recently in dogs (Vernon, 1962; Kaneko *et al.*, 1965). The canine malabsorption syndrome is characterized clinically by chronic diarrhea, steatorrhea, and progressive weight loss, and histopathologically by atrophy of the villi of the mucosal cells of the small intestine (Kaneko *et al.*, 1965). The canine disease has features which are similar to nontropical sprue (adult coeliac disease) of man, a disease caused by sensitivity to the protein gluten (Jeffries *et al.*, 1969; Floch, 1969). The relationship of gluten to the pathogenesis of canine intestinal malabsorption, however, is not known.

1. Malabsorption of Fat

Steatorrhea, the presence of excessive amounts of fat in the feces, is a prominent sign of intestinal malabsorption in dogs. The stools are bulky, gray or tan in color, and grossly may have an oily appearance. The normal dog excretes 3–5 gm of fat in the stool each day. This level of fecal fat is quite constant and is independent of dietary fat intake over a wide range from 15 to 48 gm/day (Heersma and Annegers, 1948). In intestinal malabsorption the ability to absorb fat is decreased and fecal fat excretion increases significantly. Under these conditions, the amount of fecal fat excreted becomes proportional to dietary intake.

Steatorrhea may be documented qualitatively by staining the fresh stool with a lipophilic stain such as Sudan III and observing increased numbers of oil droplets under light microscopy. In experienced hands this method is a highly reliable diagnostic procedure (Drummey *et al.*, 1961). A quantitative estimate of the degree of steatorrhea may be obtained using a dietary balance method in which fat intake and fecal excretion are measured simultaneously over a 2- or 3-day period. Fecal fat is determined using the technique of van de Kamer *et al.* (1949) which employs ether extraction of fecal lipid and titration of fatty acids. The results are expressed as grams of neutral fat excreted per 24 hours.

2. Malabsorption of Other Nutrients

In addition to malabsorption of fat, the canine malabsorption syndrome is associated with decreased absorption of other nutrients. These defects in absorption are responsible for the progressive malnutrition which is a cardinal feature of the disease. There may be malabsorption of vitamin D and/or calcium resulting in osteomalacia. The anemia sometimes observed may be the result of malabsorption of iron or of the B vitamins which are required for normal erythropoiesis. Glucose malabsorption has been clearly documented by Kaneko *et al.* (1965) and it is likely that amino acids, which are absorbed at a similar level of the small intestine and by similar transport mechanisms, are also malabsorbed. Carbohydrate and fat malabsorption unquestionably are responsible for the caloric deficit observed and amino acid malabsorption may contribute to the development of hypoalbuminemia, although this is thought to be due primarily to increased intestinal loss of plasma protein (see Section IV,C).

3. Differential Diagnostic Considerations

The diagnosis of primary or idiopathic canine malabsorption can be made only after appropriate diagnostic procedures have excluded the presence of (1) other inflammatory, neoplastic, or parasitic diseases of the intestine, and (2) the diseases of the pancreas or liver which result in defective intraluminal digestion. The presence of parasitic infection is determined by examining the feces for parasite ova. Other inflammatory or neoplastic diseases of the intestine may be suggested on the basis of clinical or radiological examination but a definitive diagnosis usually depends on histopathological examination of an intestinal biopsy specimen.

Both primary and secondary intestinal malabsorption must be differentiated from those diseases in which there is decreased intraluminal hydrolysis of nutrients. The latter are due most frequently to pancreatic exocrine insufficiency, the result of such diseases as chronic pancreatitis or juvenile pancreatic atrophy (N. V. Anderson and Low, 1965a,b). In these diseases, degradation of the major dietary constituents is reduced because of a primary lack of pancreatic enzymes. Intraluminal hydrolysis of fat may also be decreased because of a deficiency of bile salts caused either by decreased hepatic secretion or because of bile duct obstruction. Under certain experimental conditions, diversion of bile flow in the dog actually has a quantitatively small effect on fat absorption (Wells et al., 1955).

The problems of pancreatic exocrine deficiency are discussed in detail elsewhere in this text (Chapter 6, Volume I). The most simple and perhaps most widely used test to differentiate intestinal malabsorption from pancreatic exocrine insufficiency is that described by Jasper (1954). The test is employed to detect reduction in trypsinlike activity in the feces of dogs with decreased pancreatic exocrine secretion (Grossman, 1962). There is wide variation in normal activity making interpretation of the test difficult (Frankland, 1969). The test reveals only the presence or absence of hydrolysis of gelatin and does not differentiate between gelatinase activity produced by intestinal bacteria from that secreted by the pancreas. There is evidence in some species that trypsin is almost completely destroyed by bacteria during its passage through the intestine and that the proteinase activity of the feces is primarily of bacterial origin (Borgström et al., 1959). Despite these theoretical objections, the test has been of clinical diagnostic value in our hands. Fecal gelatinase activity has been detected consistently in cases of intestinal malabsorption and is almost always absent when severe pancreatic exocrine insufficiency is present. Gelatinase activity may be found, however, in the feces of dogs with moderate degrees of pancreatic insufficiency.

4. Tests of Intestinal Absorption

a. OLEIC ACID AND TRIOLEIN ABSORPTION.   Several tests have been developed for the clinical evaluation of intestinal absorptive capacity. The absorption of

[^{131}I] oleic acid and [^{131}I] triolein have been studied extensively in normal dogs (Turner, 1958; Michaelson *et al.*, 1960) and Kaneko *et al.* (1965) have used this test to study dogs with intestinal malabsorption. The day before administration of the ^{131}I-labeled compound, a small amount of Lugol's iodine solution is administered to block thyroidal uptake of the isotope. Tracer amounts of the test substances are mixed with nonradioactive carrier and are administered orally. Absorption is determined by measuring the radioactivity of the plasma at intervals following administration and calculating the percent of the dose absorbed based on plasma volume.

It is possible to use the results of these two tests, when performed in sequence, to differentiate between steatorrhea caused by a deficiency of pancreatic enzymes and that caused by a primary defect in absorption (Kallfelz *et al.*, 1968). If steatorrhea

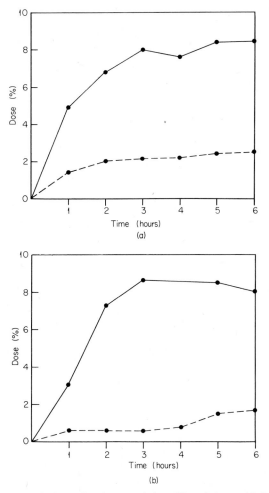

Fig. 10. (a) [^{131}I] Oleic acid absorption in normal dogs (3) and dogs with intestinal malabsorption (2). Absorption is expressed as percent of the dose present in the plasma at intervals following administration. (——) Normal; (———) intestinal malabsorption. (From Kaneko *et al.*, 1965.)   (b) [^{131}I] Triolein absorption in normal dogs (3) and in dogs with intestinal malabsorption (2). Absorption is expressed as percent of the dose present in the plasma at intervals following administration. (——) Normal; (———) intestinal malabsorption. (From Kaneko *et al.*, 1965.)

is caused by a lack of pancreatic lipase, oleic acid absorption will be normal, whereas that of triolein, which requires lipolysis for absorption, will be significantly reduced. The absorption of both compounds is reduced in intestinal malabsorption (Fig. 10a and b). The results of this test also may vary depending on the rate of intestinal motility (Tennant et al., 1969b).

   b. GLUCOSE ABSORPTION.   The absorption of glucose can be measured by means of an oral glucose tolerance test in which a test dose of glucose is given by mouth and the blood glucose level measured at intervals for 3–4 hours following administration. In canine malabsorption, the blood glucose level does not rise normally because of reduced absorption (Kaneko et al., 1965). The major disadvantage of relying on this test alone is that it does not differentiate between decreased intestinal absorption and increased tissue uptake following absorption. This problem can be minimized by comparing results of the oral glucose tolerance test with those obtained with the intravenous tolerance test. The results of these tests, however, must be interpreted carefully and in relation to other clinical and laboratory findings.

   c. D-XYLOSE ABSORPTION.   The absorption of D-xylose also can be used to evaluate intestinal function. D-Xylose is not metabolized by the body to any significant degree and the problems of evaluating tissue utilization which occur with glucose are eliminated. Because of the large amounts of D-xylose used in the test, absorption is independent of active transport processes and the rate of absorption is proportional to luminal concentration.

   A D-xylose absorption test for dogs has been described by Van Kruiningen (1968). In this procedure, a standard 25-gm dose of D-xylose is administered by stomach tube. During the 5-hour period following administration, the dog is confined in a metabolism cage and urine is collected quantitatively. At the end of the 5-hour test period, the urine remaining in the bladder is removed by catheter and the total quantity excreted in 5 hours is determined. Normal dogs excreted an average of 12.2 gm during the test period with a range of 9.1–16.5 gm. The results obtained by this method are dependent not only on the rate of intestinal absorption but also on the rate of renal excretion and it is necessary, therefore, to know that kidney function is normal.

   Recently, we have used an oral xylose tolerance test for the clinical evaluation of intestinal absorption. Dogs are fasted overnight, a blood sample is obtained, and D-xylose is administered by stomach tube at the rate of 0.5 gm/kg. A control test is performed on a normal dog simultaneously with each dog with signs of intestinal malabsorption. The first blood sample is obtained one-half hour after administration. The second sample is obtained 1 hour following administration, and additional samples are taken at hourly intervals for 5 hours. The xylose concentration in the blood is determined by the method of Roe and Rice (1948). Maximum blood levels almost always are reached at 1 hour after administration of the test dose. In preliminary studies of four dogs with the malabsorption syndrome, maximum blood xylose levels averaged 58% of corresponding control values.

D. PROTEIN-LOSING ENTEROPATHY

   Albumin, γ-globulin, and other plasma proteins are present in normal gastrointestinal secretions. Because protein usually undergoes complete degradation within the intestinal lumen, it has been suggested that the gastrointestinal tract must have a physiological role in the catabolism of plasma proteins. The quantitative significance of this pathway, however, has been the subject of considerable controversy. Some investigators have concluded that as much as 50% or more of the normal catabolism of albumin (Glenert et al., 1961, 1962; R. M. Campbell et al., 1961; Wetterfors, 1964, 1965; Wetterfors et al, 1965) and γ-globulin (Andersen et al., 1963) occurs in the gastrointestinal tract. Others believe that the physiological role of the intestine in plasma protein catabolism is far less significant accounting for only about 10% of the total catabolism (Waldmann et al., 1967, 1969; Katz et al., 1960; Franks et al., 1963a,b).

Regardless of the questions of the quantitative role of the gastrointestinal tract in plasma protein catabolism, it is well established that normal intestinal losses are increased significantly in a variety of gastrointestinal diseases which are referred to collectively as *protein-losing enteropathies*. The increased loss causes hypoproteinemia (especially hypoalbuminemia) which may be observed in various types of chronic enteric diseases. The excessive losses are produced by ulcerations or other mucosal changes which alter permeability or by obstruction of lymphatic drainage from the intestine. If severe, hypoalbuminemia may result in retention of fluid with development of ascites and subcutaneous edema of pendant areas.

Excessive plasma protein loss has now been demonstrated in swine with chronic ileitis (Nielsen, 1966), in calves with acute enteric infections (Marsh et al., 1969), in cattle with parasitic or other inflammatory abomasal disease (Halliday et al., 1968; Nielsen and Nansen, 1967) and in Johne's disease (Patterson et al., 1967; Nielsen and Andersen, 1967). In addition to the classical mucosal and submucosal lesions of Johne's disease, Nielsen and Andersen (1967) have demonstrated the presence of secondary intestinal lymphangiectasia. R. S. F. Campbell et al. (1968) recently reported a case of primary canine intestinal lymphangiectasia with hypoalbuminemia. Farrow and Penny (1969) have also reported primary protein-losing enteropathy in the dog. Increased intestinal protein loss is the most likely explanation for the hypoalbuminemia associated with certain other enteric diseases including intestinal malabsorption (Kaneko et al., 1965; Vernon, 1962) and lymphoma of the intestine.

TABLE IV   ALTERATIONS IN SERUM PROTEINS OF DOGS WITH ULCERATIVE COLITIS[a]

	Mean[b] (gm/100 ml)	Range[b] (gm/100 ml)	Normal values[c] (gm/100 ml)
Total serum protein	5.98	4.40–9.10	5.90–6.70
Albumin	2.44	1.14–4.83	3.00–3.70
α-Globulin	0.92	0.39–1.50	0.86
β-Globulin	1.08	0.60–1.86	1.30
γ-Globulin	1.53	0.46–4.60	0.60–0.90
A/G ratio	1.00	0.17–2.45	1.00

[a] Ewing et al. (1969).
[b] 36 observations on 29 affected dogs.
[c] Dimopoullos (1963).

E. CANINE ULCERATIVE COLITIS

Canine ulcerative colitis was described originally in the report of Cello (1964). Since that time, ulcerative colitis and its variant form, granulomatous colitis of Boxer dogs, has been reported by several investigators (Van Kruiningen *et al.*, 1965; Kennedy and Cello, 1966; S. A. Koch and Skelley, 1967; Sander and Langham, 1968). The disease causes chronic, intractable diarrhea which is often hemorrhagic. In addition to diarrhea, afflicted dogs may vomit and are often emaciated. Fever is usually not present.

Biochemical manifestations of ulcerative colitis depend upon duration and severity of illness, degree of colorectal involvement, and the presence of systemic complications. In severe cases of long duration with extensive colorectal involvement, hypoalbuminemia and hyper-γ-globulinemia (Table IV) are sometimes observed. The pathogenesis of hypoalbuminemia probably involves increased loss of plasma through the denuded and inflamed colorectal mucosa. Hyper-γ-globulinemia is probably an associated response to chronic inflammation.

F. DISTURBANCES IN RUMEN FUNCTION

The digestive process of ruminants differs greatly from that of other animals because of microbial digestion and metabolism within the rumen. Short-chain fatty acids—acetic, propionic, and butyric acids—are major end products of rumen fermentation and represent the chief dietary source of energy for ruminants (Hungate *et al.*, 1961). The polysaccharide cellulose, which is not digested by most simple-stomached animals, is readily utilized by ruminants because of the activity of cellulytic bacteria. Significant quantities of nonprotein nitrogen can also be utilized for protein synthesis by ruminal bacteria, and the bacterial protein subsequently used to meet the protein requirements of the animal. Maintenance of bacterial fermentation within the rumen also presents certain unusual hazards to ruminant animals. When rapid changes in food intake occur, the products of fermentation can be released more rapidly than they can be removed. Acute rumen tympany and acute rumen indigestion are diseases which result from such abrupt changes in diet (Hungate, 1966, 1968).

1. Acute Rumen Indigestion (Rumen Overload)

Acute rumen indigestion occurs in sheep or cattle on a high roughage diet when they inadvertently are allowed access to large amounts of readily fermentable carbohydrate such as grain. *Streptococcus bovis* is the rumen microorganism chiefly responsible for rapid fermentation and for production of large quantities of lactic acid (Hungate *et al.* 1952; Krogh, 1963a,b).

As lactic acid accumulates, the rumen pH falls and rumen atony develops. The excessive lactic acid produced results in development of metabolic acidosis with significant reduction in plasma bicarbonate ion concentration. The urine pH may fall from a normal value of 8.0 to as low as 5.0. Fluid continues to accumulate in the rumen causing hemoconcentration which may lead ultimately to hypovolemic shock and death (Hyldgaard-Jensen and Simesen, 1966). If affected animals survive the initial period of explosive fermentation, a chemical rumenitis, caused by lactic acid, may develop. Secondary mycotic rumenitis may also occur and be fatal. Hepatic abscesses also may result from severe rumenitis.

2.   Acute Rumen Tympany (Bloat)

The rumen of mature cattle can produce 1.2–2.0 liters gas/min (Hungate et al., 1965). The gas is composed primarily of carbon dioxide and methane which are products of rumen fermentation. Carbon dioxide is also released when salivary bicarbonate is acted upon by organic acids within the rumen. Under normal conditions, these large amounts of gas are continually removed by eructation.

Any factor which interferes with eructation can produce acute tympany of the rumen (bloat) leading to rapid death. Interruption of the normal eructation reflex or mechanical obstruction of the esophagus are examples. Bloat is most frequently observed, however, in cattle consuming large quantities of fresh legumes or in feedlot cattle on high concentrate rations. The primary factor in these more common types of bloat is a change in the ruminal contents to a foamy or frothy character. Gas is trapped in small bubbles within the rumen and cannot be eliminated by eructation.

The chemical changes which cause foam to form within the rumen are not completely clear. Recent reports (Nichols, 1966; Nichols and Deese, 1966) suggest that plant pectin and pectin methyl esterase, an enzyme system also from plants, are critical factors. The enzyme acts on pectin to release pectic and galacturonic acids which greatly increase the viscosity of the rumen fluid resulting in formation of a highly stable foam. Slime-producing bacteria also have been incriminated in the pathogenesis of frothy bloat. These microorganisms produce an extracellular polysaccharide which results in stable foam formation.

Effective medical treatment and control are directed toward decreasing or preventing foam formation. This has been accomplished with certain nonionic detergents with surfactant properties which break up or prevent formation of foam within the rumen (Bartley, 1965). Another approach has been the prophylactic administration of sodium alkylaryl sulfonate which inhibits pectin methyl esterase activity, preventing foam formation by eliminating the products of this enzyme reaction (Nichols, 1963).

ACKNOWLEDGMENTS

The authors wish to express their appreciation to Mrs. Doris Harrold, Mrs. Jan Philbrick, and Mr. Mario Reina-Guerra who helped prepare this chapter.

REFERENCES

Abrams, R., and Brooks, F. P. (1960). Proc. Soc. Exptl. Biol. Med. **104**, 278.
Ailhaud, G., Samuel, D., Lazdunski, M., and Desnuelle, P. (1964). Biochim. Biophys. Acta **84**, 643.
Alpers, D. H. (1969). J. Biol. Chem. **244**, 1238.
Alpers, D. H., and Isselbacher, K. J. (1967). J. Biol. Chem. **242**, 5617.
Altamirano, M. (1963). J. Physiol. (London) **168**, 787.
Alvarado, F. (1966a). Science **151**, 1010.
Alvarado, F. (1966b). Biochim. Biophys. Acta **112**, 292.

Alvarado, F., and Crane, R. K. (1962). *Biochim. Biophys. Acta* **56**, 170.

Andersen, S. B., Glenert, J., and Wallevik, K. (1963), *J. Clin. Invest.* **42**, 1873.

Anderson, J. C., Barton, M. A., Gregory, R. A., Hardy, P. M., Kenner, G. W., Macleod, J. K., Preston, J., Sheppard, R. C., and Morley, J. S. (1964). *Nature* **204**, 933.

Anderson, N. V., and Low, D. G. (1965a). *Animal Hosp.* **1**, 101.

Anderson, N. V., and Low, D. G. (1965b). *Animal Hosp.* **1**, 189.

Auricchio, S., Semenza, G., and Rubino, A. (1965). *Biochim. Biophys. Acta* **96**, 498.

Bachrach, W. H. (1953). *Physiol. Rev.* **33**, 566.

Barry, B. A., Matthews, J., and Smyth, D. H. (1961). *J. Physiol.* **157**, (*London*) 279.

Bartley, E. E. (1965). *J. Am. Vet. Med. Assoc.* **147**, 1397.

Bell, N. H. (1966). *Proc. Soc. Exptl. Biol. Med.* **123**, 529.

Ben Abdeljlil, A., and Desnuelle, P. (1964). *Biochim. Biophys. Acta* **81**, 136.

Benzonana, G., and Desnuelle, P. (1965). *Biochim. Biophys. Acta* **105**, 121.

Berger, E. Y., Kanzaki, G., Homer, M. A., and Steele, J. M. (1959). *Am. J. Physiol.* **196**, 74.

Bertolini, M., and Pigman, W. (1967). *J. Biol. Chem.* **242**, 3776.

Bhavanandan, V. P., Buddecke, E., Carubelli, R., and Gottschalk, A. (1964). *Biochem. Biophys. Res. Commun.* **16**, 353.

Bieri, J. G., and Pollard, C. J. (1954). *Brit. J. Nutr.* **8**, 32.

Bihler, I., and Crane, R. K. (1962). *Biochim. Biophys. Acta* **59**, 78.

Bihler, I., Hawkins, K. A., and Crane, R. K. (1962). *Biochim. Biophys. Acta* **59**, 94.

Bloom, B., Chaikoff, I. L., and Reinhardt, W. O. (1951). *Am. J. Physiol.* **166**, 451.

Bodanszky, A., Ondetti, M. A., Mutt, V., and Bodanszky, M. (1969). *J. Am. Chem. Soc.* **91**, 944.

Borgström, B. (1954). *Biochim. Biophys. Acta* **13**, 149.

Borgström, B. (1964a). *J. Lipid Res.* **5**, 522.

Borgström, B. (1964b). *Biochim Biophys. Acta* **106**, 171.

Borgström, B., Dahlqvist, A., Gustafsson, B. E., Lundh, G., and Malmquist, J. (1959). *Proc. Soc. Exptl. Biol. Med.* **102**, 154.

Boucher, W. B., and Abt, D. (1968). *J. Am. Vet. Med. Assoc.* **153**, 76.

Brambell, F. W. R. (1958). *Biol. Rev.* **33**, 488.

Bremer, J. (1956). *Biochem. J.* **63**, 507.

Brindley, D. N., and Hübscher, G. (1965). *Biochim. Biophys. Acta* **106**, 495.

Bro-Rasmussen, F., Killmann, S.-A., and Thaysen, J. H. (1956). *Acta Physiol. Scand.* **37**, 97.

Brown, J. R., and Hartley, B. S. (1966). *Biochem. J.* **101**, 214.

Bywater, R. J., and Penhale, W. J. (1969). *Res. Vet. Sci.* **10**, 591.

Campbell, R. M., Cuthbertson, D. P., Mackie, W., McFarlane, A. S., Phillipson, A. T., and Sudsaneh, S. (1961). *J. Physiol. (London)* **158**, 113.

Campbell, R. S. F., Brobst, D. F., and Bisgard, G. (1968). *J. Am. Vet. Med. Assoc.* **153**, 1050.

Cello, R. M. (1964). *Mod. Vet. Pract.* **45**, 35.

Clark, B., and Hübscher, G. (1960). *Nature* **185**, 35.

Clark, B., and Hübscher, G. (1961). *Biochim. Biophys. Acta* **46**, 479.

Clark, B., and Hübscher, G. (1962). *Nature* **195**, 599.

Clarkson, T. W., Cross, A. C., and Toole, S. R. (1961). *Am. J. Physiol.* **200**, 1233.

Code, C. F., Bass, P., McClary, G. B., Newnum, R. L., and Orvis, A. L. (1960). *Am. J. Physiol.* **199**, 281.

Cori, C. F. (1925). *J. Biol. Chem.* **66**, 691.

Crane, R. K. (1965). *Federation Proc.* **24**, 1000.

Crane, R. K., Forstner, G., and Eichholz, A. (1965). *Biochim. Biophys. Acta* **109**, 467.

Csáky, T. Z. (1961). *Am. J. Physiol.* **201**, 999.

Csáky, T. Z. (1963). *Federation Proc.* **22**, 3.

Csáky, T. Z., and Hara, Y. (1965). *Am. J. Physiol.* **209**, 467.

Csáky, T. Z., and Ho, P. M. (1966). *Life Sci.* **5**, 1025.

Csáky, T. Z., and Lassen, U. V. (1964). *Biochim. Biophys. Acta* **82**, 215.

Curran, P. F. (1960). *J. Gen. Physiol.* **43**, 1137.

Curran, P. F. (1965). *Federation Proc.* **24**, 993.

Curran, P. F., and Schultz, S. G. (1968). *In* "Handbook of Physiology" (Am. Physiol. Soc., J. Field, ed.), Sect. 6, Vol. III, p. 1217. Williams & Wilkins, Baltimore, Maryland.

Dahlqvist, A. (1961). *Nature* **190**, 31.

Dalton, R. G., Fisher, E. W., and McIntyre, W. I. M. (1965). *Brit. Vet. J.* **121**, 34.

Danforth, E., and Moore, R. O. (1959). *Endocrinology* **65**, 118.

Danielsson, H. (1963). *Advan. Lipid Res.* **1**, 335.

Darrow, D. C. (1964). "A Guide to Learning Fluid Therapy." Thomas, Springfield, Illinois.

Davenport, H. W. (1966). "Physiology of the Digestive Tract," 2nd ed. Year Book Publ., Chicago, Illinois.

Davie, E. W., and Neurath, H. (1955). *J. Biol. Chem.* **212**, 515.

Dawson, A. M., and Isselbacher, K. J. (1960). *J. Clin. Invest.* **39**, 150.

Deutsch, H. F., and Smith, V. R. (1957). *Am. J. Physiol.* **191**, 271.

Dietschy, J. M., Salomon, H. S., and Siperstein, M. D. (1966). *J. Clin. Invest.* **45**, 832.

Dimopoullos, G. T. (1963). *In* "Clinical Biochemistry of Domestic Animals" (C. E. Cornelius and J. J. Kaneko, eds.), p. 109. Academic Press, New York.

Dowling, J. E., and Wald, G. (1958). *Proc. Natl. Acad. Sci. U.S.* **44**, 648.

Drummey, G. D., Benson, J. A., and Jones, C. M. (1961). *New Engl. J. Med.* **264**, 85.

Dukes, H. H. (1955). "The Physiology of Domestic Animals," 7th ed. Cornell Univ. Press (Comstock), Ithaca, New York.

Eichholz, A. (1967). *Biochim. Biophys. Acta* **135**, 475.

Eichholz, A. (1968). *Biochim. Biophys. Acta* **163**, 101.

Eichholz, A., and Crane, R. K. (1965). *J. Cell Biol.* **26**, 687.

Emas, S., and Grossman, M. I. (1967). *Gastroenterology* **52**, 29.

Espersen, G. (1961). *Nord. Veterinarmed* **13**, Suppl. I, p. 7.

Espersen, G., and Simesen, M. G. (1961). *Nord. Veterinarmed* **13**, 147.

Ewing, G. O., Gomez, J. A., and Cello, R. M. (1969). Unpublished data.

Farrow, B. R. H., and Penny, R. (1969). *J. Small Animal Pract.* **10**, 513.

Faust, R. G., Wu, S. L., and Faggard, M. L. (1967). *Science* **155**, 1261.

Fisher, E. W. (1965). *Brit. Vet. J.* **121**, 132.

Fisher, E. W., and McEwan, A. D. (1967). *Brit. Vet. J.* **123**, 4.

Fisher, R. B., and Parsons, D. S. (1953). *J. Physiol. (London)* **119**, 224.

Floch, M. H. (1969). *Am. J. Clin. Nutr.* **22**, 327.

Fordtran, J. S., Rector, F. C., and Carter, N. W. (1968). *J. Clin. Invest.* **47**, 884.

Forstner, C. G., Sabesin, S. M., and Isselbacher, K. J. (1968). *Biochem. J.* **106**, 381.

Frankland, A. L. (1969). *J. Small Animal Pract.* **10**, 531.

Franks, J. J., Mosser, E. L., and Anstadt, G. L. (1963a). *J. Gen. Physiol.* **46**, 415.

Franks, J. J., Edwards, K. W., Lackey, W. W., and Fitzgerald, J. B. (1963b). *J. Gen. Physiol.* **46**, 427.

Ganguly, J., and Murthy, S. K. (1967). *In* "The Vitamins" (W. H. Sebrell, Jr. and R. S. Harris, eds.), 2nd ed., Vol. 1, p. 125. Academic Press, New York.

Gilman, A., and Koelle, E. S. (1960). *Am. J. Physiol.* **199**, 1025.

Glenert, J., Jarnum, S., and Riemer, S. (1961). *Acta Chir. Scand.* **121**, 242.

Glenert, J., Jarnum, S., and Riemer, S. (1962). *Acta Chir. Scand.* **124**, 63.

Gottschalk, A. (1966). *In* "Glycoproteins. Their Composition, Structure, and Function" (A. Gottschalk, ed.), p. 20, Elsevier, Amsterdam.

Gottschalk, A., and Fazekas de St. Groth, S. (1960). *Biochim. Biophys. Acta* **43**, 513.

Gottschalk, A., and Thomas, M. A. W. (1961). *Biochim Biophys. Acta* **46**, 91.

Gray, J. S., and Bucher, G. R. (1941). *Am. J. Physiol.* **133**, 542.

Gregory, R. A. (1966). *Gastroenterology* **51**, 953.

Gregory, R. A. (1967). *In* "Handbook of Physiology" (Am. Physiol. Soc., J. Field, ed.) Sect. 6, Vol. II, p. 827. Williams & Wilkins, Baltimore, Maryland.

Gregory, R. A., and Tracy, H. J. (1964). *Gut* **5**, 103.

Gregory, R. A., Hardy, P. M., Jones, D. S., Kenner, G. W., and Sheppard, R. C. (1964). *Nature* **204**, 931.

Grim, E. (1962). *Am. J. Digest. Diseases* **7**, 17.

Grossman, M. I. (1958). *Gastroenterology* **34**, 1159.

Grossman, M. I. (1962). *Proc. Soc. Exptl. Biol. Med.* **110**, 41.

Gustafsson, B. E., and Norman, A. (1962). *Proc. Soc. Exptl. Biol. Med.* **110**, 387.

Gustafsson, B. E., and Norman, A. (1969a). *Brit. J. Nutr.* **23**, 429.

Gustafsson, B. E., and Norman, A. (1969b). *Brit. J. Nutr.* **23**, 627.

Gustafsson, B. E., Bergström, S., Lindstedt, S., and Norman, A. (1957). *Proc. Soc. Exptl. Biol. Med.* **94**, 467.

Gustafsson, B. E., Midtvedt, T., and Norman, A. (1966). *J. Exptl. Med.* **123**, 413.

Haden, R. L., and Orr, T. G. (1923). *J. Exptl. Med.* **37**, 377.

Haden, R. L., and Orr, T. G. (1924). *J. Exptl. Med.* **38**, 55.

Haessler, H. A., and Isselbacher, K. J. (1963). *Biochim. Biophys. Acta* **73**, 427.

Hakim, A. A., and Lifson, N. (1964). *Am. J. Physiol.* **206**, 1315.

Hakim, A., Lester, R. G., and Lifson, N. (1963). *J. Appl. Physiol.* **18**, 409.

Halliday, G. J., Mulligan, W., and Dalton, R. G. (1968). *Res. Vet. Sci.* **9**, 224.

Harris, J. B., and Edelman, I. S. (1964). *Am. J. Physiol.* **206**, 769.

Hartley, B. S., and Kauffman, D. L. (1966). *Biochem. J.* **101**, 229.

Hartley, B. S., Brown, J. R., Kauffman, D. L., and Smillie, L. B. (1965). *Nature* **207**, 1157.

Hartman, P. A., Hays, V. W., Baker, R. O., Neagle, L. H., and Catron, D. V. (1961). *J. Animal Sci.* **20**, 114.

Haslewood, G. A. D. (1964). *Biol. Rev.* **39**, 537.

Hatch, F. T., Aso, Y., Hagopian, L. M., and Rubenstein, J. J. (1966). *J. Biol. Chem.* **241**. 1655.

Heersma, J. R., and Annegers, J. H. (1948). *Am. J. Physiol.* **153**, 143.

Heizer, W. D., and Laster, L. (1969). *Biochim. Biophys. Acta* **185**, 409.

Herriott, R. M. (1938). *J. Gen. Physiol.* **21**, 501.

Herriott, R. M. (1962). *J. Gen. Physiol.* **45**, 57.

Hindle, W., and Code, C. F. (1962). *Am. J. Physiol.* **203**, 215.

Hirschowitz, B. I. (1966). *Am. J. Digest. Diseases* **11**, 183.

Hirschowitz, B. I., and Sachs, G. (1965). *Am. J. Physiol.* **209**, 452.

Hjerpe, C., and Tennant, B. (1968). Unpublished observations.

Hladky, S. B. (1965). *Bull. Math. Biophys.* **27**, 79.

Hofmann, A. F. (1963). *Biochem. J.* **89**, 57.

Hofmann, A. F. (1966). *Gastroenterology* **50**, 56.

Hofmann. A. F., and Small, D. M. (1967). *Ann. Rev. Med.* **18**, 333.

Hsu, L., and Tappel, A. L. (1965). *Biochim. Biophys. Acta* **101**, 83.

Huber, J. T., Jacobson, N. L., Allen, R. S., and Hartman, P. A. (1961). *J. Dairy Sci.* **44**, 1494.

Hungate, R. E. (1966). "The Rumen and its Microbes." Academic Press, New York.

Hungate, R. E. (1968). *In* "Handbook of Physiology" (Am. Physiol. Soc., J. Field, Ed.), Sect. 6, Vol. V, p. 2725. Williams & Wilkins, Baltimore, Maryland.

Hungate, R. E., Dougherty, R. W., Bryant, M. P., and Cello, R. M. (1952). *Cornell Vet.* **42**, 423.

Hungate, R. E., Mah, R. A., and Simesen, M. (1961). *Appl. Microbiol.* **9**, 554.

Hungate, R. E., Fletcher, D. W., Dougherty, R. W., and Barrentine, B. F. (1965). *Appl. Microbiol.* **13**, 161.

Hyldgaard-Jensen, J., and Simesen, M. G. (1966). *Nord. Veterinarmed.* **18**, 73.

Ingraham, R. C., and Visscher, M. B. (1936). *Am. J. Physiol.* **114**, 676.

Isselbacher, K. J. (1966). *Gastroenterology* **50**, 78.

Isselbacher, K. J. (1967). *Federation Proc.* **26**, 1420.

Isselbacher, K. J., and Budz, D. M. (1963). *Nature* **200**, 364.

Janowitz, H. D., Colcher, H., and Hollander, F. (1952). *Am. J. Physiol.* **171**, 325.

Jasper, D. E. (1954). *North Am. Vet.* **35**, 523.

Jeffries, G. H., Weser, E., and Sleisenger, M. H. (1969). *Gastroenterology* **56**, 777.

Johnston, J. M. (1968). *In* "Handbook of Physiology" (Am. Physiol. Soc., J. Field, ed.), Sect. 6, Vol. III, p. 1353. Williams & Wilkins, Baltimore, Maryland.

Johnston, J. M., and Borgström, B. (1964). *Biochim. Biophys. Acta* **84**, 412.

Kallfelz, F. A., Norrdin, R. W., and Neal, T. M. (1968). *J. Am. Vet. Med. Assoc.* **153**, 43.

Kalser, M. H. (1964). *In* "Gastroenterology" (H. L. Bockus, ed.), Vol. II, p. 423. Saunders, Philadelphia, Pennsylvania.

Kaneko, J. J., Moulton, J. E., Brodey, R. S., and Perryman, V. D. (1965). *J. Am. Vet. Med. Assoc.* **146**, 463.

Katz, J., Rosenfeld, S., and Sellers, A. L. (1960). *Am. J. Physiol.* **200**, 1301.

Keller, P. J. (1968). *In* "Handbook of Physiology" (Am. Physiol. Soc., J. Field, ed.), Sect. 6, Vol. V, p. 2605. Williams & Wilkins, Baltimore, Maryland.

Kennedy, P. C., and Cello, R. M. (1966). *Gastroenterology* **51**, 926.
Kern, F., and Borgström, B. (1965). *Biochim. Biophys. Acta* **98**, 520.
Koch, A. R., Brazeau, P., and Gilman, A. (1956). *Am. J. Physiol.* **186**, 350.
Koch, S. A., and Skelley, J. F. (1967). *J. Am. Vet. Med. Assoc.* **150**, 22.
Kohler, E. M. (1968). *Am. J. Vet. Res.* **29**, 2263.
Kohn, P., Dawes, E. D., and Duke, J. W. (1965). *Biochim. Biophys. Acta* **107**, 358.
Kolínská, J., and Semenza, G. (1967). *Biochim. Biophys. Acta* **146**, 181.
Krogh, N. (1963a). *Acta Vet. Scand.* **4**, 27.
Krogh, N. (1963b). *Acta Vet. Scand.* **4**, 41.
Lack, L., and Weiner, I. M. (1961). *Am. J. Physiol.* **200**, 313.
Lack, L., and Weiner, I. M. (1963). *Federation Proc.* **22**, 1334.
Lack, L., and Weiner, I. M. (1966). *Am. J. Physiol.* **210**, 1142.
Laskowski, M., Haessler, H. A., Miech, R. P., Peanasky, R. J., and Laskowski, M. (1958). *Science* **127**, 1115.
Laurent, T. C., and Persson, H. (1965). *Biochim Biophys. Acta* **106**, 616.
Leaf, A., and Santos, R. F. (1961). *New Engl. J. Med.* **264**, 335.
Lecce, J. G. (1966). *Biol. Neonatorum* [N.S.] **9**, 50.
Lecce, J. G., and Morgan, D. O. (1962). *J. Nutr.* **78**, 263.
Lecce, J. G., Morgan, D. O., and Matrone, G. (1964). *J. Nutr.* **84**, 43.
Levenson, S. M., Rosen, H., and Upjohn, H. L. (1959). *Proc. Soc. Exptl. Biol. Med.* **101**, 178.
Lindemann, B., and Solomon, A. K. (1962). *J. Gen. Physiol.* **45**, 801.
Lindstedt, S., and Samuelsson, B. (1959). *J. Biol. Chem.* **234**, 2026.
McGuire, E. J., and Roseman, S. (1967). *J. Biol. Chem.* **242**, 3745.
Mahadevan, S., Sastry, P. S., and Ganguly, J. (1963). *Biochem. J.* **88**, 531.
Mahadevan, S., Ayyoub, N. I., and Roels, O. A. (1966). *J. Biol. Chem.* **241**, 57.
Malathi, P. (1967). *Gastroenterology* **52**, 1106.
Marsh, C. L., Mebus, C. A., and Underdahl, N. R. (1969). *Am. J. Vet. Res.* **30**, 163.
Matthews, D. M., and Laster, L. (1965). *Gut* **6**, 411.
Mattson, F. H., and Volpenhein, R. A. (1962). *J. Lipid Res.* **3**, 281.
Mattson, F. H., and Volpenhein, R. A. (1964). *J. Biol. Chem.* **239**, 2772.
Mattson, F. H., and Volpenhein, R. A. (1966). *J. Lipid Res.* **7**, 536.
Mattson, F. H., Benedict, J. H., Martin, J. B., and Beck, L. W. (1952). *J. Nutr.* **48**, 335.
Michaelson, S. M., El-Tamami, M. Y., Thomson, R. A. E., and Howland, J. W. (1960). *Am. J. Vet. Res.* **21**, 364.
Midtvedt, T., and Norman, A. (1967). *Acta Pathol. Microbiol. Scand.* **71**, 629.
Murthy, S. K., and Ganguly, J. (1962). *Biochem. J.* **83**, 460.
Mutt, V., and Jorpes, J. E. (1967). *Recent Progr. Hormone Res.* **23**, 483.
Nasset, E. S., and Ju, J. S. (1961). *J. Nutr.* **74**, 461.
Neurath, H., Rupley, J. A., and Dreyer, W. J. (1956). *Arch. Biochem. Biophys.* **65**, 243.
Newey, H., and Smyth, D. H. (1959). *J. Physiol.* (*London*) **145**, 48.
Newey, H., and Smyth, D. H. (1960). *J. Physiol.* (*London*) **152**, 367.
Newey, H., and Smyth, D. H. (1964). *Nature* **202**, 400.
Nichols, R. E. (1963). *J. Am. Vet. Med. Assoc.* **143**, 998.
Nichols, R. E. (1966). *Am. J. Vet. Res.* **27**, 369.
Nichols, R. E., and Deese, D. (1966). *Am. J. Vet. Res.* **27**, 623.
Nielsen, K. (1966). *Acta Vet. Scand.* **7**, 321.
Nielsen, K., and Andersen, S. (1967). *Nord. Veterinarmed.* **19**, 31.
Nielsen, K., and Nansen, P. (1967). *Can. J. Comp. Med. Vet. Sci.* **31**, 106.
Ockner, R. K., Hughes, F. B., and Isselbacher, K. J. (1969). *J. Clin. Invest.* **48**, 2367.
Olson, J. A. (1961). *J. Biol. Chem.* **236**, 349.
Palay, S. L., and Karlin, L. J. (1959). *J. Biophys. Biochem. Cytol.* **5**, 363.
Parsons, B. J., Smyth, D. H., and Taylor, C. B. (1958). *J. Physiol.* (*London*) **144**, 387.
Parsons, D. S., and Wingate, D. L. (1961). *Biochim. Biophys. Acta* **46**, 170.
Patterson, D. S. P., Allen, W. M., and Lloyd, M. K. (1967). *Vet. Record* **81**, 717.
Patterson, D. S. P., Allen, W. M., Berrett, S., Ivins, L. N., and Sweasey, D. (1968). *Res. Vet. Sci.* **9**, 117.

Payne, L. C., and Marsh, C. L. (1962a). *J. Nutr.* **76**, 151.
Payne, L. C., and Marsh, C. L. (1962b). *Federation Proc.* **21**, 909.
Peric-Golia, L., and Socic, H. (1968). *Am. J. Physiol.* **215**, 1284.
Phillips, R. W., and Knox, K. L. (1969). *J. Comp. Lab. Med.* **3**, 1.
Playoust, M. R., and Isselbacher, K. J. (1964). *J. Clin. Invest.* **43**, 878.
Playoust, M. R., Lack, L., and Weiner, I. M. (1965). *Am. J. Physiol.* **208**, 363.
Powell, D. W., Malawer, S. J., and Plotkin, G. R. (1968). *Am. J. Physiol.* **215**, 1226.
Rao, G. A., and Johnston, J. M. (1966). *Biochim. Biophys. Acta* **125**, 465.
Redman, C. M., Siekevitz, P., and Palade, G. E. (1966). *J. Biol. Chem.* **241**, 1150.
Rhodes, J. B., Eichholz, A., and Crane, R. K. (1967). *Biochim. Biophys. Acta* **135**, 959.
Riklis, E., and Quastel, J. H. (1958). *Can. J. Biochem. Physiol.* **36**, 347.
Roe, J. H., and Rice, E. W. (1948). *J. Biol. Chem.* **173**, 507.
Ryle, A. P. (1965). *Biochem. J.* **96**, 6.
Ryle, A. P., and Hamilton, M. P. (1966). *Biochem. J.* **101**, 176.
Ryle, A. P., and Porter, R. R. (1959). *Biochem. J.* **73**, 75.
Sabesin, S. M., and Isselbacher, K. J. (1965). *Science* **147**, 1149.
Sander, C. H., and Langham, R. F. (1968). *A. M. A. Arch. Pathol.* **85**, 94.
Sarda, L., and Desnuelle, P. (1958). *Biochim. Biophys. Acta* **30**, 513.
Sari, H., Entressangles, B., and Desnuelle, P. (1966). *Biochim. Biophys. Acta* **125**, 597.
Saunders, S. J., and Isselbacher, K. J. (1965). *Biochim. Biophys. Acta* **102**, 397.
Saunders, S. J., and Isselbacher, K. J. (1966). *Gastroenterology* **50**, 586.
Schachter, D., Finkelstein, J. D., and Kowarski, S. (1964). *J. Clin. Invest.* **43**, 787.
Schultz, S. G., and Zalusky, R. (1964). *J. Gen. Physiol.* **47**, 1043.
Senior, J. R., and Isselbacher, K. J. (1962). *J. Biol. Chem.* **237**, 1454.
Skála, I., and Hrubá, F. (1964). *Am. J. Physiol.* **206**, 458.
Skou, J. C. (1965). *Physiol. Rev.* **45**, 596.
Smith, H. W., and Halls, S. (1967). *J. Pathol. Bacteriol.* **93**, 531.
Strauss, E. W. (1966). *J. Lipid Res.* **7**, 307.
Tasker, J. B. (1967). *Cornell Vet.* **57**, 668.
Taylor, W. H. (1959a). *Biochem. J.* **71**, 73.
Taylor, W. H. (1959b). *Biochem. J.* **71**, 373.
Taylor, W. H. (1968). *In* "Handbook of Physiology" (Am. Physiol. Soc., J. Field., ed.), Sect. 6, Vol. V, p. 2567. Williams & Wilkins, Baltimore, Maryland.
Tennant, B., Harrold, D., and Reina-Guerra, M. (1968). *Cornell Vet.* **58**, 136.
Tennant, B., Harrold, D., Reina-Guerra, M., and Laben, R. C. (1969a). *Am. J. Vet. Res.* **30**, 345.
Tennant, B., Reina-Guerra, M., Harrold, D., and Goldman, M. (1969b). *J. Nutr.* **97**, 65.
Tennant, B., Harrold, D., and Reina-Guerra, M. (1970). Unpublished data.
Thompson, G. R., Ockner, R. K., and Isselbacher, K. J. (1969). *J. Clin. Invest.* **48**, 87.
Thompson, J. C. (1969). *Ann. Rev. Med.* **20**, 291.
Tracy, H. J., and Gregory, R. A. (1964). *Nature* **204**, 935.
Turner, D. A. (1958). *Am. J. Digest. Diseases* **3**, 594.
Ugolev, A. M. (1965). *Physiol. Rev.* **45**, 555.
Ussing, H. H. (1947). *Nature* **160**, 262.
Vahouny, G. V., and Treadwell, C. R. (1964). *Proc. Soc. Exptl. Biol. Med.* **116**, 496.
Vahouny, G. V., Weersing, S., and Treadwell, C. R. (1965). *Biochim. Biophys. Acta* **98**, 607.
Vallee, B. L., Stein, E. A., Summerwell, W. N., and Fischer, E. H. (1959). *J. Biol. Chem.* **234**, 2901.
van de Kamer, J. H., ten Bokkel Huinink, H., and Weyers, H. A. (1949). *J. Biol. Chem.* **177**, 347.
Van Kruiningen, H. J. (1968). *In* "Current Veterinary Therapy" (R. W. Kirk, ed.), 3rd ed., p. 521. Saunders, Philadelphia, Pennsylvania.
Van Kruiningen, H. J., Mohtali, R. J., Strandberg, J. D., and Kirk, R. W. (1965). *Pathol. Vet. (Basel)* **2**, 521.
Vernon, D. F. (1962). *J. Am. Vet. Med. Assoc.* **140**, 1062.
Waldmann, T. A., Morell, A. G., Wochner, R. D., Strober, W., and Sternlieb, I. (1967). *J. Clin. Invest.* **46**, 10.
Waldmann, T. A., Wochner, R. D., and Strober, W. (1969). *Am. J. Med.* **46**, 275.
Walker, D. M. (1959). *J. Agr. Sci.* **52**, 357.

Wasserman, R. H., and Taylor, A. N. (1966). *Science* **152**, 791.

Wasserman, R. H., and Taylor, A. N. (1968). *J. Biol. Chem.* **243**, 3987.

Wasserman, R. H., Corradino, R. A., and Taylor, A. N. (1968). *J. Biol. Chem.* **243**, 3978.

Weiner, I. M., and Lack, L. (1962). *Am. J. Physiol.* **202**, 155.

Weiner, I. M., and Lack, L. (1968). *In* "Handbook of Physiology" (Am. Physiol. Soc., J. Field, ed.), Sect. 6, Vol. III, p. 1439. Williams & Wilkins, Baltimore, Maryland.

Wells, M. H., Shingleton, W. W., and Saunders, A. P. (1955). *Proc. Soc. Exptl. Biol. Med.* **90**, 717.

Wetterfors, J. (1964). *Acta Med. Scand.* **176**, 787.

Wetterfors, J. (1965). *Acta Med. Scand.* **177**, 243.

Wetterfors, J., Liljedahl, S.-O., Plantin, L.-O., and Birke, G. (1965). *Acta Med. Scand.* **177**, 227

Wheeler, H. O., and Mancusi-Ungaro, P. L. (1966). *Am. J. Physiol.* **210**, 1153.

Wiggans, D. S., and Johnston, J. M. (1959). *Biochim. Biophys. Acta* **32**, 69.

Wilson, T. H. (1962). "Intestinal Absorption." Saunders, Philadelphia, Pennsylvania.

Windmueller, H. G., and Levy, R. I. (1968). *J. Biol. Chem.* **243**, 4878.

Wiseman, G. (1968). *In* "Handbook of Physiology" (Am. Physiol. Soc. J. Field, ed.), Sect. 6, Vol. III, p. 1277. Williams & Wilkins, Baltimore, Maryland.

Wollenweber, J., Kottke, B. A., and Owen, C. A., Jr. (1965). *Clin. Res.* **13**, 410.

Zachman, R. D., and Olson, J. A. (1963). *J. Biol. Chem.* **238**, 541.

Zilversmit, D. B. (1965). *J. Clin. Invest.* **44**, 1610.

4   Skeletal Muscle

George H. Cardinet, III

I. INTRODUCTION

The skeletal muscle mass comprises 30–50% of the body weight; hence skeletal muscle cells (fibers) constitute the largest mass of cells in the body which have similar morphological and physiological properties. The protoplasmic properties of contractility and conductility which characterize the muscle fiber are the expression of the functional properties of the sarcoplasmic organelles. Studies of the muscle fiber have provided excellent examples of the integration of form and function whereby molecular and organelle structure and function can be directly related to cellular morphology and function, which in turn can be related to the morphology and function of the organ and organism.

Owing to the contractile property of the skeletal muscle fiber, the function of skeletal muscle is generally described to be contraction. This definition of skeletal muscle function is of course correct, but it represents an oversimplification and unfortunately has resulted too often in the view that all muscles of the body are a homogeneous mass of contractile cells. Skeletal muscles of the body might more appropriately be considered as organs. The resultant action of contraction differs between muscles of the body, and the precise manner in which different muscles contract also differs. In addition, skeletal muscles differ in their vascular supply, nerve supply, and constituent fiber populations, all of which confer differences in their morphology and function. Singly, or in concert with other muscles, skeletal muscles function in virtually all systems of the body.

An attempt will be made in this chapter to outline the great diversity that exists in skeletal muscle. By so doing, it is hoped that the knowledge and techniques developed, especially during the past 20 years, will find their rightful introduction and application into neuromuscular disorders of clinical veterinary medicine.

There are, no doubt, numerous neuromuscular disorders in domestic animals that are still unrecognized and the observations made almost 20 years ago by Innes (1951) seem worthy of citing here.

> ... I have drawn attention before to the fact that no diseases are recognized until they are found by looking with great care. One need only scan the veterinary literature of the last twenty years for this to be confirmed, and a long list of conditions could be compiled which might have been discovered years previously if more meticulous methods of pathological examinations had been used. Veterinary pathology has still a long road to travel before it achieves the profundity of human pathology, and this is not said in any deprecatory sense of past achievements. There are many reasons why this is so, but lack of volume of material studied and inattention to the lessons to be learnt from medical work have played a part. In veterinary work, unfortunately, also the question of economics always intrudes, and in the end we are constantly influenced by a consideration of what is, or is not, important.
>
> In conducting autopsy examinations of animals there is usually an immense amount of bias in selection of tissues for histological work; in the case of skeletal muscles (from my own experience) no doubt they are mostly ignored unless macroscopical changes are very obvious. Perhaps this article may help to focus attention on the pathology of muscular disorders.

Since 1951, some advances have been made. Most notable have been the comparative biomedical investigations resulting from the recognition and description of hereditary muscular dystrophies in the mouse (Michelson et al., 1955), chicken (Asmundson and Julian, 1956), and hamster (Homburger et al., 1962). However, in domestic animals which are more usually considered of clinical importance, the status of neuromuscular disease remains essentially unchanged.

II.   THE SARCOPLASMIC ORGANELLES AND MUSCULAR CONTRACTION

A. EXCITATION–CONDUCTION

The morphology of skeletal muscle will not be extensively reviewed here and the reader is referred to any current histology text for details (e.g., Bloom and Fawcett, 1968; Ham, 1969). The cell or plasma membrane of the skeletal muscle fiber (sarcolemma) is specialized for conduction. A specialization of the sarcolemma exists at the site of union between the muscle fiber and its motor neuron, the myoneural junction. Associated with the conduction of an impulse in the motor neuron and subsequent release of acetylcholine at the myoneural junction, the sarcolemma is depolarized and a wave of depolarization is spread over the sarco-lemma away from the myoneural junction. This depolarization is propagated into the depths of the muscle fiber by the transverse tubules. These membrane organelles, invaginations of the sarcolemma, enter the fiber transverse to the long axis, and their lumina are open to the intercellular spaces.

Within the muscle fiber, the transverse tubules become closely associated with another membrane organelle, the sarcoplasmic reticulum, which consists of a series of vesicles and tubules which surround the myofibrils. By some mechanism the depolarization of the transverse tubules results in the release of calcium from the sarcoplasmic reticulum into the sarcoplasm surrounding the myofibrils. The calcium initiates a series of events whereby the interaction of ATP, actin, and myosin results in contraction.

B. Contraction

Muscular contraction results in the transformation of chemical energy into me-chanical energy or work. This involves the filamentous organelles actin and myosin. According to the sliding-filament model of contraction (H. E. Huxley and Hanson,

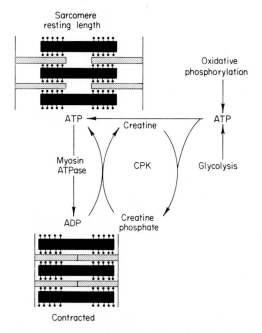

Fig. 1. Muscular contraction involves the shortening of sarcomeres by sliding of the overlapping arrays of thick (myosin) and thin (actin) myofilaments. The energy for contraction is derived from the hydrolysis of ATP in the presence of an ATPase associated with the cross bridges of the myosin filaments. The ATP is generated by the energy metabolism of the muscle fiber, principally by anaerobic glycolysis or oxidative phosphorylation. The utilization of ATP may be direct from these sources or indirect from the phosphorylation of ADP from creatine phosphate by creatine phosphokinase (CPK).

1954; A. F. Huxley and Niedergerke, 1954) shortening is achieved by the sliding of overlapping arrays of the myofilaments actin and myosin. Associated with the myosin filaments are projections or cross bridges which attach to the actin filaments and the generating force for sliding of the filaments is postulated to be due to changes in the angle of attachment of the cross bridges (H. E. Huxley, 1969).

The energy for muscular contraction is derived from the hydrolysis of adenosine triphosphate (ATP) into adenosine diphosphate (ADP) and inorganic phosphate. This reaction occurs in the presence of an ATPase associated with the cross bridges of the myosin filaments and the calcium liberated from the sarcoplasmic reticulum during excitation. Adenosine triphosphate is produced in mitochondria by oxidative phosphorylation and in the sarcoplasm by glycolysis. Muscle may use ATP directly from these sources or indirectly from the phosphorylation of ADP from the breakdown of creatine phosphate by creatine phosphokinase (Davies, 1965). The events associated with muscular contraction are summarized (Fig. 1).

III. HETEROGENEITY OF SKELETAL MUSCLE

A. Gross Muscle Coloration

Differences in gross coloration of muscles have been recognized for a long time and early observations have been reviewed by Needham (1926). Not only is a variation in color noted between species of animals but also between individual muscles within the same individual. The color of some muscles range from deep red to pale, whereas other muscles exhibit intermediate shades of coloration. Early workers believed that the differences in coloration were due to differences in the content of blood within the muscles; however, it was later shown that the red coloration was due to the presence of myoglobin. The terms red and white were introduced to distinguish between muscles based on their gross coloration. Subsequently, numerous biochemical, histochemical and physiological studies have been conducted with selected muscles from a variety of species. As a result the terms red and white have come to imply more specific meaning, relating to physiological properties and populations of types of muscle fibers within a muscle.

B. Physiological Properties

Muscle coloration was observed to be associated with significant differences in the physiological properties of muscular contraction (Ranvier, 1873, 1874, 1880). It was demonstrated that the speed of contraction of red muscles was slower than white muscles, and a number of other investigations tended to support Ranvier's observations in a variety of animals (Kronecker and Stirling, 1878; Lee et al., 1916; Denny-Brown, 1929). In addition, redness of a muscle was associated with (1) the development of tetanus at lower frequencies of stimulation, (2) the development of smaller twitch tensions, and (3) a greater resistance to fatigue. Conversely, white muscles required greater frequencies of stimulation for the development of tetanus, developed larger twitch tensions, and tended to fatigue quickly. Hence, muscles were found to differ in their physiological properties of contraction and the terminology of slow and fast muscles evolved. Moreover, since speed of contraction was closely associated with gross muscle coloration, the terms red and white came to be used interchangeably with slow and fast, respectively. There are exceptions, however, to this association of gross coloration with physiological properties of contraction which will be discussed shortly.

The morphological and functional unit of skeletal muscle is the motor unit. The motor unit consists of (1) the motor neuron whose cell body lies in the anterior or ventral horn of the spinal cord and whose axon extends along the anterior or ventral root and peripheral nerve, (2) the neuromuscular junctions, and (3) the muscle fibres innervated by the neuron. There are different types of motor neurons based on their rates of discharge: (1) phasic motor neurons with a fast discharge rate and (2) tonic motor neurons with a slow rate (Granit et al., 1957). In addition, the phasic motor neuron is characterized by shorter after-hyperpolarization potentials, faster conduction velocities, and larger axons than the tonic motor neuron (Eccles et al., 1958). Investigations of these parameters in motor neurons of slow-red and fast-white muscles indicate that tonic motor neurons supply slow-red muscles and phasic motor neurons supply fast-white muscles (Eccles et al., 1958). Thus, there are at least two types of motor units which differ in their physiological properties and motor neuron innervation. Based on isometric twitch characteristics, a third type of motor unit has also been described which is intermediate in its physiological characteristics to fast and slow motor units (Close, 1967).

C. QUANTITATIVE BIOCHEMISTRY

Quantitative differences in enzyme activities and various substrate concentrations have been reported between red and white muscles. These biochemical differences between red and white muscles have tended to reflect differences in their principal metabolic pathways active in the generation of energy (ATP) for muscular contraction. In general, the results of these studies indicate that white muscles are biochemically suited to derive energy for contraction by substrate phosphorylation via anaerobic glycolysis. White muscles tend to have higher glycogen and creatine phosphate concentrations as well as higher activities for the enzymes associated with glycolysis. Red muscles, on the other hand, have higher myoglobin concentrations and appear to be better suited to derive their energy by oxidative phosphorylation via the respiratory chain following the oxidation of glucose, fatty acids, and ketone bodies via the Krebs cycle (D. E. Green, 1951; Lawrie, 1952; 1953; Ogata, 1960; Domonkos, 1961; Domonkos and Latzkovits, 1961a,b; George and Talesara, 1961; Beatty et al., 1963, 1966b, 1967; Blanchaer, 1964; Dawson and Romanul, 1964; George and Bokdawala, 1964; George and Iype, 1964; Dawson and Kaplan, 1965; Cosmos, 1966; Cosmos and Butler, 1967; Beecher et al., 1968; Gutmann, 1968).

Whereas anaerobic glycolysis appears to be the principal metabolic pathway of carbohydrates in white muscles, red muscles of the guinea pig, rat, and monkey have greater activities for glycogen synthetase (Stubbs and Blanchaer, 1965; Bocek and Beatty, 1966), and studies with ^{14}C-glucose indicate a greater incorporation of glucose into glycogen (Bocek et. al., 1966). Another exception is the activity of hexokinase which is higher in red muscles of the chicken and guinea pig (Cardinet, 1967; Peter et al., 1968). The significance of these findings remains to be elucidated and it may be that glycogen is metabolized differently in red and white muscle.

Aerobic glycolysis via the pentose cycle does not appear to be a principal metabolic pathway in skeletal muscle (Glock and McLean, 1954; M. R. Green and Landau, 1965; Beatty *et al.*, 1966a,c).

The role of amino acids in the energy metabolism of muscle is uncertain. Transaminase activities are higher in red muscle of the chicken (Cardinet, 1967). Also, amino acid uptake, incorporation, and turnover in skeletal muscle protein is greater in red muscle (Goldberg, 1967, Gutmann, 1968). The differences in energy-yielding metabolic pathways of red and white muscles are summarized (Fig. 2).

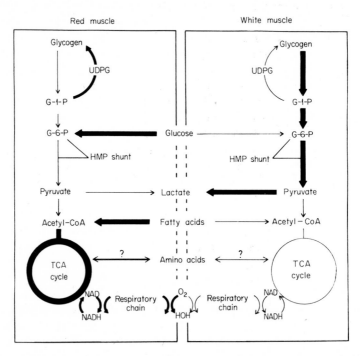

Fig. 2. Schematic representation of some differences in the energy metabolism of red and white muscles. In red muscles, energy for contraction is derived primarily by oxidative phosphorylation resulting from the oxidation of carbohydrates, fatty acids, and perhaps amino acids via the tricarboxylic acid cycle (TCA). White muscles derive their energy primarily via anaerobic glycolysis by the degradation of glycogen to lactate. Aerobic glycolysis (hexose monophosphate shunt) is a minor pathway in both muscles.

In addition to differences between red-slow and white-fast muscles in their metabolism for the generation of ATP, differences have also been demonstrated in their utilization of ATP for contraction. Myosins isolated from red and white muscles of the rabbit differ qualitatively and quantitatively with respect to their ATPase activities. Red-slow and white-fast muscles contain similar amounts of myosin, however, the ATPase activities of slow muscles are lower than in fast muscles and their pH dependency and liability in acid and alkaline conditions differ (Barany *et al.*, 1965; Seidel, 1967). Further, studies have established a direct relationship between the speed of contraction and myosin–ATPase activity (Barany, 1967).

Therefore, it is possible that the rate of ATP hydrolysis is the rate-limiting step which determines the speed of contraction (Barany, 1967; Mommaerts, 1969).

D. HISTOLOGY AND HISTOCHEMISTRY

Different types of muscle fibers were recognized by early microscopists. By examination of unstained sections or in combination with various lipid stains, two basic types of muscle fibers were described. One type of fiber was dark or opaque and contained numerous granules and lipid droplets between the myofibrils. The other type of fiber was light or translucent and contained few granules and lipid droplets. These fibers were referred to as dark and light muscle fibers, respectively. In addition, fibers intermediate to dark and light fibers, were described (Bullard, 1912–1913). The most common finding was that mammalian muscles contained variable percentages of dark and light fibers and therefore were mixed with respect to their muscle fiber-type composition. However, in certain instances such as in the rabbit, guinea pig, and chicken some muscles were found to contain predominately dark fibers and their gross coloration was red, while other muscles were found to contain predominately light fibers and their gross coloration was white. Although there was no unanimous agreement by early investigators, the tendency for fibers of red muscles to be darker than the fibers of white muscles led to the designation of dark and light fibers as red and white fibers, respectively. Histochemical and biochemical studies of red and white muscles have further tended to support the concept that gross muscle coloration is associated with the muscle fiber-type composition of a muscle (Nachmias and Padykula, 1958; Dubowitz and Pearse, 1960; Stein and Padykula, 1962; Romanul, 1964; Beatty et al., 1966b; Bocek and Beatty, 1966; Cosmos and Butler, 1967; Gauthier, 1969).

With the development and introduction of histochemical techniques to studies of muscle, the heterogeneity of muscle fibers became more obvious. Since these techniques localized enzyme systems at the cellular level, their application involved implications of biochemical and functional heterogeneity of fibers which had been suggested by the early microscopists. Histochemical studies of succinic dehydrogenase (SDH), nicotinamide adenine dinucleotide diaphorase (NADD), and nicotinamide adenine dinucleotide phosphate diaphorase (NADPD), demonstrated that the red or dark granular fibers had higher activities for these enzymes than the white or less granular light fibers (Padykula, 1952; Wachstein and Meisel, 1955; Nachmias and Padykula, 1958; Dubowitz and Pearse, 1960). In conjunction with electron microscopic observations the activities of these enzymes were localized to mitochondria. The granules and higher activities of these enzymes in the dark or red fibers correspond to greater numbers of mitochondria. Studies of red and white muscle fibers of the rat diaphragm and semitendinosus have revealed that the mitochondria of red fibers are large with abundant cristae, while the white fibers have fewer mitochondria which are smaller and have fewer cristae. Associated with the large mitochondria of the red fibers are lipid inclusions. Therefore, the granules and lipid droplets described by early microscopists correspond to mitochondria and lipid inclusions, respectively (Padykula and Gauthier, 1963, 1967; Gauthier and Padykula, 1966; Gauthier, 1969). Similar differences exist in red and white muscle fibers of the chicken (Fig. 3).

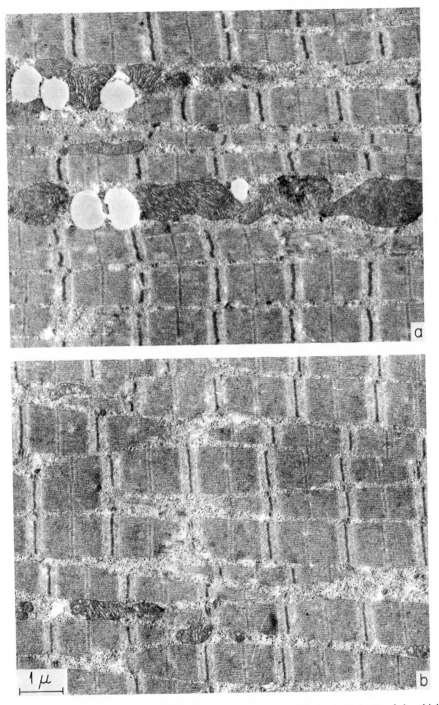

Fig. 3. Electron micrographs of a red muscle fiber (*a*) and white muscle fiber (*b*) of the chicken. The mitochondria of the red fiber are large and numerous with lipid inclusions associated with them. The mitochondria of the white fiber are much smaller, less numerous, and lipid inclusions are usually not observed.

A reciprocal histochemical profile for red and white fibers was observed between mitochondrial enzymes and phosphorylase, an indicator of anaerobic glycolysis (Dubowitz and Pearse, 1960). Red fibers with high mitochondrial enzyme activities had low phosphorylase activities while the reverse was true of white fibers and these authors introduced a classification of fibers where red and white fibers were designated as type I and type II fibers, respectively. Owing to the fact that various intermediate histochemical reactions of fibers exist between the extreme or classical characteristics described for red or type I fibers and white or type II fibers, other classifications have been proposed. Stein and Padykula (1962) proposed a classification of A, B, and C fibers based on their SDH reactions; this classification roughly corresponds with the classification of white, intermediate, and red muscle fibers, respectively. As many as eight fiber types have been described in rat muscle where esterase activity was found to be more precisely reciprocal with phosphorylase activity, suggesting a reciprocity between anaerobic glycolysis and lipid metabolism (Romanul, 1964).

Type I and type II fibers may also be differentiated by their myosin ATPase reactions (Engel, 1962, 1965). Of all the histochemical techniques applied, the myofibrillar ATPase reaction tends to separate fibers more definitely into two types though some intermediate fibers are still observed. The histochemical method for the detection of myosin ATPase (Padykula and Herman, 1955a,b) utilizes an alkaline pH incubating medium and therefore favors the type of myosin–ATPase activity of fast-white muscle. If myosin ATPase activity is rate-limiting in the speed of shortening, this histochemical method should be the most specific for the identification and association of muscle fibers types with contraction speed.

Histochemical localization of glycogen synthetase has varied. In human muscle its activity has been usually parallel with that of phosphorylase in type II or white fibers (Engel, 1962) but reciprocal and higher in type I or red fibers of rat and monkey muscle (R. Hess and Pearse, 1961; Bocek and Beatty, 1966) which is in agreement with quantitative results in the rat and monkey.

Owing to the fact that gross coloration is associated with the fiber-type composition of a muscle and its contraction speed, muscle fiber types have been equated with speed of contraction. Therefore, red or type I fibers have become referred to as slow or tonic, and white or type II fibers as fast or phasic. Until recently, this concept has been primarily based on indirect evidence, and while most evidence tends to support this concept, there are exceptions to this general view. Studies of the diaphragm muscle in small mammals (Gauthier and Padykula, 1966) and thyroarytenoid muscle in the rabbit (Hall-Craggs, 1968) indicate that in some red muscles the speed of contraction is fast rather than slow. Since these muscles contain fibers with certain characteristics of red muscle fibers based on mitochondrial enzyme histochemistry, it must be concluded that not all red fibres are slow.

More direct evidence in support of speed of contraction and muscle fiber types has been advanced by studies of isolated motor units in conjunction with histochemical analyses (Edstrom and Kugelberg, 1968). It was demonstrated that motor units were largely composed of a single muscle fiber type. Thus, fast motor units were composed of white, type II or type A muscle fibers; slow motor units were comprised of red, type I or type C muscle fibers; and motor units of intermediate speed were composed of intermediate or type B muscle fibers (Fig. 4).

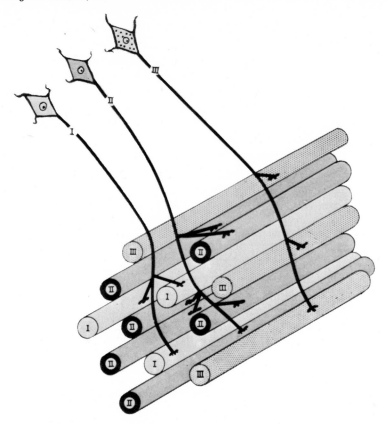

Fig. 4. Schematic representation of skeletal muscle motor units. Motor units appear to have a homogeneous fiber-type composition whereby slow contracting motor units are composed of type I muscle fibers; fast contracting motor units are composed of type II fibers; and motor units with intermediate contraction speeds are composed of intermediate type fibers which are designated III in this illustration (based on study of Edstrom and Kugelberg, 1968).

The general histochemical classification and associated properties of muscle fiber types is summarized (Table I) and illustrated (Fig. 5). Such a classification is the result of investigations from a variety of species as well as individual muscles within a single species. It must be emphasized that numerous variations are to be found and direct extrapolation of results from species to species or muscle to muscle are not always valid.

IV. NEURAL TROPHIC INFLUENCES ON MUSCLE

Trophic influences of nerve on muscle may be defined as those functions of the nerve that affect or regulate the metabolism of the muscle (Guth, 1968). This definition should encompass structural and physiological properties as well, since the structure of the muscle fiber and its organelles, physiological properties, and biochemical properties are all interdependent.

TABLE I   SOME GENERAL HISTOCHEMICAL, MORPHOLOGICAL, AND PHYSIOLOGICAL
PROPERTIES OF MUSCLE FIBERS

Property	Muscle fiber	
	Type I	Type II
Fiber size (usually)	Smaller	Larger
References to color	Red	White
	Dark	Light
Mitochondria	Large and numerous	Small and few
Myoglobin	High	Low
Oxidative enzymes		
SDH	High	Low
NADD	High	Low
NAPDD	High	Low
Lipid	High	Low
Esterase	High	Low
Phosphorylase	Low	High
Glycogen	Low	High
Myosin–ATPase (alkaline)	Low	High
Speed of contraction	Slow	Fast
Function	Tonic or sustained activity	Phasic or rapid activity

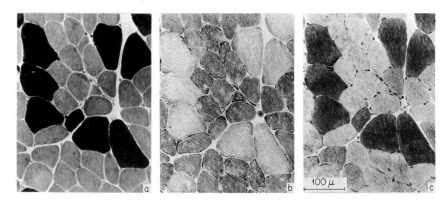

Fig. 5. Serial sections of skeletal muscle incubated for the histochemical localization of (a) myosin–ATPase, (b) NADD, and (c) phosphorylase. Type I muscle fibers are darker staining for NADD and lighter staining for myosin–ATPase and phosphorylase. Conversely, type II fibers are darker staining for myosin–ATPase and phosphorylase, and lighter staining for NADD. In this example the fibers tend to be sharply separated into the fiber-type classifications of type I or type II fibers; however, some intermediate activities may be noted.

The implication of neuronal influences on muscle integrity have long been recognized by studies of denervation whereby numerous morphological, physiological, and biochemical changes result (Gutmann, 1962). More precise implications have evolved where the influence of the motor neuron on speed of contraction and muscle fibers types has been demonstrated in a series of experiments where nerves to fast and slow muscles have been cross-united (Buller et al., 1960; Buller and

Lewis, 1965; Close, 1965; Romanul and Van Der Meulen, 1966, 1967; Dubowitz, 1967; Robbins *et al.*, 1969). In this experimental design, motor neurons which normally innervate slow muscles come to innervate muscles which are normally fast, while motor neurons which normally innervate fast muscles come to innervate muscles which are normally slow. These experiments have resulted in a reversal of contraction speed, i.e., fast muscles become slow and slow muscles become fast. Accompanying these changes in the speed of contraction is a corresponding change in the enzyme profiles of the muscle fibers. Hence, slow muscles which have fiber populations with histochemical characteristics of high oxidative, low glycolytic, and low myosin ATPase activities become changed to fiber populations with low oxidative, high glycolytic, and high myosin ATPase activities when innervated by a nerve which normally innervates a fast muscle. Converse changes occur by cross union of a fast muscle with the nerve of a slow muscle (Romanul and Van Der Meulen, 1966, 1967; Dubowitz, 1967; Robbins *et al.*, 1969). Therefore, the neuron influences (1) the type of energy metabolism in a muscle fiber and all the structural changes in fiber organelles that this implies, and (2) the physiological properties of contraction. The changes in speed brought about by neural influence presumably has a direct effect on the contractile material, thereby determining the intrinsic speed of shortening (Close, 1965). In view of the suggestion that myosin ATPase is the rate-limiting reaction in contraction speed it may be that the neural influence specifically affects the type of myosin ATPase in a fiber.

Precisely how motor neurons exert their influence on muscle fibers is unknown. Two general postulates exist: (1) the influence of motor neurons is due to the frequency of the impulse discharge (Vrbova, 1963; Salmons and Vrbova, 1969), or (2) the influence of motor neurons is mediated by specific chemical substances liberated by the neuron (Buller *et al.*, 1960). However mediated, the evidence suggests that the nerve directs the expression of the genetic complement in muscle fibers, and that the muscle fiber maintains the potential for differentiation and re-differentiation at the direction of the nervous system.

V. SERUM ENZYME DETERMINATIONS IN THE DIAGNOSIS OF NEUROMUSCULAR DISORDERS

A. General Principles

A valuable adjunct to the clinical diagnosis of neuromuscular diseases is the utilization of serum enzyme determinations. This involves the detection of enzymes in the serum or plasma which are normally confined to muscle fibers and whose activities or concentrations are usually low in the serum or plasma. Necrosis and lysis of muscle fibers is an example of a process which results in elevated serum activities of intracellular enzymes. Elevations in serum enzyme activities may also occur in association with increased cell permeability (leakage), increased enzyme production by the parenchymal cells, obstructions to normal enzyme excretory routes, increased amount of enzyme-forming tissue and delayed removal or in-activation of enzyme (Cornelius, 1967) and perhaps cell secretion.

B. Serum Glutamic Oxalacetic Transaminase (SGOT)

The most widely used serum enzyme determination in neuromuscular diseases of domestic animals has been that for serum glutamic oxalacetic transaminase (SGOT). Some of the normal values reported for domestic animals are summarized (Table II). Normal values do not appear to be greatly different between sexes although reported values for cows (Cornelius et al., 1959a) are somewhat higher than values for bulls (Roussel and Stallcup, 1966). Differences associated with age have been reported in sheep (Lagace et al., 1961) and seasonal differences in bulls (Roussel and Stallcup, 1966). Also, physical activity is associated with higher values in horses (Cornelius et al., 1963; Cardinet et al., 1963, 1967).

Elevations of SGOT activities have been reported in white muscle disease of lambs and calves (Blincoe and Dye, 1958; Kuttler and Marble, 1958; Swingle et al., 1959; Blincoe and Marble, 1960), tying-up and paralytic myoglobinuria in horses (Cornelius et al., 1963; Cardinet et al., 1963, 1967), hereditary muscular dystrophy in chickens (Cornelius et al., 1959b), and myodegeneration due to ingestion of toxic plants in cattle (Henson et al., 1965). Although the use of SGOT determinations have proven valuable as a diagnostic aid, the enzyme lacks organ specificity since in addition to high concentrations in skeletal and cardiac muscle, GOT activities

TABLE II   NORMAL VALUES OF SERUM GLUTAMIC OXALACETIC TRANSAMINASE (SGOT) IN
VARIOUS DOMESTIC ANIMALS

Species	Comment	SGOT activity (Sigma-Frankel units/ml)			References
		Mean	Standard deviation	Range	
Bovine	Bull, 1–97 wk	23.7	± 17.3	—	Roussel and Stallcup (1966)
	Cows, 2–10 yr	43.8	± 5.7	—	Cornelius et al. (1959a)
	Calves, 7–27 dy	23.6	± 3.7	—	Cornelius et al. (1959a)
Canine	>9 mo	22.7	± 5.4	—	Cornelius et al. (1959a)
	<2 yr	26.6	± 1.6	—	Hibbs and Coles (1965)
	4–12 mo	22.1	± 5.5	12–28	Crawley and Swenson (1965)
	1–5 yr	25.8	± 7.8	13–53	Crawley and Swenson (1965)
	>5 yr	22.4	± 5.2	14–30	Crawley and Swenson (1965)
Equine	Unexercised, not in training	165	± 33.8	—	Cornelius et al. (1959a)
	>1 yr	186	± 52	120–336	Cornelius et al. (1963)
		151	± 18.0	110–190	Cardinet et al. (1963)
		178	± 52	99–354	Cardinet et al. (1967)
	Exercised, in	346	±157	100–950	Cornelius et al. (1963)
	training >1 yr	250	± 31	185–320	Cardinet et al. (1963)
Feline	>1 mo	19.0	± 4.8	12–27	Cornelius and Kaneko (1960)
Ovine	Lambs, 7–35 dy	56	± 31	—	Blincoe and Marble (1960)
	0–4 wk	—	—	43–53	Lagace et al. (1961)
	5–8 wk	—	—	<126	Lagace et al. (1961)
	>10 wk	—	—	<81	Lagace et al. (1961)
Porcine	1–3 yr	31.1	± 14.1	—	Cornelius et al. (1959a)
Gallus domesticus	6 mo	370	±186	—	Cornelius (1960)

are high in the liver as well as other organs (Cornelius *et al.*, 1959a; Nagode *et al.*, 1966; Cardinet *et al.*, 1967).

C. Serum Creatine Phosphokinase (SCPK)

An enzyme widely used as a diagnostic aid in neuromuscular disorders of man is creatine phosphokinase (CPK). The use of serum determinations of this enzyme (SCPK) offers greater promise of organ specificity than other enzyme determinations employed to date, in diseases of muscle. In muscle, this enzyme functions in making ATP available for contraction by the phosphorylation of ADP from creatine phosphate (Fig. 1). Analyses of tissues from various animals indicate significant activities of CPK in skeletal and cardiac muscle, low activities in brain and insignificant activities in most other organs, especially the liver (Oliver, 1955; Tanzer and Gilvarg, 1959; Colombo *et al.*, 1962; Eppenberger *et al.*, 1962; Cardinet *et al.*, 1967). Therefore, elevations in SCPK activities would be more specific for diseases of skeletal and/or cardiac muscle than SGOT. Some normal values for SCPK have been determined in domestic animals (Table III). There are variations in normal values with regards to age, sex, and physical activity. Therefore, case histories regarding age, sex, and physical activity are important in evaluating levels of activity.

TABLE III NORMAL VALUES OF SERUM CREATINE PHOPHOKINASE (SCPK) IN SOME DOMESTIC ANIMALS

Species	Comment		SCPK activity IU/liter[a]			References
			Mean	Standard deviation	Range	
Canine	0–4 mo	males	4.7	±0.3	1.2–8.2	Cardinet (1969)
		females	3.0	±0.2	1.2–5.5	
	4–6 mo	males	2.4	±0.2	0.1–6.6	
		females	1.8	±0.2	0.4–6.2	
	6–12 mo	males	1.8	±0.2	0.4–5.6	
		females	0.8	±0.2	0.0–7.5	
	> 12 mo	males	1.2	±0.3	0.2–2.6	
		females	0.8	±0.1	0.0–1.8	
Caprine		females	0.9	±0.9	0.0–2.5	Cardinet (1969)
Equine	Unexercised, not in training 3–12 yr		1.3	±0.9	0.0–3.6	Cardinet *et al.* (1967)
Feline		males	1.7	±1.1	0.4–3.4	Cardinet (1969)
		females	1.9	±1.3	0.0–4.5	
Ovine		males	0.8	±0.6	0.0–2.9	Cardinet (1969)
		females	0.5	±0.3	0.0–0.9	
Gallus Domesticus	27–134 days		38.1 to 59.1	—	—	Holliday *et al.* (1965)
	1 yr	males	109	—	—	
		females	50	—	—	

[a]Enzyme activities determined by method of Tanzer and Gilvarg (1959). Determinations in chicken carried out in presence of cysteine.

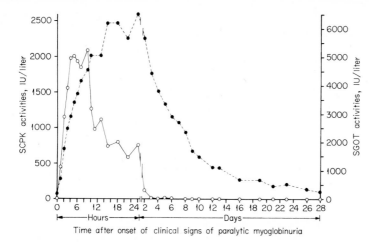

Fig. 6.   Differences in the time course of elevations in SGOT and SCPK activities due to muscle necrosis (equine paralytic myoglobinuria). The SGOT activities remain elevated for much longer periods than SCPK. (○) CPK; (●) SGOT. (From Cardinet et al., 1967.)

Elevations in SCPK activities have been reported in hereditary muscular dystrophy of chickens (Holliday et al., 1965), myodegeneration due to ingestion of toxic plants in cattle (Henson et al., 1965), and paralytic myoglobinuria in horses (Gerber, 1964; Cardinet et al., 1967). In a comparative study, the behavior of SGOT and SCPK activities are distinctly different during the course of equine paralytic myoglobinuria (Fig. 6). Elevations in SGOT activities were present for weeks after the onset of clinical disease while SCPK activities remained elevated for only a few days. The course of elevations of these enzymes in this disease can be directly attributed to different disappearance rates of their activity in the plasma (Fig. 7).

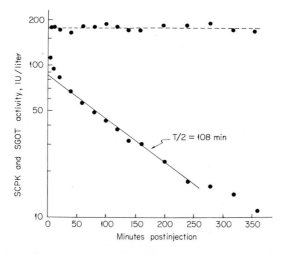

Fig. 7.   Disappearance of SGOT and SCPK activities in the serum of a horse following the intravenous injection of GOT and CPK. The differences in the course of serum elevations of these two enzymes due to necrosis in the horse is the result of differences in their disappearance rates in the serum. (——) SCPK; (– – –) SGOT. (From Cardinet et al., 1967.)

While SCPK is more specific for muscle necrosis than SGOT, the simultaneous determinations of SGOT and SCPK are potentially valuable diagnostic and prognostic aids owing to the different disappearance rates of their plasma activities: (1) elevated SCPK activities indicate that muscle necrosis is active or had recently occurred, (2) persistent elevations of SCPK would indicate that muscle necrosis was progressively active, and (3) elevated SGOT due to muscle necrosis accompanied by decreasing or normal SCPK activities would indicate that muscle necrosis was no longer active. It has not been established that there are similar differences in the disappearance rates of SGOT and SCPK activities in the plasma of other animals. Therefore, it is not possible to say that the same assessment of muscle necrosis with the simultaneous determination of SGOT and SCPK activities can be applied to the other species.

Elevations in SCPK activities have been reported in polioencephalomalacia and focal symmetrical encephalomalacia of sheep and it has been suggested that SCPK determinations may be of value in diseases of the central nervous system (Smith and Healy, 1968). However, in diseases of the central nervous system which involve motor function, elevations of SCPK may be from skeletal muscle rather than from the central nervous system. This appears to be the case in central nervous system disorders in man (Cao et al., 1969).

The normal SCPK values presented (Table III) were determined by the method of Tanzer and Gilvarg (1959). Except for the values reported for the chicken, the assays were conducted without the addition of cysteine to the incubating medium. Storage of sera at $0–5°$ C results in a loss of activity. The addition of cysteine to the incubating medium (final concentration about 12 mM) results in higher values of serum activities, and the losses due to storage are minimized (Okinaka et al., 1964; Weismann et al., 1966; J. W. Hess et al., 1968). The cysteine reactivates the SCPK activity loss during storage; therefore, the addition of cysteine to the incubating media appears to be the method of choice and necessitates normal values to be established where cysteine is added to the incubating medium. Other sulfhydryl compounds can be substituted for cysteine with the same result, e.g., glutathione.

Diseases of muscle are usually classified as to their origin or primary lesion. Myogenic diseases are those where the primary affect of the disease process is considered to be in the muscle fiber itself, while neurogenic diseases result in secondary changes to the muscle fiber as a result of alterations in its innervation. While SCPK determinations may be specific for diseases of muscle, they do not provide information relative to the origin of the disease process; however, elevations of SCPK are generally higher in myogenic than neurogenic diseases. More precise information regarding the origin of muscle diseases is possible by the use histological and histochemical examination of muscle biopsies.

VI.   MUSCLE BIOPSY AND HISTOCHEMISTRY IN THE DIAGNOSIS OF NEUROMUSCULAR DISORDERS

A. GENERAL CONSIDERATIONS

The use of muscle biopsies allows examination of muscle fibers, neuromuscular junctions, peripheral nerve branches, connective tissue and blood vessels. As discussed, histochemical examination of skeletal muscle provides information relative to morphological, biochemical, and implied physiological properties of muscle fibers. Therefore, the application of histochemical techniques in conjunction with routine light microscopic examination of muscle biopsies offers the potential to evaluate and integrate the morphological, biochemical, and physiological manifestations of neuromuscular diseases. The application of histochemical techniques have become essential diagnostic procedures in neuromuscular disorders of man and it has been possible to distinguish some differences in the histochemical reactions and properties of muscle in myogenic and neurogenic diseases. For reviews of histochemical investigations in neuromuscular disorders of man the reader is referred to Engel (1962, 1965, 1967) and Dubowitz (1966, 1968).

These techniques have not been extensively applied to neuromuscular disorders in animals except for the hereditary muscular dystrophies of the mouse (Fahimi and Roy, 1966; Bajusz, 1965) and chicken (Cosmos, 1966; Cosmos and Butler, 1967; Cardinet, 1967). In these diseases, the dystrophic process appears to affect white muscles more extensively than red muscles. The value of histochemical techniques applied to neuromuscular disorders in animals can be illustrated in the recent description of a developmental myopathy in the dog (Cardinet et al., 1969). This disease was characterized by a large variation in the size of muscle fibers in the pectineus muscle. The extent of the lesions varied and in many cases the lesions were easily overlooked by routine examination of hematoxylin-eosin stained sections. When histochemical techniques were applied, the lesion was readily recognized and revealed more precise information about the nature of the disease. The disease was characterized by hypotrophy of type II muscle fibers (Fig. 8), with diminished glycogen content and lower phosphorylase activity in the affected type II fibers. Based on current knowledge of muscle fiber types and neural regulation of their properties, it was postulated that this disease might be neurogenic in origin, perhaps a lack of neural trophic factor(s) which regulate the growth and differentiation of muscle fibers. This disease and the implications of its origin would probably have gone unrecognized if the method of examination had been limited to conventional light microscopy. There are, no doubt, numerous neuromuscular disorders in domestic animals which remain to be recognized, and the application of histochemistry offers the potential for their recognition as well as furthering our knowledge of diseases currently recognized but not investigated by histochemical methods.

B. Histochemical Methods

The following methods are employed in this laboratory for the routine examination of muscle biopsies and are recommended. The outlined techniques are not the only methods available and specific cases may warrant the use of other methods. Extensive discussions of histochemical techniques are available (Pearse, 1960; Barka and Anderson, 1963).

Biopsy and fresh necropsy samples of muscle are cut transversely and mounted on thin moistened pieces of cork. The small blocks of tissue are quenched in 2-methylbutane cooled in liquid nitrogen. The 2-methylbutane is cooled to near its freezing point ($-160°C$) to insure rapid freezing of the tissue. This is a critical step in prepar-

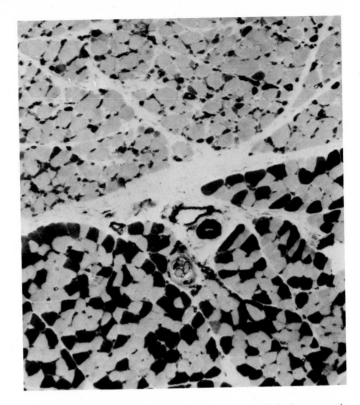

Fig. 8.   Type II muscle fiber hypotrophy in the canine. Fasciculi in lower portion of field have normal sized type I (light-staining) and type II (dark-staining) fibers. Fasciculi at top or upper portion have fibers with wide variations in sizes; type I fibers tend to be normal in size or hypertropic, while type II fibers are all hypotropic. Myosin–ATPase. × 120.

ing muscle samples for frozen sectioning since muscle is very susceptible to the development of freezing artifacts. The samples are then transferred to a cryostat, appropriately mounted, and serially sectioned (8–12 μ thick) at -15 to $-20°$ C. Sections are picked up on coverslips and air dried. Where indicated, any one of several hematoxylin–eosin and PAS staining techniques may be employed.

Section	Method	Value
1	Hematoxylin–eosin	General morphology and histopathology
2	Myosin–ATPase	Differentiation of fibre types; assessment of fiber type involvement and/or changes in localization due to disease
3	NADD or SDH	Differentiation of fiber types; assessment of fiber type involvement and/or changes in localization due to disease
4	Phosphorylase	Differentiation of fiber types; assessment of fiber type involvement and/or changes in localization due to disease
5	PAS–hematoxylin	Assessment of glycogen content and good resolution of myelinated axons of intramuscular nerve branches
6	Esterase	Differentiation of fiber types; assessment of fiber type involvement and/or changes in localization due to disease; localization of myoneural junctions.

Where indicated, additional sections may be specially stained for connective tissue (e.g., Van Gieson stain) and acid phosphatases (Barka and Anderson, 1962).

Myosin–ATPase Method (Padykula and Herman, 1955a,b)

1. Prepare fresh incubating medium with the following stock solutions and substrate in the order listed:

Sodium barbital, 0.1 M	2.0 ml
Calcium chloride, 2%	1.0 ml
Distilled water	7.0 ml
Adenosine triphosphate	15.2 mg

   Adjust pH to 9.4 to 9.6 with 1 N NaOH

2. Use unfixed sections or sections fixed in formalin (pH 7.0 at 4°C) for 5 minutes and rinsed in distilled water. Incubate sections for 5–30 minutes at 37°C. Test sections should be used with each trial and checked during the course of the incubation to determine the optimum incubation time.

3. Rinse sections three to four times with 1% calcium chloride.

4. Transfer sections to 2% cobaltous chloride for 5 minutes.

5. Rinse with distilled water.

6. Develop color with dilute ammonium sulfide solution (2 ml of 20–24% stock solution in 100 ml distilled water).

7. Wash, dehydrate, clear in xylol, and mount with synthetic media.

NADD, NADPD, and SDH Methods (Scarpelli et al., 1958; Pearse, 1960)

1. Prepare fresh incubating media with the following stock solutions and substrates in the order listed:

   A. *NADD or NADPD*

MTT, 3-(4,5-dimethylthiazolyl-2)-2,5-diphenyltetrazolium bromide, 1 mg/ml	2.5 ml
Tris(hydroxymethyl)aminomethane buffer, 0.1 M (pH 7.4)	2.5 ml
Cobaltous chloride, 0.5 M	0.5 ml
Distilled water	4.5 ml
NADH or NADPH	10 mg

   B. *SDH*

MTT, 1 mg/ml	2.5 ml
Tris buffer, 0.1 M	2.5 ml
Cobaltous chloride, 0.5 M	0.5 ml
Distilled water	3.5 ml
Sodium succinate, 0.06 M	1.0 ml

   Adjust pH to 7.0 to 7.1 with 1 N NaOH or HCl as required.

2. Incubate unfixed sections for 15–60 minutes at 37°C.

3. Rinse in distilled water and fix in formalin.
4. Wash sections well and mount in glycerin jelly (15 gm gelatin) dissolved in heated distilled water to which 100 ml glycerol is added and mixed thoroughly.

Phosphorylase Method (Takeuchi and Kuriaki, 1955; Takeuchi, 1956)

1. Prepare fresh incubating medium with the following stock solutions and substrates:

Glucose-1-phosphate	50 mg
Muscle adenylic acid (AMP)	10 mg
Glycogen	2 mg
Sucrose	2.5 gm
Acetate buffer, 0.2 M (pH 5.7)	10 ml
Distilled water	10 ml
Ethanol, 95%	5 ml
Insulin, 40 units/ml	0.25 ml

Adjust pH to 5.7 with 1 N NaOH or HCl as necessary
2. Incubate unfixed sections for 15–30 minutes at 37° C.
3. Wash sections with 40% ethanol, 3–4 times rapidly.
4. Rinse with absolute ethanol and air-dry sections.
5. Color may be developed with dilute iodine solution or PAS stain. Native glycogen does not stain with iodine; however, color developed by staining of newly formed glycogen during incubation is not permanent. Sections stained with PAS may be counterstained with hematoxylin.
6. Mount iodine-stained sections in glycerin jelly. PAS–hematoxylin stained sections may be dehydrated in ethanol, cleared in xylol, and mounted with synthetic media.

Esterase Method (Barka and Anderson, 1963)

1. Prepare fresh incubating medium with the following stock solutions and substrates in order of listing:

α-Naphthol acetate, dissolved in 0.5 ml acetone	5 mg
Monosodium phosphate, 0.15 M	20 ml
Hexazonium pararosanilin freshly prepared	1.6 ml

(Prepared from 0.8 ml, 4% sodium nitrite, and 0.8 ml stock solution of 2 gm pararosanilin dissolved in 50 ml of 2 N HCl with heating)

Adjust pH to 7.2 with 0.15 M disodium phosphate.
2. Incubate unfixed sections for 10–30 minutes at 37°C.
3. Wash with distilled water and fix in formalin.
4. Sections may be dehydrated with ethanol, cleared with xylol, and mounted with synthetic media.

REFERENCES

Asmundson, V. S., and Julian, L. M. (1956). *J. Heredity* **47**, 248.

Bajusz, E. (1965). *In* "Muscle" (W. M. Paul *et al.*, eds.), pp. 555–563. Pergamon Press, Oxford.

Barany, M. (1967). *J. Gen. Physiol.* **50**, 197.

Barany, M., Barany, K., Reckard, T., and Volpe, A. (1965). *Arch. Biochem. Biophys.* **109**, 185.

Barka, T., and Anderson, P. J. (1962). *J. Histochem. Cytochem.* **10**, 741.

Barka, T., and Anderson, P. J. (1963). "Histochemistry." Harper, New York.

Beatty, C. H., Peterson, R. D., and Bocek, R.M. (1963). *Am. J. Physiol.* **204**, 939.

Beatty, C. H., Basinger, G. M., and Bocek, R. M. (1966a). *Arch. Biochem. Biophys.* **117**, 275.

Beatty, C. H., Basinger, G. M., Dully, C. C., and Bocek, R. M. (1966b). *J. Histochem. Cytochem.* **14**, 590.

Beatty, C. H., Peterson, R. D., Basinger, G. M., and Bocek, R. M. (1966c). *Am. J. Physiol.* **210**, 404.

Beatty, C. H., Basinger, G. M., and Bocek, R. M. (1967). *J. Histochem. Cytochem.* **15**, 93.

Beecher, G. R., Kastenschmidt, L. L., Cassens, R. G., Hoekstra, W. G., and Briskey, E. J. (1968). *J. Food Sci.* **33**, 84.

Blanchaer, M. C. (1964). *Am. J. Physiol.* **206**, 1015.

Blincoe, C., and Dye, W. B. (1958). *J. Animal Sci.* **17**, 224.

Blincoe, C., and Marble, D. W. (1960). *Am. J. Vet. Res.* **21**, 866.

Bloom, W., and Fawcett, D. W. (1968). "A Textbook of Histology." Saunders, Philadelphia, Pennsylvania.

Bocek, R. M., and Beatty, C. H. (1966). *J. Histochem. Cytochem.* **14**, 549.

Bocek, R. M., Peterson, R. D., and Beatty, C. H. (1966). *Am. J. Physiol.* **210**, 1101.

Bullard, H. H. (1912–1913). *Am. J. Anat.* **14**, 1.

Buller, A. J., Eccles, J. C., and Eccles, R. M. (1960). *J. Physiol. (London)* **150**, 417.

Buller, A. J., and Lewis, D. M. (1965). *J. Physiol. (London)* **178**, 343.

Cao, A., De Vigiliis, S., Lippi, C., and Trabalza, N. (1969). *Clin. Chim. Acta* **23**, 475.

Cardinet, G. H. (1967). *Dissertation Abstr.* **27**, 3362-B.

Cardinet, G. H. (1969). Unpublished observations.

Cardinet, G. H., Fowler, M. E., and Tyler, W. S. (1963). *Am. J. Vet. Res.* **24**, 980.

Cardinet, G. H., Littrell, J. F., and Freedland R. A. (1967). *Res. Vet. Sci.* **8**, 219.

Cardinet, G. H., Wallace, L. J., Fedde, M. R., Guffy, M. M., and Bardens, J. W. (1969). *Arch. Neurol.* **21**, 620–630.

Close, R. (1965). *Nature* **206**, 831.

Close, R. (1967). *In* "Exploratory Concepts in Muscular Dystrophy and Related Disorders" (A. T. Milhorat, ed.), pp. 142–150, Excerpta Med. Found., Amsterdam.

Colombo, J. P., Richterich, R., and Rossi, E. (1962). *Klin. Wochschr.* **40**, 37.

Cornelius, C. E. (1960). *Calif. Vet.* **13**, No. 6, 22.

Cornelius, C. E. (1967). *Proc. Am. Animal Hosp. Assoc.* p. 82.

Cornelius, C. E., and Kaneko, J. J. (1960). *J. Am. Vet. Med. Assoc.* **137**, 62.

Cornelius, C. E., Bishop, J., Switzer, J., and Rhode, E. A. (1959a). *Cornell Vet.* **49**, 116.

Cornelius, C. E., Law, G. R., Julian, L. M., and Asmundson, V. S. (1959b). *Proc. Soc. Exptl. Biol. Med.* **101**, 41.

Cornelius, C. E., Burnham, L. G., and Hill, H. E. (1963). *J. Am. Vet. Med. Assoc.* **142**, 639.

Cosmos, E. (1966). *Develop. Biol.* **13**, 163.

Cosmos, E., and Butler, J. (1967). *In* "Exploratory Concepts in Muscular Dystrophy and Related Disorders" (A. T. Milhorat, ed.), pp. 197–204. Excerpta Med. Found., Amsterdam.

Crawley, G. J., and Swenson, M. J. (1965). *Am. J, Vet. Res.* **26**, 1468.

Davies, R. E. (1965). *In* "Muscle" (W. M. Paul *et al.*, eds.), pp. 49–69. Pergamon Press, Oxford.

Dawson, D. M., and Kaplan, N. O. (1965). *J. Biol. Chem.* **240**, 3215.

Dawson, D. M., and Romanul, F. C. A. (1964). *Arch. Neurol.* **11**, 369.

Denny-Brown, D. E. (1929). *Proc. Roy. Soc.* **B104**, 371.

Domonkos, J. (1961). *Arch. Biochem. Biophys.* **95**, 138.

Domonkos, J., and Latzkovitz, L. (1961a). *Arch. Biochem. Biophys.* **95**, 144.

Domonkos, J., and Latzkovitz, L. (1961b). *Arch. Biochem. Biophys.* **95**, 147.

Dubowitz, V. (1966). *J. Neurol., Neurosurg., Psychiat.* [N. S.] **29**, 23.

Dubowitz, V. (1967). *J. Physiol. (London)* **193**, 481.

Dubowitz, V. (1968). "Developing and Diseased Muscle." Spastics Intern. Med. Publ., London

Dubowitz, V., and Pearse, A. G. E. (1960). *Histochemie* **2**, 105.

Eccles, J. C., Eccles, R. M., and Lundberg, A. (1958). *J. Physiol (London)* **142**, 275.

Edstrom, L., and Kugelberg, E. (1968). *J. Neurol., Neurosurg., Psychiat.* [N.S.] **31**, 424.

Engel, W. K. (1962). *Neurology* **12**, 778.

Engel, W. K. (1965). In "Neurohistochemistry" (C. W. M. Adams, ed.), pp. 622–672. Elsevier, Amsterdam.

Engel, W. K. (1967). *Pediat. Clin. North Am.* **14**, 963.

Eppenberger, H. M., von Fellenberg, R., Richterich, R., and Aebi, H. (1962). *Enzymol. Biol. Clin.* **2**, 139.

Fahimi, H. D., and Roy, P. (1966). *Science* **152**, 1761.

Gauthier, G. F. (1969). *Z. Zellforsch. Mikroskop. Anat.* **95**, 462.

Gauthier, G. F., and Padykula, H. A. (1966). *J. Cell Biol.* **28**, 333.

George, J. C., and Bokdawala, F. D. (1964). *J. Animal Morphol. Physiol.* **11**, 124.

George, J. C., and Iype, P. T. (1964). *Pavo* **2**, 84.

George, J. C., and Talesara, C. L. (1961). *J. Cellular Comp. Physiol.* **58**, 253.

Gerber, H. (1964). *Zentr. Veterinaermed.* **11**, 135.

Glock, G. E., and McLean, P. (1954). *Biochem. J.* **56**, 171.

Goldberg. A. L. (1967). *Nature* **216**, 1219.

Granit, R., Phillips, C. G., Skoglund, S., and Steg, G. (1957). *J. Neurophysiol.* **20**, 470.

Green, D. E. (1951). In "Enzymes and Enzyme Systems" (J. T. Edsall, ed.), pp. 15–46. Harvard Univ. Press,Cambridge, Massachusetts.

Green, M. R., and Landau, B. R. (1965). *Arch. Biochem. Biophys.* **111**, 569.

Guth, L. (1968). *Physiol. Rev.* **48,** 645.

Gutmann, E. (1962). "The Denervated Muscle." Publ. House Czech. Acad. Sci., Prague.

Gutmann, E. (1968). *Symp. Biol. Hung.* **8**, 56.

Hall-Craggs, E. C. B. (1968). *J. Anat.* **102**, 241.

Ham, A. W. (1969). "Histology." Lippincott, Philadelphia, Pennsylvania.

Henson, J. B., Dollahite, J. W., Bridges, C. H., and Rao, R. R. (1965). *J. Am. Vet. Med. Assoc.* **147**, 142.

Hess, J. W., Murdock, K. L., and Natho, G. J. W. (1968). *Am. J. Clin. Pathol.* **50**, 89.

Hess, R., and Pearse, A. G. E. (1961). *Proc. Soc. Exptl. Biol. Med.* **107**, 569.

Hibbs, C. M., and Coles, E. H. (1965). *Proc. Soc. Exptl. Biol. Med.* **118**, 1059.

Holliday, T. A., Asmundson, V. S., and Julian, L. M. (1965). *Enzymol. Biol. Clin.* **5**, 209.

Homburger, F., Baker, J. R., Nixon, G. W., and Wilgram, G. (1962). *Arch. Internal Med.* **110**, 660.

Huxley, A. F., and Niedergerke, R. (1954). *Nature* **173**, 971.

Huxley, H. E. (1969). *Science* **164**, 1356.

Huxley, H. E., and Hanson, J. (1954). *Nature* **173**, 973.

Innes, J. R. (1951). *Brit. Vet. J.* **107**, 131.

Kronecker, H., and Stirling, W. (1878). *Arch. Anat. Physiol., Physiol. Abt.* **2**, 1.

Kuttler, K. L., and Marble, D. W. (1958). *Am. J. Vet. Res.* **19**, 632.

Lagace, A., Bell, D. S., Moxon, A. L., and Pounden, W. B. (1961). *Am. J. Vet. Res.* **22**, 686.

Lawrie, R. A. (1952). *Nature* **170**, 122.

Lawrie, R. A. (1953). *Biochem. J.* **55**, 298.

Lee, F. S., Guenther, A. E., and Meleney, H. E. (1916). *Am. J. Physiol.* **40**, 446.

Michelson, A. M., Russell, E. S., and Harman, P. J. (1955). *Proc. Natl. Acad. Sci. VS* **41**, 1079.

Mommaerts, W. F. H. M. (1969). *Physiol. Rev.* **49**, 427.

Nachmias, V. T., and Padykula, H. A. (1958). *J. Biophys. Biochem. Cytol.* **1**, 47.

Nagode, L. A., Frajola, W. J., and Loeb, W. F. (1966). *Am. J. Vet. Res.* **27**, 1385.

Needham, D. M. (1926). *Physiol. Rev.* **6**, 1.

Ogata, T. (1960). *J. Biochem. (Tokyo)* **6**, 726.

Okinaka, S., Sugita, H., Momoi, H., Toyokura, Y., Watanabe, T., Ebashi, F., and Ebashi, S. (1964). *J. Lab. Clin. Med.* **64**, 299.

Oliver, I. T. (1955). *Biochem. J.* **61**, 116.

Padykula, H. A. (1952). *Am. J. Anat.* **91**, 107.

Padykula, H. A., and Gauthier, G. F. (1963). *J. Cell Biol.* **18**, 87.

Padykula, H. A., and Gauthier, G. F. (1967). In "Exploratory Concepts in Muscular Dystrophy and Related Disorders" (A. T. Milhorat, ed.), pp. 117–127. Excerpta Med. Found., Amsterdam.

Padykula, H. A., and Herman, E. (1955a). *J. Histochem. Cytochem.* **3**, 161.

Padykula, H. A., and Herman, E. (1955b). *J. Histochem. Cytochem.* **3**, 170.

Pearse, A. G. E. (1960). "Histochemistry, Theoretical and Applied" Little, Brown, Boston, Massachusetts.

Peter, J. B., Jeffress, R. N., and Lamb, D. R. (1968). *Science* **160**, 200.

Ranvier, L. (1873). *Compt. Rend.* **77**, 1030.

Ranvier, L. (1874). *Arch. Physiol. Normal. Pathol.* [2] **1**, 5.

Ranvier, L. (1880). "Leçons d'anatomie générale sur les systèmes musculaires." De La Haye, Paris.

Robbins, N., Karpati, G., and Engel, W. K. (1969). *Arch. Neurol.* **20**, 318.

Romanul, F. C. A. (1964). *Arch. Neurol.* **11**, 355.

Romanul, F. C. A., and Van Der Meulen, J. P. (1966). *Nature* **212**, 1369.

Romanul, F. C. A., and Van Der Meulen, J. P. (1967). *Arch. Neurol.* **17**, 387.

Roussel, J. D., and Stallcup, O. T. (1966). *Am. J. Vet. Res.* **27**, 1527.

Salmons, S., and Vrbova, G. (1969). *J. Physiol. (London)* **201**, 535.

Scarpelli, D. G., Hess, R., and Pearse, A. G. E. (1958). *J. Biophys. Biochem. Cytol.* **4**, 747.

Seidel, J. C. (1967). *J. Biol. Chem.* **242**, 5623.

Smith, J. B., and Healy, P. J. (1968) *Clin. Chim. Acta* **21**, 295.

Stein, J. M., and Padykula, H. A. (1962). *Am. J. Anat.* **110**, 103.

Stubbs, S. G., and Blanchaer, M. C. (1965). *Can. J. Biochem.* **43**, 463.

Swingle, K. F., Young, S., and Dang, H. C. (1959). *Am. J. Vet. Res.* **20**, 75.

Takeuchi, T. (1956). *J. Histochem. Cytochem.* **4**, 84.

Takeuchi, T., and Kuriaki, H. (1955). *J. Histochem. Cytochem.* **3**, 153.

Tanzer, M. L., and Gilvarg, C. (1959). *J. Biol. Chem.* **234**, 3201.

Vrbova, G. (1963). *J. Physiol. (London)* **169**, 513.

Wachstein, M., and Meisel, E. (1955). *J. Biophys. Biochem. Cytol.* **1**, 483.

Weismann, U., Colombo, J. P., Adam, A., and Richterich, R. (1966). *Enzymol. Biol. Clin.* **7**, 266.

5   Hemostasis and Blood Coagulation

W. Jean Dodds and J. J. Kaneko

I.   INTRODUCTION

Hemostasis may be defined as the process by which hemorrhage of whatever cause is arrested. The complete process is associated with initial control of bleeding from the injured vessel to the final arrest of bleeding. Hemostasis is a complex mechanism of physiological and biochemical events which terminate in the formation of a stable plug which seals off the blood vessel. The entire process involves at least three major factors: blood coagulation, the vessel wall, and blood platelets. The coagulation mechanism has been the subject of most intensive investigations in man and animals for many years. In domestic animals, these have been largely confined to their research applications. With the increasing awareness of hemorrhagic disease in domestic animals, knowledge of the hemostatic mechanisms and the clinical bio-chemical events in coagulation assumes added importance.

II. HEMOSTASIS

A. THE BLOOD VESSEL

When a blood vessel is injured or severed, a brief local reflex vasoconstriction occurs which may be sufficient in the case of minor injury to slow the escape of blood. At the same time, adhesion of platelets to exposed collagen fibres in the vessel wall initiates hemostasis. Interaction of the platelet mass with collagen causes focal release of adenosine diphosphate (ADP) at the point of injury, as well as other constituents such as serotonin, histamine, and platelet phospholipids. The next step involves the action of the released ADP on other platelets in the ambient fluid. ADP causes platelet aggregation so that a large mass or aggregate forms over the injured area. At the same time, the injured tissue and altered platelets release thromboplastins which initiate the blood coagulation mechanism and fibrin formation. Finally, there is a fusion of the platelet mass with the fibrin formed by coagulation to form an effective stable plug.

B. THE BLOOD PLATELET

Blood platelets are cellular particles produced by megakaryocytes mainly of the bone marrow. The lung has also been mentioned as a possible source of platelets. The megakaryocyte is a large (25–50 μ) cell with a polyploid nucleus which is extremely pleomorphic. As the cell matures, pseudopods form and platelets bud off at the extremities. The normal platelet seen in a Wright stained blood film is from 1 to 4 μ in diameter and is spherical, oval, or rod-shaped. The cytoplasm is pale blue and contains reddish granules. Circulating platelets are disc shaped.

The role of the blood platelet in hemostasis is as important as that of the coagulation mechanism. Platelets are involved together with the blood vessel wall and the contact activated coagulation factors (XI and XII) in the initiation of the hemostatic process. A decrease in the number of circulating platelets (thrombocytopenia) or the presence of abnormal nonfunctioning platelets (thrombasthenia, thrombocyto-pathia) will impair hemostasis. In some instances, an excess of platelets (thrombocy-tosis or thrombocythemia) can produce inadequate hemostasis but usually this condition promotes clotting and may predispose a patient to thrombosis. An ex-cellent review of the role of platelets in coagulation processes and vascular disease is discussed by Rowsell (1969).

Platelets promote hemostasis in several ways. When a blood vessel is injured, they accumulate at the site of injury. They adhere to the vessel wall, then to each other and lastly become involved in the coagulation process. Upon exposure of platelets to collagen fibers of the vessel wall certain active constituents are re-leased from the platelet (serotonin, histamines, ADP). The release of ADP into the ambient fluid causes the adherence and aggregation of surrounding platelets to the area. The mechanism whereby ADP induces platelet aggregation is not understood, but is thought to require fibrinogen and calcium ions. Recent studies have suggested that the reaction cannot take place unless adequate energy (glucose) is available to the platelet (Kinlough et al., 1969). The platelets also undergo a series of reactions mediated by thrombin and connective tissue which produces marked structural changes. This process has been called "viscous metamorphosis" of platelets. The thrombin associated with viscous metamorphosis and evolved from tissue injury rapidly activates the coagulation mechanism. Once fibrin has formed around the platelet aggregate, a stable hemostatic plug is produced.

The platelet is essential for normal blood coagulation since it is required for the intrinsic or intravascular coagulation pathway. The phospholipid released from platelets (platelet factor 3) serves an important function in the activation sequence of coagulation. Platelets release their phospholipid when they are activated by such factors as collagen, ADP, and thrombin.

Recent investigations have shown that the platelet can carry out several synthetic processes independently even though it lacks a nucleus. Platelets synthesize proteins by using preformed messenger RNA and ribosomes from the megakaryocyte and synthesis can continue for 2–3 days. This would account for the short survival time or life span of circulating platelets. In addition, platelets have an active glycolytic pathway and synthesize sugars and fatty acids (Marcus and Zucker, 1965). Another function of platelets that deserves mention is their ability to phagocytize particles (e.g., viruses, latex, immune complexes, iron) (Glynn et al., 1965).

A deficiency of circulating platelets (thrombocytopenia) can be hereditary or acquired. The most common form of this disease occurs as a result of hypersensitivity to drugs, bacteria, viruses, etc. and is known as idiopathic thrombocytopenic purpura (ITP) if the causative agent cannot be established. This condition was once considered to be an autoimmune phenomenon. It is now known, however, that the platelet is sensitized by an agent which attaches itself on the platelet as a hapten and it is the platelet–hapten combination against which the body makes antibodies. This means that the destruction of platelets by this "auto"-antibody is self-limiting as soon as the incitant is removed. A serious hemorrhagic diathesis can result from thrombocytopenia and prompt treatment with platelet transfusions and steroid therapy is necessary. In some cases, the primary site of platelet destruction in this disease is the spleen and splenectomy would be indicated. Acquired thrombocytopenia also accompanies many systemic diseases especially those involving the bone marrow (e.g., leukemias).

Idiopathic thrombocytopenic purpura is a well-recognized syndrome in domestic animals. It is most often recognized in dogs, and certain breeds such as middle-aged, obese, miniature poodles seem predisposed. Most of these animals present a picture of profound depression, bruises, and petechiae of the mucous membranes. Diagnosis is based upon a platelet count. If the animal is anemic, *fresh* whole blood transfusions will help replace both red blood cells and platelets. Platelet concentrates or fresh platelet-rich plasma are indicated in severe cases and low level corticosteroid therapy should be instituted to increase platelet production from the bone marrow. If the patient recovers sufficiently but has repeated relapses, splenectomy should be considered.

Abnormally functioning platelets are seen both as hereditary and acquired traits. In this case, the number of circulating platelets may be normal but their function impaired. Hereditary cases are autosomal and can be classified as thrombopathias or thrombasthenias (Glanzmann's disease). There are various platelet function tests which can distinguish these two syndromes. In general, however, platelet function defects may be manifested by some or all of the following: abnormal silicone clotting times; abnormal prothrombin consumption; long bleeding times; defective clot retraction; reduced platelet factor 3 availability; low platelet fibrinogen concentration; defective platelet aggregation with ADP, thrombin, or collagen; abnormal platelet adhesiveness; and bizarre platelet morphology (Marcus and Zucker, 1965). It is also possible that thrombopathia and thrombasthenia may actually be the extremes of a spectrum of platelet function abnormalities and that various intermediate types which display a mixture of the characteristics of both forms exist. One such mixed form, thrombasthenic-thrombopathy, will be discussed later. A comprehensive review of the literature concerning patients with hereditary platelet disorders was made by Caen et al. (1966).

C. The Blood Coagulation Mechanism

1. General

Blood coagulation is a complex series of reactions involving the various coagula-

TABLE I BLOOD CLOTTING FACTORS AND SYNONYMS

International classification[a]	Synonyms
Factor I	Fibrinogen
Factor II	Prothrombin
Factor III	Tissue thromboplastin
Factor IV	Calcium
Factor V	Proaccelerin
	Labile factor, accelerator globulin (AcG)
Factor VII	Proconvertin
	Serum prothrombin conversion accelerator (SPCA), stable factor, autoprothrombin I
Factor VIII	Antihemophilic factor (AHF)
	Antihemophilic globulin (AHG), platelet cofactor I, plasma thromboplastic factor A
Factor IX	Christmas factor
	Plasma thromboplastin component (PTC), platelet cofactor II, autoprothrombin II, plasma thromboplastic factor B
Factor X	Stuart factor
	Stuart-Prower factor
Factor XI	Plasma thromboplastin antecedent (PTA)
Factor XII	Hageman factor
Factor XIII	Fibrin stabilizing factor (FSF)
	Fibrinase, Laki-Lorand factor

[a]As recommended by the International Committee for the Nomenclature of Blood Clotting Factors (1962). The most commonly used synonym is capitalized for each factor.

tion factors, designated in the International Nomenclature by Roman numerals. These factors and their common synonyms are listed in Table 1. The most widely accepted theory of coagulation is based upon the concept that these clotting factors are present in an inactive or zymogen form and that they are activated sequentially to form enzymes by a "cascade" (MacFarlane, 1964) or "waterfall" (Davie and Ratnoff, 1964) mechanism. Esnouf (1968) has proposed that this original mechanism should be revised slightly in the light of recent evidence. Two systems exist in coagulation: an intrinsic or intravascular mechanism essential for clot formation and an extrinsic or tissue system that enchances the reactions. From Fig. 1, it can be seen that these two systems converge at the level of factor X activation and proceed down a common pathway to the formation of fibrin. A simplified version of the process is given in Fig. 2.

Calcium (factor IV) participates in a number of steps in the coagulation process (Fig. 1). The widespread use of chelating agents as anticoagulants is based upon their binding affinity for calcium ions. A summary of the detailed role of calcium in activating specific coagulation steps has been recently published (Davie et al., 1969).

The clotting mechanism can be best described as a series of sequential activating steps that produce a plasma thromboplastic and/or a tissue thromboplastic component, both of which can convert prothrombin to thrombin in the presence of calcium ions. The enzymically active factors are protein in nature and, in general, each of the sequential activations are enzymic hydrolyses of the inactive precursor forms. It

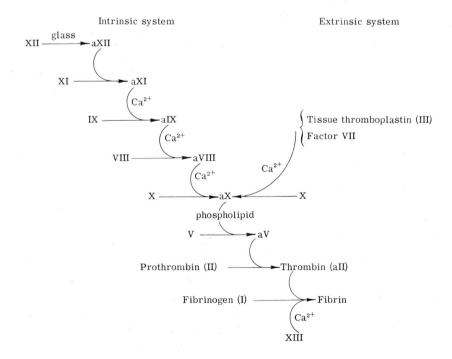

Fig. 1. The intrinsic and extrinsic systems of the blood clotting mechanism. See Table I for nomenclature.

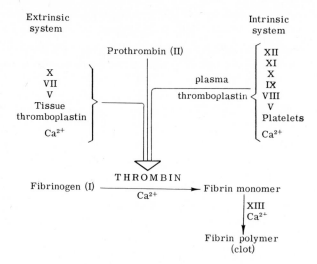

Fig. 2. Summary of the factors involved in blood coagulation and the final reaction. See Table I for nomenclature.

should be noted that factor III (tissue thromboplastin) does not take part in the intrinsic system and that there is no factor VI designated in the nomenclature. The active enzyme, thrombin, then acts upon fibrinogen and converts it to insoluble fibrin. The final stage also requires calcium ions and factor XIII to produce a stable clot. The formation of this clot is also the endpoint in most of the tests for coagulation defects.

The following sections briefly outline some of the current and salient aspects of the individual clotting factors. Each has been the subject of extensive research and the reader is referred to the several excellent reviews (Ratnoff, 1966a; Biggs and Mac Farlane, 1962, Davie *et al.*, 1969) for greater detail.

D. THE INTRINSIC SYSTEM

1. Hageman Factor (Factor XII)

Hageman factor (factor XII) is involved in the initial stage of clotting through the "contact activation" process. Factor XII has a molecular weight of 82,000, is not adsorbed by $Al(OH)_3$, $BaSO_4$, or $Ca_3(PO_4)_2$, is adsorbed with kaolin and celite, is stable at $56°C$ and various pH's, and is a sialoglycoprotein. Hageman factor is activated by glass, collagen, skin, stearate, ellagic and uric acids, and most foreign surfaces. Factor XII activation is inhibited by cytochrome C, lysozyme, ribonuclease, and spermine. This factor is reported to be required for some of the complement reactions (C' esterase), for the Schwartzman reaction, and for activation of the fibrinolytic mechanism. It is also said to enhance vessel permeability and to convert plasma kallikreinogen to kallikrein, the enzyme that elaborates plasma kinins (Nossel, 1969; Ratnoff, 1966b). It should be emphasized here that most of the properties and functions of Hageman factor also apply to PTA (factor XI) which plays an equal role in the initial activation stages of coagulation.

Deficiency of factor XII does not usually produce any clinical problem. The defect occurs in both sexes and is manifested by a prolonged clotting time in glass tubes, and lack of correction when plasma is mixed with that of a known Hageman-deficient patient. Most affected patients do not bleed spontaneously and rarely have problems following injury or surgical procedures. The defect is usually picked up by accident during a coagulation work-up of a patient. Birds (chickens, ducks, pigeons) are known to lack Hageman factor, as do some horses and marine mammals (porpoises) (Rowsell, 1969; Lewis, 1969). No reports of hereditary factor XII deficiency in domestic animals have been made.

2. Plasma Thromboplastin Antecedent (Factor XI)

Plasma thromboplastin antecedent (PTA or factor XI) is involved in the early stages of coagulation along with Hageman factor. It does not appear to require Ca^{2+} for its activity. Factor XI is probably a β_2-globulin (Rosenthal, 1955) of molecular weight estimated to be 100,000–200,000 and with a half-life of 40–84 hours (Rosenthal and Sloan, 1965) in the circulation. Horowitz and Fujimoto (1965), on the other hand, reported half-life survivals of only 10 hours in two patients. Factor XI is present in both serum and plasma, and is stable at $-20°C$ for up to 2 years, and at room temperature for over 4 months. Factor XI levels in plasma from patients with either mild or moderate deficiency tend to increase on storage at $-20°C$ but not if the patient is very severely deficient in factor XI. The increase in PTA activity of deficient plasma upon storage makes it unreliable as a reagent for factor XI assay. Fortunately, however, several reliable artificial factor XI-deficient substrates have been developed by celite adsorption of normal plasma (Horowitz et al., 1963). An excellent review of the role of factors IX, XI, XII, and platelets in the early stages of coagulation was made recently by Nossel (1969). There is some disagreement concerning the adsorbability of factor XI to products such as $Al(OH)_3$, $BaSO_4$, kaolin, celite. Recent evidence suggests that it is adsorbable depending upon the concentration of adsorbing agent used.

A deficiency of factor XI has been called hemophilia C, which is a misnomer because the inheritance pattern of factor XI deficiency is autosomal and not X-linked as are the other two forms of hemophilia. In addition, the deficiency state paradoxically does not usually produce severe hemorrhagic problems (Edson et al., 1967).

Congenital deficiences of factor XI are classified as severe if PTA levels are less than 10%, moderate from 10–20%, and mild from 20–70%. A recent report describes a family of cows with factor XI deficiency (Kociba et al., 1969). In the propositus, the defect occurred concomitantly with lymphoblastic leukemia. To our knowledge this is the first report of PTA deficiency in animals, although some avians are thought to lack factor XI. The defect is manifest in the laboratory by abnormal intrinsic coagulation tests: clotting time, partial thromboplastin time, and thromboplastin generation time.

3. Christmas Factor (Factor IX)

Christmas factor (PTC or factor IX) is a protein of 60,000–80,000 molecular weight that is present in both plasma and serum. Its activity increases in serum over that in plasma and is also increased by contact with glass. It is relatively heat labile and is adsorbed from plasma or serum by $Al(OH)_3$, $BaSO_4$, and $Ca_3(PO_4)_2$. Factor IX is a β-globulin, is stable to storage and is synthesized by the liver, spleen, and possibly other sites (Dodds, 1969a). Factor IX activation takes place in the presence of activated factor XI and Ca^{2+} accelerates the reaction but is not an absolute requirement. Heparin inhibits subsequent activation of the coagulation sequence by combining with activated factor IX (Nossel, 1969). The turnover time (18–36 hours) of factor IX in the circulation is longer than that of factor VIII (9–16 hours) (Rizza and Biggs, 1969).

Hereditary and acquired deficiencies of factor IX have been well documented. Previous to 1952, factor IX deficiency was not distinguishable from factor VIII deficiency. Following the discovery of this entity in the boy, Stephen Christmas (Biggs *et al.*, 1952) from which the names Christmas disease and Christmas factor evolved, factor IX deficiency was called hemophilia B (Aggeler *et al.*, 1952) to separate it from factor VIII deficiency (hemophilia A). Like factor VIII deficiency, this disease has an X-linked inheritance pattern. Treatment regimes for hemophilia B patients are less vigorous than those required for hemophilia A and new factor IX concentrates have become available and recently reviewed by Rizza and Biggs (1969).

Factor IX deficiency has been reported in Cairn terriers (Rowsell *et al.*, 1960), black and tan Coonhounds (Dodds, 1968; Rowsell, 1969), and in Saint Bernards (Dodds *et al.*, 1969). In the smaller breeds, factor IX deficiency does not cause many spontaneous problems, whereas in larger dogs with the defect, serious hemorrhage is as common as with canine factor VIII deficiency (Dodds, 1968). *In vivo* hemostatic studies in factor IX-deficient dogs revealed a delayed secondary bleeding time with poor stability of the initial primary hemostatic plug (Hovig *et al.*, 1968) as was also seen with factor VIII deficiency. Treatment and management of dogs with hemophilia B has been described (Dodds, 1968).

Acquired factor IX deficiencies occur from anticoagulant therapy of patients to reduce the risk of intravascular thrombosis, in animals ingesting rat poison, and in cases that develop spontaneous factor IX inhibitors. As with factor VIII deficiency, it is now recognized that two types of factor IX deficiency occur; the common form lacking factor IX protein and a variant inhibitor form with a factor IX molecule that is biologically inactive. These inhibitors have been studied by a number of investigators (Roberts *et al.*, 1966; Denson *et al.*, 1968).

4. Antihemophilic Factor (Factor VIII)

There is a voluminous clinical and research literature concerning the antihemophilic factor (AHF, AHG, or factor VIII) which is well outside the scope of the current review. The following summarizes some of the more salient points of factor VIII and its two deficiency states, hemophilia A and von Willebrand's disease.

Factor VIII is a large protein with MW estimates up to 2,000,000 found in normal plasma at levels of about 50–200 units/ml. The factor VIII level in plasma fluctuates greatly upon exercise, adrenalin response, pregnancy, central nervous stimulation, and oral contraceptives (Biggs and MacFarlane, 1962; Iversen and Waaler, 1966). Factor VIII migrates in the α_2- and β_2-globulin fractions. In plasma, it is closely associated with fibrinogen so that most purified factor VIII fractions are still contaminated with fibrinogen. Factor VIII is stable for only short periods of time at room temperature or at 4°C. For maximum stability it should be quick frozen and kept at −20°C or lower. It is stabile to heat of 56°C for up to 15 minutes, but this thermolability is extremely variable. Factor VIII is not adsorbed by $Al(OH)_3$ or $BaSO_4$, is activated by thrombin, and inactivated by plasmin. The use of plasma and various purified factor VIII preparations (Pool and Shannon, 1965) in the treatment of hemophilia is well known and an excellent summary has been recently published by Rizza and Biggs (1969).

This factor is known to have a short survival time *in vivo* (9–16 hours) and transfusions of patients with a deficiency of AHF should be made two or three times daily in order to maintain the level of AHF above that critical for hemostasis (20%). Factor VIII is synthesized primarily in the liver but also in the spleen (Weaver *et al.*, 1964; Norman *et al.*, 1967; Dodds, 1969a,d). There is some suggestion by several investigators that factor VIII may also be synthesized in the kidney (Dodds, 1969a; Barrow and Graham, 1968) and by organs containing reticuloendothelial cells (Marchioro *et al.*, 1969). The finding that factor VIII is synthesized by the spleen has incited some discussion and experiments on the use of splenic transplants in "curing" hemophilia. At this time only data from experimental transplants between hemophilic and normal dogs have been obtained and with variable results (Norman *et al.*, 1968; Marchioro *et al.*, 1969). Modern treatment methods using factor VIII concentrates continue to be effective and the number of side effects or complications minimal.

Hereditary and acquired deficiencies of factor VIII are well documented. The most common hereditary deficiency produces hemophilia A which accounts for about 80% of the cases of congenital bleeding disease in North America. Hemophilia A is inherited as an X-linked recessive trait which means that it is carried by the female, transmitted to her daughters and manifested in her sons. Statistically, 50% of the daughters of a carrier mother will also be carriers and 50% of her sons will be affected with hemophilia provided that their father is normal. It is possible, however, with this mode of inheritance to produce true hemophilic females. The instance occurs when a carrier female has progeny by a hemophilic male. Half of their daughters will be carriers and half will have hemophilia. Many reviews are available concerning hemophilia in man (Rizza and Biggs, 1969) and hemophilia in animals is also well recognized. It was first described in dogs by Field *et al.* (1946) and has now been studied extensively by a number of investigators (Dodds, 1968). Hemophilia A is now known in nearly all breeds of dogs. Hemophilia A also occurs in horses (R. D. Archer, 1961; Sanger *et al.*, 1964), cats, and cattle.

It has been postulated that hemophilia A was caused by a lack of factor VIII. Recent evidence, however, indicates that while this appears to be true of the majority of hemophiliacs, some have an abnormal circulating factor VIII that is biologically inactive though antigenically similar to factor VIII (Feinstein *et al.*, 1969; Hoyer and Breckenridge, 1968). It is possible that this same condition exists in canine hemophilia although it has not been found in the Albany colony of hemophilic dogs (Dodds, 1969b). The treatment and management of animals with hemophilia A has been recently outlined (Dodds, 1968).

The second hereditary factor VIII deficiency that deserves mention is known as von Willebrand's disease (VWD). This disease differs from hemophilia A in several important aspects. It occurs in both sexes as an autosomal characteristic. The factor VIII deficiency varies in severity from < 1% factor VIII to mild cases with 40–60% factor VIII. Patients with von Willebrand's disease have long bleeding times and abnormal platelet adhesiveness. The most unusual feature of this disease, however, is the phenomenon seen when von Willebrand's patients are transfused with either normal or factor VIII-deficient plasma; they begin to synthesize their own factor VIII for a period of 24 to 48 hours. Pregnancy seems to correct the deficiency in affected women, so that their factor VIII level becomes more normal with each successive pregnancy. These findings have led to the hypothesis that there is a von Willebrand's stimulating material in normal plasma which is missing in patients with VWD and is probably a precursor of circulating factor VIII (Chan *et al.*, 1968). A good review of this clinical entity was made by Larrieu *et al.* (1968). Some of our recent experiments with isolated perfused rabbit organs have demonstrated the synthesis of a stimulating factor in the liver that directly enhances factor VIII synthesis in the spleen, a phenomenon somewhat analogous to the effect of von Willebrand's stimulating factor (Dodds, 1969d). Von Willebrand's disease has been recognized for some years in swine (Bogart and Muhrer, 1942) and has recently been studied in a family of German Shepherds (Dodds, 1969c).

Acquired deficiencies of factor VIII occur most often as a result of intravascular coagulation, the "defibrination syndrome," and also as a result of the development of a circulating factor VIII inhibitor. Factor VIII inhibitors develop spontaneously in a wide variety of instances: in hemophiliacs following sensitization from multiple transfusions, in postpartum women, in autoimmune disease such as lupus and ulcerative colitis (Bloom *et al.*, 1966; Roberts *et al.*, 1965). The antibodies produced are IgG immunoglobulins and some of them appear to be monotypic (Shapiro, 1967; Hougie, 1967). Usually, they are self-limiting and disappear as quickly as they appeared. In hemophiliacs, the development of inhibitors is a serious threat which may prevent successful treatment of bleeding episodes.

E. THE EXTRINSIC SYSTEM

1. *Tissue Thromboplastin (Factor III)*

Thromboplastin is a species-specific factor extracted from tissue juice and is a potent activator of the extrinsic coagulation mechanism. The species specificity of tissue extract disappears if it is first incubated with homologous serum (Irsigler *et al.*, 1965). Purified human brain thromboplastin is more accurate and effective for use as a universal activator in coagulation tests than either bovine or rabbit brain thromboplastins, but for practical purposes these are satisfactory. Thromboplastin accelerates the clotting of blood or plasma in the presence of factor VII and calcium according to the scheme on Fig. 1.

2. *Proconvertin (Factor VII)*

Factor VII is a stable, extrinsic (tissue) coagulation factor that is apparently not required for intrinsic (intravascular) coagulation. It is present in both plasma and serum. It has the most rapid turnover rate of any coagulation factor and a half-life of 2–4 hours (Dodds *et al.*, 1967). It seems surprising that a factor not essential for primary hemostasis would be biosynthesized so rapidly. Extensive studies on the structure, metabolism, and function of factor VII have been conducted by Prydz (1965) who estimates the molecular weight of factor VII as 48,000 in serum and 63,000 in plasma.

Congenital deficiencies of factor VII (hypoproconvertinemia) have been reported and well studied in both man and animals. Affected patients (male or female) rarely have serious bleeding episodes although they tend to bruise severely when injured. The exact role of factor VII in the circulation is not understood but it does not appear to be essential for life. A comprehensive review of human factor VII deficiency has been reported by Owen *et al.*(1964). Two instances of congenital factor VII deficiency in animals have been reported and both were in Beagle dogs, one from Canada (Mustard *et al.*, 1962) and the other from England (Garner *et al.*, 1967). In both instances, the disease was mild and with autosomal inheritance. Affected dogs have less than 5% factor VII and heterozygotes have about 50% factor VII. The defect is detected by the presence of a long prothrombin time, normal Russell's viper venom time and a prolonged factor VII assay using known factor VII-deficient plasma. There is also a tendency for factor VII-deficient animals to have a prolonged serum prothrombin consumption time (Dodds, 1969b). Other coagulation tests are normal with this disease. Acquired factor VII deficiency most frequently is seen with liver disease or from treatment of patients with warfarin anticoagulants. It also occurs in animals that ingest rat poison.

F. The Common System

1. Stuart Factor (Factor X)

The Stuart factor is activated by activated factor VIII of the intrinsic system or by the extrinsic system and it in turn activates proaccelerin, factor V. Factor X is an α-globulin (Biggs and MacFarlane, 1962) of MW about 60,000–80,000 which is synthesized in the liver in the presence of vitamin K. It is present in both plasma and serum. A number of compounds such as viper venom promote the activation of Stuart factor. In the intrinsic pathway activated factor VIII activates the Stuart factor in the presence of calcium and phospholipid (from platelets). In the extrinsic pathway, tissue thromboplastin (factor III) and factor VII in the presence of calcium promote the activation of Stuart factor. Thus, the intrinsic and extrinsic pathways of coagulation converge at the step involving the activation of factor X to proceed via a common pathway to fibrin formation. Factor X is destroyed by heating to 56°C and is stable when frozen at -20°C or lower for several months. Its activity disappears from blood that is clotted with an excess of brain extract, and can be adsorbed out of plasma by $Al(OH)_3$, $BaSO_4$, and $Ca_3(PO_4)_2$.

Congenital deficiencies of factor X are rare; their frequency is comparable to that of factor VII deficiency. Hougie *et al.* (1957) described one of the original families with this defect. Domestic animals, however, have not yet been reported to have this disease.

Acquired factor X deficiency is seen with liver disease, anticoagulant therapy, vitamin K deficiency, and rat poisoning—conditions which affect all the factors of the prothrombin complex.

2. Proaccelerin (Factor V)

This factor is required for both the intrinsic (intravascular) and extrinsic (tissue system) coagulation pathways. Factor V accelerates the production of thrombin from prothrombin in the presence of tissue extract and calcium chloride. Activated factor X converts factor V in the presence of phospholipid to activated factor V, the final prothrombin converting principle (Newcomb and Hoshida, 1965). Factor V is an extremely labile material and disappears from plasma as it ages.

Hereditary deficiencies of factor V (parahemophilia) are extremely rare. The defect occurs in both sexes and produces a moderate to severe hemorrhagic diathesis. There is a report of a family with elevated levels of factor V which produces a tendency to thrombosis (Gaston, 1966). Very little information is available concerning factor V in animals (Irfan, 1967) and there are no reports of congenital factor V deficiency in any animal species. Factor V deficiency is manifested in the laboratory by prolongation of the prothrombin time, partial thromboplastin time, whole blood clotting time, and shortened prothrombin consumption time in serum. Acquired factor V deficiency occurs with the intravascular coagulation syndromes.

3. Prothrombin (Factor II)

Prothrombin is a protein of molecular weight about 68,000. It is an α-globulin and present in the plasma at a concentration of 300 Iowa units/ml. It is converted to the active enzyme, thrombin, by the action of several factors known as plasma or tissue thromboplastins (Fig. 1). These various prothrombin activators are a complex mixture of substances. Prothrombin is synthesized primarily by the liver and has a turnover time of 10–12 hours (Anderson and Barnhart, 1964). Both the biosynthesis and release of prothrombin require the action of vitamin K. Warfarin (a coumarin derivative), the ingredient found in rat poison, blocks prothrombin synthesis at an intermediate step which can be overcome by the administration of vitamin K_1 (Dulock and Kolinen, 1968). The exact role of vitamin K in prothrombin synthesis is unknown but it may possibly function as a coenzyme in its synthesis. Vitamin K is also a known requirement for three other factors, factors VII, IX, and X.

Hereditary defects of prothrombin have been reported in man. The hereditary form occurs in families as an autosomal characteristic, appears to be a dysprothrombinemia, and produces mild to moderate bleeding problems (Shapiro, 1969). Guinea pigs are reported to have natural hypoprothrombinemia (Mayer et al., 1965) and a prothrombin complex deficiency and has been reported in a family of inbred mice (Meier et al., 1962). A suspected instance of vitamin K mediated prothrombin deficiency in a Labrador dog has been investigated and the animal placed on continuous oral vitamin K therapy (Dodds, 1969b). The most common causes of acquired prothrombin defects in man and animals are related to the use of dicumarol as an oral anticoagulant for the control of intravascular thrombosis in man, the accidental ingestion of rat poison in animals, and advanced liver disease in all species. Defects in prothrombin are manifested by a long clotting time and abnormal one-stage pro-thrombin assay. Quantitation of the defect can be made with a two-stage prothrombin test.

4. Fibrinogen (Factor I)

Fibrinogen is the substrate for thrombin and the precursor of fibrin. The estimated molecular weight of this protein is 340,000 and is probably composed of three pairs of peptide chains $\alpha(A)$, $\beta(B)$, and γ. Following the action of thrombin upon fibrin-ogen, two major fibrinopeptides (A and B) are split off and a fibrin monomer re-mains. Fibrin monomers are then polymerized to form insoluble fibrin by a reaction which requires the interactions of fibrin stabilizing factor (factor XIII) and calcium ions (Forman et al., 1968). Fibrinogen is also required as a cofactor in the platelet aggregation responses in vivo and in vitro. The major site of fibrinogen biosynthesis is the liver and the turnover time of fibrinogen has been estimated at 50 hours with a biologic half-life of 36 hours (Miller et al., 1964). Heparin, a well-known antico-agulant, is thought to act by inhibiting the action of thrombin upon fibrinogen and also by blocking the activation of factor IX by activated factor XI.

Hereditary and acquired deficiencies of fibrinogen are well known. These can be caused by a complete lack of fibrinogen (afibrinogenemia), a reduced level of fibrin-ogen (hypofibrinogenemia), or an abnormal fibrinogen (dysfibrinogenemia) (For-man et al., 1968; McKenzie and Fowler, 1968). The hereditary fibrinogen defects produce a mild to moderate bleeding diathesis and have an autosomal inheritance pattern.

Fibrinogen defects (quantitative or qualitative) are demonstrated in the labora-tory by a complete failure to clot in any of the usual (clotting time, partial thrombo-plastin time, etc.) coagulation tests. Blood or plasma will also fail to clot when thrombin is added to it, and plasma forms no precipitate when heated to 56°C for 10 or 15 minutes. The formation of this precipitate is the basis for a rapid method of fibrinogen estimation (Kaneko and Smith, 1967). Abnormal platelet function tests have also been reported with fibrinogen defects and this has been attributed to the role of fibrinogen as a platelet cofactor (Inceman et al., 1966).

5. Fibrin Stabilizing Factor (Factor XIII, FSF)

Discovered in 1948, this factor is the latest one to be designated a Roman numeral according to the International Committee classification. A very small amount (2–10%) of factor XIII is sufficient for adequate hemostasis. The half-life of this factor appears to be 4–7 days. FSF is a thrombin-labile protein, requires calcium ions for its activity, is an α_2-globulin, is found in plasma and platelets but only a trace is left in serum. It can be inhibited by several metals (Ag, Pb, Zn) and by snake venoms. The molecular weight is estimated at 350,000 and the molecule contains 3 subunits. The similarity of the molecule to fibrinogen has been noted by several investigators (Alami et al., 1968). The function of factor XIII is to convert unstable soluble fibrin monomer in the presence of calcium ions to insoluble stable fibrin polymer. It is thought to do this by forming crosslinkages between adjacent fibrin strands (Lorand et al., 1962).

Patients with factor XIII deficiency usually have a history of bleeding problems. This fact is amazing when one considers that so little FSF is required for fibrin cross-linkage and stabilization. Patients have poor wound healing, bleed at delivery, bruise easily, develop hematomas, and bleed after minor surgery especially dental extractions. The laboratory test that is diagnostic of FSF deficiency is based on the principle that FSF-deficient fibrin will dissolve when mixed with either 5 M urea or 1–2% monoiodoacetic acid. The deficiency appears in both sexes and reduction of plasma factor XIII levels is said to occur during pregnancy (Coopland et al., 1969). Factor XIII deficiency has not been reported in animals.

6. Fibrinolysins

In addition to the coagulation mechanism, plasma contains a group of enzymes designated as the fibrinolytic system. For details concerning this process, the review by Fearnley (1969) should be consulted. Briefly, the mechanism involves the conversion of the inactive substrate plasminogen by activator substances to the active enzyme plasmin. Plasmin then acts upon fibrin to break it down into fibrin-split products. Plasminogen is a β-globulin of MW 143,000. Many substances can be activator substances but the most widely studied plasminogen activators are streptokinase from β-hemolytic streptococci and urokinase, the activator found in urine. Other activators are niacin, chloroform, and Hageman factor (Ratnoff, 1966b). Activators of plasminogen are present in the blood, the vessel wall, body fluids, and in most tissues. Plasmin, the active fibrinolytic enzyme has a molecular weight of 108,000–125,000, and can hydrolyze a number of proteins such as fibrin, fibrinogen, factor V, gelatin, casein, esters of arginine, and lysine. Plasmin is normally absent from blood and body fluids because there are at least two known types of antiplasmins found in circulating blood which inactivate free plasmin.

Inadequate fibrinolysis becomes important in the control and prevention of thrombotic episodes. For this reason, patients with chronic thrombophlebitis or other thromboses are treated with fibrinolytic agents such as streptokinase and urokinase in order to reverse or contain the process. Overactive fibrinolysis occurs in man and animals and can produce hemorrhagic problems (Rowsell, 1969). The fibrinolytic mechanism also plays a vital role in the "defibrination syndrome" that accompanies intravascular coagulation.

G. New Clotting Factors

Several new coagulation factors have recently been recognized but have not yet been designated with Roman numerals in the International Nomenclature. The Fletcher factor was first described by Hathaway et al. (1965). This new factor is closely related to the contact factors of coagulation (XI and XII). Deficiency of Fletcher factor produces a very prolonged partial thromboplastin time and abnormal thromboplastin generation. This abnormality is corrected in vitro by fresh Al(OH)₃ plasma, by serum, and by mixing affected plasma with factor VIII-, IX-, XI-, or XII-deficient plasmas.

The thorium vulnerable factor is another factor which is present in serum and required for intrinsic thromboplastin generation. It is adsorbable by $BaSo_4$, reduced in liver disease, activated by trypsin, and is heat labile. It could be identical to activated factor IX (Alexander, 1966).

The "Dynia" factor was first reported in 1966 and 1967 (Pechet et al., 1967). This clotting factor is located in the first phase of coagulation, between the activations of factors IX and X. The defect of the Dynia factor is corrected by normal plasma, serum, $Al(OH)_3$ and $BaSO_4$ adsorbed plasma. It produces abnormal intrinsic coagulation activity.

Additional new clotting factors are discussed by Pechet et al. (1967) and include such factors as prephase accelator, Nishimine factor, and Tatsumi factor which is thought to be the same as thorium vulnerable factor.

III. LABORATORY DIAGNOSIS OF COAGULATION DISORDERS

A. General

The importance of proper collection and preparation of blood samples for laboratory diagnosis of coagulation disorders cannot be overemphasized. Scrupulous cleanliness and avoidance of rough handling or rough surfaces must be adhered to in order to obtain satisfactory results. Smooth surfaces are necessary to prevent activation of factor XII (Hageman factor) and to inhibit spontaneous platelet clumping. Therefore, plastic, vaseline-coated or siliconized glassware, syringes, and test tubes should be used in all sample preparations and testing procedures.

Blood must be taken by careful venipuncture to avoid contamination with tissue juices which will activate the coagulation system in about 10 seconds. Trisodium citrate or sodium oxalate are the anticoagulants of choice for coagulation studies. A standard technique is to use 1 part 3.8% trisodium citrate to 9 parts blood. Heparin which inhibits thrombin action, also interferes with the assay of coagulation factors, while EDTA inhibits platelet interactions so that neither of these anticoagulants is applicable to coagulation studies.

The anticoagulated blood should be centrifuged immediately at about 2500 rpm for 15 minutes to obtain platelet-poor plasma. Very slow spinning (800 rpm for 5–10 minutes) or rapid spinning for a short period (1500 rpm for 2–3 minutes) will give platelet-rich plasma for platelet function tests. Plasma should be drawn off and tested immediately or frozen at $-20°C$ for assay at a more convenient time. Coagulation factors are quite temperature-sensitive so that plasma for assay should be kept chilled in an ice bath. Frozen samples should be thawed but once all tests performed as soon as possible. Repeated freezing and thawing will destroy coagulation activity. Platelet assays must of course be made only with fresh samples for freezing will disrupt the platelet membrane.

There are a large variety of tests available for the diagnosis of different coagulation disorders. It is well to remember that the endpoint in almost all the tests is formation of the fibrin clot. The conditions are adjusted so that the limiting factor(s) is the factor being tested. Table II outlines selected tests for the classification and differentiation of hemorrhagic disorders.

TABLE II LABORATORY TESTS FOR DIAGNOSIS OF HEMORRHAGIC DISEASE

1. Platelet function tests:
   Platelet count
   Russell's viper venom time
   Platelet aggregation and clot retraction
   Whole blood clotting time
2. Prothrombin complex or extrinsic tests:
   Prothrombin time
   Russell's viper venom time
3. Plasma thromboplastin or intrinsic tests:
   Whole blood clotting time
   Partial thromboplastin time
   Prothrombin consumption time

B. PLATELET COUNTING AND EVALUATION

1. Direct Counting

The preparation and counting of platelets are done in the same manner as red blood cell counting, except that the filled chamber is allowed to set in a moist environment for 15–20 minutes. Simple diluents such as 2% disodium EDTA in 0.8% saline, or 1% ammonium oxalate work well. The number of platelets in the five small squares of the hemacytometer chamber is counted and then multiplied by a factor of 10,000. Other methods used are the (1) Rees-Ecker diluting fluid instead of EDTA, (2) phase contrast microscopy, (3) Unopette* method, and (4) the electronic counter methods. The normal range as determined by the direct method is between 175,000/mm³ and 500,000/mm³ in most animals and less than 100,000/mm³ can usually be considered clinically significant.

2. Indirect Counting

The indirect method of platelet estimation is the more practicable of the platelet counting methods and lends itself to screening use. It may be performed from the stained blood smear, which has been prepared for routine hematological examination of blood. The simplest procedure is to note the number of platelets per oil immersion field. The finding of three or less would suggest a thrombocytopenic condition. If the total red cell count or the white cell count is known, the number of platelets may be compared to the number of red or white cells in the smear, e.g., no. of platelets/100 WBC. This relative number may be transposed into the absolute number simply by:

$$\frac{\text{No. of platelets}}{100 \text{ WBC}} \times \text{WBC ct} = \text{no. of platelets}$$

*Becton-Dickinson, Rutherford, New Jersey.

3.   Clot Retraction

Under normal circumstances, whole blood clots retract from the sides of a container resulting in the separation of a transparent serum and the compacted clot. This reaction is mainly a function of the quantity and quality of intact platelets. The test is performed by placing 5 ml of blood in a conical centrifuge tube stoppered with a stopper in which a coiled copper wire is embedded, all previously warmed to 37°C in a water bath. Formation of a clot and separation from the walls is checked at 2 and 4 hours and again at 24 hours. At 24 hours, the normal clot has retracted into a compact mass which clings to and is readily removed by the stopper with its coiled wire. Another simple and more sensitive method was recently developed by F. B. Taylor and Zucker (1969). One ml of fresh whole blood is taken by plastic syringe and added to 9 ml of cold buffered saline. Two ml of this diluted mixture is transferred by a cold plastic pipet to a small glass test tube containing 1 unit of thrombin* (0.1 ml of a 10 unit/ml solution) and cooled in an ice bath. The contents of the tube are mixed by inversion and kept in the ice bath or refrigerator for 30 minutes. After 30 minutes, the samples are transferred to a 37°C water bath for 1 hour and then checked. Control samples must be performed simultaneously and the test permits repetition four times with the 10 ml of diluted blood.

4.   Other Indicators of Platelet Function

In addition to platelet counting, platelet function can be tested by the Russell's viper venom time (RVVT) test which depends upon functional platelets. One of the most sensitive indicators of platelet function is the ability of platelets to aggregate when tested *in vitro* with various agents such as ADP, thrombin, collagen suspension, and adrenaline. Because platelet aggregation tests require special equipment, one of the clot retraction assays has been modified (Dodds, 1969b) so that it will also measure platelet aggregation. The test is a practical and reliable indicator of platelet function. About 6 ml of fresh citrated blood are required from both the patient and a normal control. Platelet-rich plasma for the test is prepared from the blood by slow spinning, as described above, in polycarbonate or other plastic test tubes. For the actual assay, maximum platelet activation is required and 0.4 ml of the platelet rich plasma is placed into a plain glass test tube. Thrombin* (0.1 ml of a 10 unit/ml solution) is then added, and the tube is tilted gently back and forth under a lamp until platelet aggregation commences. This procedure takes about 30 seconds and produces a snowflake effect in the sample. Following aggregation, clotting occurs and incubation for 1 hour at 37°C will allow for retraction. Record this retraction as 1–4 +. There is a good correlation between the degree of aggregation and subsequent clot retraction. Abnormal results will occur if platelet numbers or function is reduced. A platelet count on the sample prior to the test will rule out thrombocytopenia as the cause for abnormal retraction. A severe defect in platelet number or function will prolong the whole blood clotting time when measured in plastic or siliconized test tubes (noncontact-activated), whereas it will probably not

---

*Parke-Davis, Detroit, Mich.

show up if the blood is clotted in a plain glass (contact-activated) tube. Abnormal platelet adhesiveness can occur with platelet defects although it is also associated with von Willebrand's disease.

C. Bleeding Time (Duke Method)

A moderately deep skin (or mucous membrane) puncture is made with a No. 11 Bard-Parker blade so that a free flow of blood is obtained. Pressure should not be used to obtain the free flow. At 30-second intervals, the drops of blood are removed by absorbing with a piece of filter paper and the time at which bleeding ceases is noted. In domestic animals, the Duke bleeding time varies between 1 and 5 minutes by this method. In man, this method has been found to be less sensitive than the Ivy bleeding time. The most accurate way to standardize bleeding time determinations in animals, however, involves direct microscopic observation of incised cutaneous vessels in an anesthetized subject (Hovig et al., 1968). This method is not applicable to clinical practice. Long bleeding times occur with platelet defects, vascular lesions, capillary fragility, and von Willebrand's disease.

D. Clotting Time

The wide range of values for bleeding times and coagulation times in normal animals are usually caused by variations in technique and temperature. Of these, temperature is of the utmost importance, particularly in coagulation time determinations, and it cannot be stressed too strongly that normal controls should be run together with the patient.

The coagulation time determination may be performed easily and quickly by either of two procedures. In the capillary method, a skin puncture is made similar to the bleeding time method. After wiping off the first drop of blood, blood is taken up into a capillary tube about 15 cm long by 1–1.5 mm diameter. At intervals of 1 minute, the tube is broken off at 1–2 cm pieces. When coagulation occurs, fibrin strands will be seen between the broken ends and the time is noted. By this method, the horse and cow exhibit coagulation times varying between 3 and 15 minutes. The other domestic species vary between 1 and 5 minutes.

In the more accurate tube method of Lee and White, 3 ml of venous blood is drawn into a clean dry disposable plastic syringe. It is important that the vein be entered quickly and cleanly to avoid contamination by tissue juice and to avoid air bubbles due to exessive suction. One ml of blood is delivered into each of three 13-mm (I.D.) test tubes which are then placed in a 37°C water bath. After 2 minutes, the first of the three tubes is gently tilted at 30-second intervals until the tube can be inverted without spillage of blood. At this time, tilting of the second tube is commenced and when this tube has clotted, the third tube is used. Timing is begun when blood first enters the syringe and the endpoint is reached when the blood in the third tube has clotted. The value of the Lee-White test has been questioned but according to Quick (1966), the test used as described gives excellent reproducible results. Coagulation times by this method are noticeably longer than the capillary method in all the domestic animals. In the horse and cow, times of 4–15 minutes have been recorded, while in the dog a normal range of 11–16 minutes is reported (Kaneko *et al.*, 1967). An alternate method employs four 10×75 mm test tubes (two glass and two plastic or silicone-coated glass). One ml of blood is placed in each of the four tubes and coagulation is timed as above. The clotting time in plastic or silicone-coated tubes will be about twice that of the glass tube. With this method, normal values for dogs range from 3 to 12 minutes in glass and 6 to 20 minutes, in plastic or silicone. The advantage of this technique is that platelet defects can be revealed by the plastic or silicone clotting time.

E. Fibrinogen

Of the clotting factors shown in Fig. 1, only fibrinogen can be assayed directly. Thrombin can be added to the system and the fibrin formed can be measured chemically or gravimetrically. By adding thrombin to the system, all phases of the clotting sequence are effectively bypassed and a measure of the time required for the clot to form (thrombin time test) is also a measure of the amount of fibrinogen. A very rapid direct method of fibrinogen determination based upon its precipitation at 56°C has recently been reported (Kaneko and Smith, 1967). The method uses the hand refractometer routinely employed for plasma protein determinations. Two 75-mm microhematocrit tubes are each filled with blood containing EDTA as anticoagulant, sealed and centrifuged for 5 minutes in a microhematocrit centrifuge. The plasma protein concentration is determined in one tube using the hand refractometer. The second tube is placed in a 56°C water bath for 3 minutes. This tube is again centrifuged for 5 minutes and the plasma proteins (minus the fibrinogen) are again determined with the refractometer. The fibrinogen concentration is given by the difference in the protein concentration of the plasmas before and after heating. The fibrinogen in most animals is about 200–300 mg/100 ml plasma.

F. Prothrombin Time

In this test, the clotting time of plasma is measured in the presence of tissue thromboplastin (factor III) and Ca^{2+} (factor IV) which are added in optimal amounts. According to Fig. 1, this test measures the contributions not only of prothrombin but of factors V, VII, and X as well. Therefore, when one or more of these factors is reduced, the prothrombin time is prolonged. In most cases, however, prolongation of the prothrombin time can be associated with prothrombin deficiency. Fibrinogen concentration is also critical in this process as fibrin is the endpoint of the test. In hypo- or afibrinogenemia (60–100 mg/ml or less), clot formation may be delayed or not occur at all. Prothrombin times may also be delayed by inhibitors such as antithrombins and antithromboplastins.

The one-stage prothrombin time of Quick is performed by pipetting exactly 0.1 ml of citrated plasma into 0.2 ml of a previously prepared mixture of equal volumes of commercial (rabbit brain) thromboplastin and 0.0175 or 0.025 M $CaCl_2$ in a 37°C water bath. Timing is begun at the moment the thromboplastin–$CaCl_2$ mixture is added and the times required for visible clot formation recorded in seconds. This is a sensitive test and a few seconds prolongation represents a significant reduction in the clotting factors (Spaet, 1964). The following normal ranges may be used as a guide and a normal control plasma from the same species should be run simultaneously: dog 9–14 seconds, cattle 18–28 seconds, horses 9–12 seconds. If species-specific thromboplastins are used, however, the normal prothrombin time will be 9–14 seconds for all species.

G. Prothrombin Consumption Time

The prothrombin consumption time (PCT) test measures, in serum, the amount of prothrombin available after a clot has formed, i.e., unconsumed prothrombin. In the presence of normal amounts of intrinsic coagulation factor activity (Fig. 1), adequate amounts of plasma thromboplastin would be generated during clotting and most of the prothrombin would be utilized leaving little in the serum. The prothrombin time of this serum in the presence of added fibrinogen would be long in a *normal* sample. Deficiencies of intrinsic system coagulation factors leave an excess of prothrombin in serum after clotting, so that the prothrombin time of this serum is abnormally fast. Normal values for most species are greater than 30 seconds. Hemophiliacs have very short PCT (< 10 seconds).

H. Russell's Viper Venom Time

Russell's viper venom (Stypven)* has thromboplastic activity in high dilutions and therefore can be used in place of thromboplastin in the performance of the prothrombin time test. Its thromboplastin activity is dependent upon phospholipid (platelets), prothrombin, factors V and X. Factor VII does not affect these reactions. The RVVT is prolonged in prothrombin, factors V and X deficiencies, and platelet defects.

I. Partial Thromboplastin Time

The partial thromboplastin time (PTT) test has its basis in the observation that hemophiliac plasma clots more slowly than normal (Langdell *et al.*, 1953; Rodman *et al.*, 1958). Purified brain thromboplastin (a partial thromboplastin as opposed to tissue juice which is a complete thromboplastin) is activated by kaolin and added to plasma. The mixture is incubated for a standard interval and clotting time recorded following addition of CaCl$_2$. Normal values from standard dilution curves are determined for all species and test plasmas are assayed at the same time in several dilutions and compared to the standard. For screening purposes, the PTT of undiluted samples can be measured and compared to controls. The time it takes for normal plasma to clot in this system varies tremendously with the species and the purity of the brain thromboplastin used. For example, canine plasma will have a PTT of 18–25 seconds using commerial rabbit thromboplastin, whereas purified human brain thromboplastin gives a time of 26–35 seconds. The wider the range of clotting times in a standard dilution curve, the more sensitive the test becomes for detecting minor deficiencies. For practical purposes, however, commerial reagents are perfectly adequate. In clinical hematology, the partial thromboplastin test has replaced the TGT test for routine screening in most laboratories. If the unknown plasma shows a

*Burroughs-Wellcome, Tuckahoe, New York.

prolonged PTT, a differential PTT test can be carried out by replacement studies using plasma from patients with known deficiencies. Failure to correct the PTT to normal by a specific deficient plasma suggests a deficiency of that factor (Hicks and Pitney, 1957). Hemophilic dog plasmas have a PTT time of 50–90 seconds.

J. THROMBOPLASTIN GENERATION TIME

The thromboplastin generation time (TGT) test provides a means of detecting deficiencies of the intrinsic system of clotting. The Hicks-Pitney (1957) modification of the original method can be utilized as a rapid screening test for detection of intrinsic deficiencies. The test is essentially a progressive series of one-stage prothrombin times using the thromboplastin generated by the patient's plasma. As thromboplastin continues to be generated in the system, the prothrombin time becomes progressively shorter and shorter. A normal plasma will generate sufficient thromboplastin in 10 minutes or less to have a prothrombin time of less than 15 seconds.

IV. DISORDERS OF HEMOSTASIS

It is apparent that the vessel, the blood platelet and coagulation are all of importance for hemostasis and that the differentiation of hemorrhagic conditions requires the examination of all these functions. A valuable aid in the initial evaluation of a bleeding syndrome is to be able to establish a probable cause for the hemorrhage if one is apparent. Some of the well-recognized causes of hemorrhage are listed in Table III and have been classified as the acquired and the hereditary disorders of hemostasis.

A. ACQUIRED DEFECTS

Acquired hemorrhagic disease is much more common than the hereditary forms. In general, any significant reduction of liver function will result in a hemorrhagic tendency because the liver is the major site of synthesis of coagulation factors.

TABLE III   SOME CAUSES OF HEMORRHAGE IN ANIMALS

Acquired defects
  Trauma: accidental or from surgical intervention
  Poisoning: warfarin, moldy sweet clover, cottonseed meal, aspirin overdose
  Vitamin K deficiency, scurvy, absorptive failure
  Liver disease: obstructive jaundice, infectious canine hepatitis, tumors, liver failure
  Thrombocytopenia: idiopathic, virus-induced, autoimmune disease, septicemia, splenomegaly, aplastic anemia
  Obstetrical defibrination, fibrinolytic disease
  Platelet function defects: uremia, hyperestrogenism, allergies, drugs, chronic disease, malignancy.
Hereditary defects
  Coagulation disorders: hemophilia A and B, factor VII deficiency, von Willebrand's disease, hypoprothrombinemia, hypofibrinogenemia
  Platelet disorders: thrombasthenia, thrombocytopathy

Fibrinogen deficiency in liver disease has already been discussed. For many years a hemorrhagic diathesis has been known to result from the injestion of moldy sweet clover. The anticoagulant principle in this feed was found to be a coumarin derivative and has been prepared commercially as dicoumarol and various chemical analogs (i.e., warfarin). The use of these drugs to anticoagulate patients with heart disease and as a rat poison is based upon the fact that it interferes with vitamin K metabolism and thereby prevents synthesis of the vitamin K-dependent coagulation factors (prothrombin, factors VII, IX, and X).

The prothrombin time (PT) test is the most important test to detect these factor deficiencies. In malabsorptive states or in biliary obstruction, vitamin K is poorly absorbed and the PT is prolonged. This will be corrected by a small parenteral dose of vitamin K. If the PT is prolonged due to hepatocellular disease, vitamin K will not correct it. The therapeutic use of vitamin K to counteract dicoumarol and warfarin has already been mentioned.

Recently, certain drugs have been found that predispose to hemorrhagic tendencies when used in moderate to high doses. Most of these agents impair hemostasis by inhibiting blood platelet surface reactions (O'Brien, 1968), e.g., aspirin, phenyl-butazone, promazine derivative tranquilizers. Doses of aspirin as low as $\frac{1}{2}$ tablet given to normal individuals are sufficient to prolong the bleeding time and prevent the reaction of platelets to collagen suspensions *in vitro* for 4 to 5 days (O'Brien, 1968). It is also known that high doses of aspirin are hazardous in dogs and cats because of the induction of gastric and duodenal ulceration (L. A. Taylor and Crawford, 1968). Platelet function defects produced by drugs are not in themselves dangerous to normal subjects. Caution should be taken, however, when prescribing any of these agents for animals with hemostatic defects. For example, aspirin or phenylbutazone would be contraindicated in patients suffering from warfarin poisoning, liver disease, or hemophilia.

The majority of bleeding episodes in domestic animals are related to a deficiency in the number or function of blood platelets. Defects are usually manifested by petechial hemorrhages of the mucosal surfaces, but more extensive bleeding can also occur. Thrombocytopenia frequently accompanies autoimmune diseases, such as autoimmune hemolytic disease (AHD) and systemic lupus erythrematosis (SLE). Virus infections are often associated with significant reduction in platelet numbers, and some investigators have been concerned with the effect of live virus vaccines on platelets. In children and dogs, live measles vaccine will reduce the platelet count during viremia, which occurs 5–7 days following vaccination (Oski and Naiman, 1966). Some individuals develop petechiae at this time. It is believed that sensitization of a small percentage of the population could occur so that later in life they may suffer an acute episode of thrombocytopenic purpura if they are challenged by the same antigen (Oski and Naiman, 1966). Bleeding has been associated with vaccination of swine with live hog cholera vaccine (Pilchard, 1966). Hemorrhage is a characteristic of many fatal virus diseases of swine and cattle (e.g., hog cholera, African swine fever, and rinderpest). Viral septicemias produce massive hemorrhage by affecting both the platelets and the vascular endothelium. Finally, uremic bleeding is thought to be the result of qualitative and quantitative change in the platelets which occurs with uremia and is reversible by dialysis (Stewart and Castaldi, 1967). The exact mechanism of the defect, however, is unknown.

The most dramatic and common cause of acquired fibrinogen deficiency is seen in the obstetrical defibrination sydrome. This syndrome results from intravascular coagulation and is rapidly fatal if not diagnosed accurately and treated promptly (Nilsson *et al.*, 1966; Merskey *et al.*, 1967). An acquired defibrination syndrome following obstetrical complications in a dog has been observed (Dodds, 1969b). Cortisone and ACTH are reported to decrease fibrinogen (Fearnley and Bunim, 1951). Hyperfibrinogenemia also occurs and is seen during pregnancy and in inflammation.

B. HEREDITARY DEFECTS

It was recognized about 30 years ago that hemorrhagic conditions similar to hemophilia in man could occur in animals. Early reports mention a "hemophilia-like disease of swine" (Bogart and Muhrer, 1942) which is now known to mimic von Willebrand's disease and isolated cases of bleeding in dogs in France (Tasken, 1935), England (McKenna, 1936) and the Dutch East Indies (Merkens, 1938). Field, Rickard, and Hutt (1946) reported the first extensive coagulation and genetic study in a family of Irish setters with hemophilia A (factor VIII deficiency). This defect was shown to have a sex-linked recessive inheritance pattern as does classic hemophilia of man. Hemophilia A has since been reported in German Shepherds and Collies (Rowsell, 1963), Labrador Retrievers (R. K. Archer and Bowden, 1959; Rowsell, 1969), Beagles (Brock *et al.*, 1963), Shetland Sheepdogs (Wurzel and Lawrence, 1961), Greyhounds (Sharp and Dike, 1963), Weimaraners and Chihuahuas (Kaneko *et al.*, 1967), and several other breeds such as the Vizsla and miniature poodle. Hemophilia A is also known to occur in horses (R. D. Archer, 1961; Sanger *et al.*, 1964), and has been suspected in cats.

In 1960, Rowsell *et al.* reported the first incidence of hemophilia B (factor IX deficiency or Christmas disease) in animals which they observed in Cairn Terrier dogs. There was extensive bleeding and a sex-linked inheritance pattern. Mustard *et al.* (1962) then described factor VII deficiency in Beagles. This mild hemorrhagic disease had an autosomal incompletely dominant inheritance pattern. A thrombocytopathy resembling the Glanzmann's disease type of human platelet defect was reported in a family of Otterhounds (Dodds, 1967). A canine "pseudohemophilia" which mimics von Willebrand's disease of man has recently been described in a family of German Shepherds (Dodds, 1969c). This disease is relatively common in man, and is characterized in man and animals by autosomal inheritance, prolonged bleeding time, decreased platelet adhesiveness, and variable reduction of factor VIII level. A peculiar finding, however, is that transfusion of normal or factor VIII-deficient plasma into patients with von Willebrand's disease produces unexpectedly high levels of factor VIII in their plasma within 24 hours; this activity cannot be accounted for by the factor VIII actually infused. On this basis, the existence of a "von Willebrand's stimulating factor" in plasma has been postulated (Barrow and Graham, 1964). The pigs with von Willebrand's disease (Bogart and Muhrer, 1942) have recently been reevaluated and they also respond by producing factor VIII when infused with normal pig plasma or certain of its fractions (Chan *et al.*, 1968). Hereditary hypofibrinogenemia has been diagnosed in dogs but to our knowledge has never been published.

The severe congenital coagulation disorders, such as hemophilias A and B, produce a defect in formation of plasma thromboplastin. For screening purposes, an abnormal partial thromboplastin time and whole blood clotting time will establish that a defect exists. The clotting time in plastic or silicone-coated tubes is less affected by surface and tissue activation of the sample and so is a more reliable indicator than the glass tube clotting time. In general, the glass or contact clotting time is one-half that obtained using silicone-coated or plastic (noncontact) tubes. The upper limit of normal for noncontact clotting time is 20 minutes at 37°C. Blood from carrier female hemophilic dogs usually takes more than 25 minutes (range 16–35 minutes) to clot, whereas samples from hemophilic male dogs may not clot for 1 hour or more. It must be emphasized, however, that at best the clotting time is an estimation of coagulability, and does not necessarily reflect *in vivo* hemostatic function. The response of hemophilic patients to treatment should not be monitored by clotting times for it has been shown that even saline–dextrose infusions will shorten the clotting time and yet not improve the factor VIII assay or hemostatic function (Brinkhous, 1964). The partial thromboplastin time assay is a reliable indication of intrinsic coagulation function. It can be performed during treatment of patients with plasma transfusions to follow their response. This test has been modified to quantitate any specific coagulation factor by adding human or animal plasma congenitally deficient in the factor. Such specific coagulation factor assays are more complicated and usually performed in coagulation laboratories.

It is apparent that a wide variety of hemorrhagic disorders exist in animals. It is also likely that animal models for most of the other known coagulation defects do exist and await further study. The inheritance pattern of the known hereditary disorders of coagulation are summarized in Table IV. It can be seen from this table that coagulation defects which are often thought to occur only in males, can be seen in females if the defect has an autosomal inheritance pattern. The true hemophilias, types A and B, have an X-chromosome-linked inheritance pattern, which means they are carried by the female and manifested in her sons. In addition, affected males produce only normal sons and all their daughters are carriers. By crossbreeding hemophilic male dogs with carrier females, it is possible to create hemophilic females (Brinkhous and Graham, 1950). However, such an occurrence in nature is extremely rare because of the low incidence of these defects in the random population.

TABLE IV   INHERITANCE OF HEREDITARY COAGULATION DEFECTS IN ANIMALS

Bleeding disorder	Inheritance pattern
Factor VII deficiency	Autosomal, incompletely dominant
Factor VIII deficiency (hemophilia A)	X-linked, recessive
Factor IX deficiency (hemophilia B)	X-linked, recessive
Factor XI deficiency	Autosomal
von Willebrand's disease	Autosomal
Hypofibrinogenemia	Autosomal
Thrombocytopathy; thrombasthenia	Autosomal, incompletely dominant

C. Combined Defects

The occurrence of congenital and acquired deficiencies of more than one coagulation factor in the same patient should be mentioned. Important data have been collected concerning the genetic behavior of several clotting abnormalities with reference to their linkage on the X-chromosome (i.e., linkage between the X-linked hemophilias, A and B). Several reports have been made of patients with combined hereditary factors V and VIII deficiencies (Jones *et al.*, 1962; Gobbi *et al.*, 1967), factors VIII and IX deficiencies (Robertson and Trueman, 1964), factors VIII and XI deficiencies, factors VII and IX deficiencies, and factors VII and X deficiencies (Kroll *et al.*, 1964). Isolated cases have also been reported where factors VIII, IX, and XI deficiencies coincided in the same patient. Linkage studies between the genetic loci for hemophilia A, B, and the Xg blood group system of man have determined that the hemophilia loci are located at some distance from each other on the X-chromosome (at least 12 map units apart) and that the Xg locus is at the other end of the X-chromosome 50 or more map units away for both hemophilia loci (Wall *et al.*, 1967). Crossbreeding of the various types of coagulation defective dogs have been conducted in the Albany colony and also in cooperation with the North Carolina Colony. Initial data from these studies in which factors VIII and IX deficient animals were crossbred reveal that crossover between the hemophilia A and B loci tends to occur frequently which means that the loci are far enough apart on the X-chromosome to permit recombination at random in the offspring (Dodds, 1968). Factor VII-deficient dogs have since been crossed with these factor VIII and IX crossbreeds to obtain animals with triple defects of all possible combinations (Dodds, 1969b). Factor VIII-deficient and thrombopathic dogs have also been crossbred to create a model for comparative studies with canine von Willebrand's disease (Dodds, 1969b).

Acquired multiple coagulation defects can occur from many conditions. The best known examples are seen with Warfarin (dicumarol) poisoning in animals following ingestion of rat poison or in man with overdosage in the control of intravascular thrombosis. Intravascular coagulation and defibrination also produces massive multiple coagulation defects. Vitamin K deficiency will affect synthesis of all the "prothrombin-complex" clotting factors and so induce multiple deficiencies. A hereditary deficiency in vitamin K utilization in prothrombin-complex factor synthesis has also been reported (McMillan and Roberts, 1966).

REFERENCES

Aggeler, P. M., White, S. G., Glendening, M. B., Page, E. W., Leake, T. B., and Bates, G. (1952). *Proc. Soc. Exptl. Biol. Med.* **79**, 692.

Alami, Samih, Y., Hampton, J. W., Race, G. J., and Speer, R. J. (1968). *Am. J. Med.* **44**, 1.

Alexander, B. (1966). *Thromb. Diath. Haemorrhag.* Suppl. 20, 415.

Anderson, G. F., and Barnhart, M. (1964). *Am. J. Physiol.* **206**, 929.

Archer, R. K. (1961). *Vet. Record.* **73**, 338.

Archer, R. K., and Bowden, R. S. T. (1959). *Vet. Record* **71**, 560.

Barrow, E. M., and Graham, J. B. (1964). *Progr. Hematol.* **4**, 203.

Barrow, E. M., and Graham, J. B. (1968). *Biochemistry* **7**, 3917.

Biggs, R., and MacFarlane, R. G. (1962). "Human Blood Coagulation and its Disorders," 3rd ed., Davis, Philadelphia, Pennsylvania.

Biggs, R., Douglas, A. S., MacFarlane, R. G., Dacie, J. V., Pitney, W. R., Merskey, C., and O'Brien, J. R. (1952). *Brit. Med. J.* **II**, 1378.

Bloom, A. L., Davies, A. J., and Rees, J. K. (1966). *Thromb. Diath. Haemorrhag.* **15**, 12.
Bogart, R., and Muhrer, M. E. (1942). *J. Heredity* **33**, 59.
Brinkhous, K. M. (1964). *Am. J. Clin. Pathol.* **41**, 342.
Brinkhous, K. M., and Graham, J. B. (1950). *Science* **111**, 72ɔ.
Brock, W. E., Buckner, R. G., Hampton, J. W., Bird, R. M., and Wulz, C. E. (1963). *Arch. Pathol.* **76**, 464.
Caen, J. P., Castaldi, P. A., Leclerc, J. C., Inceman, S., Larrieu, M. J., Probst, M., and Bernard, J. (1966). *Am. J. Med.* **41**, 4.
Chan, J. Y. S., Owen, C. A., Jr., Bowie, E. J. W., Didisheim, P., Thompson, J. H., Jr., Muhrer, M. E., and Zollman, P. E. (1968). *Am. J. Physiol.* **214**, 219.
Coopland, A., Alkjaersig, N., and Fletcher, A. P. (1969). *J. Lab. Clin. Med.* **73**, 144.
Davie, E. W., and Ratnoff, O. D. (1964). *Science* **145**, 1310.
Davie, E. W., Hougie, C., and Lundblad, R. L. (1969). *Recent Advan. Blood Coag.* **1**, 18.
Denson, K. W. E., Biggs, R., and Mannucci, P. M. (1968). *J. Clin. Pathol.* **21**, 160.
Dodds, W. J. (1967). *Thromb. Diath. Haemorrhag.* Suppl. 26, 241.
Dodds, W. J. (1968). *Experimentation Animale* **1**, 243.
Dodds, W. J. (1969a). *Am. J. Physiol.* **217**, 879.
Dodds, W. J. (1969b). Unpublished data.
Dodds, W. J. (1969c). Blood **34**, 842.
Dodds, W. J. (1969d). Science **166**, 882.
Dodds, W. J., Packham, M. A., Rowsell, H. C., and Mustard, J. F. (1967). *Am. J. Physiol.* **213**, 36.
Dodds, W. J., Whitney, G., and Nemerson, Y. (1969). Unpublished data.
Dulock, M. A., and Kolinen, S. N. (1968). *Thromb. Diath. Haemorrhag.* **20**, 136.
Edson, J. W., White, J. G., and Krivit, W. (1967). *Thromb. Diath. Haemorrhag.* **18**, 342.
Esnouf, M. P. (1968). *Proc. 12th Intern. Congr. Soc. Haematol., New York, 1961* p. 315.
Fearnley, G. R. (1969). *Recent Advan. Blood Coag.* **1**, 229.
Fearnley, G. R., and Bunim, J. J. (1951). *Lancet* **II**, 1113.
Feinstein, D., Chong, M. N. Y., Kasper, C. K., and Rapaport, S. I. (1969). *Science* **163**, 1071.
Field, R. A., Rickard, C. G., and Hutt, S. B. (1946). *Cornell Vet.* **36**, 283.
Forman, W. B., Ratnoff, O. D., and Boyer, M. H. (1968). *J. Lab. Clin. Med.* **72**, 455.
Garner, R., Hermoso-Perez, C., and Conning, D. M. (1967). *Nature* **216**, 1130.
Gaston, L. W. (1966). *J. Pediat.* **68**, 367.
Glynn, M. E., Movat, H. Z., Murphy, E. A., and Mustard, J. F. (1965). *J. Lab. Clin. Med.* **65**, 179.
Gobbi, F., Ascari, E., and Barbieri, U. (1967). *Thromb. Diath. Haemorrhag.* **17**, 194.
Hathaway, W. E., Belhasen, L. P., and Hathaway, H. S. (1965). *Blood* **26**, 521.
Hicks, M. D., and Pitney, W. R. (1957). *Brit. J. Haematol.* **3**, 227.
Horowitz, H. I., and Fujimoto, M. M. (1965). *Transfusion* **5**, 539.
Horowitz, H. I., Wilcox, W. P., and Fujimoto, M. M. (1963). *Blood* **22**, 35.
Hougie, C. (1967). *J. Lab. Clin. Med.* **70**, 384.
Hougie, C., Barrow, E. M., and Graham, J. B. (1957). *J. Clin. Invest.* **36**, 485.
Hovig, T., Rowsell, H. C., Dodds, W. J., Jorgensen, L., and Mustard, J. F. (1968). *Blood* **30**, 636.
Hoyer, L. W., and Breckenridge, R. T. (1968). *Blood* **32**, 962.
Inceman, S., Caen, J., and Bernard, J. (1966). *J. Lab. Clin. Med.* **68**, 21.
International Committee for the Nomenclature of Blood Clotting Factors. (1962). *J. Am. Med. Assoc.* **180**, 733.
Irfan, M. (1967). *J. Comp. Pathol.* **77**, 13.
Irsigler, K., Lechaer, K., and Deutsch, E. (1965). *Thromb. Diath. Haemorrhag.* **14**, 18.
Iversen, J. G., and Waaler, B. A. (1966). *Thromb. Diath. Haemorrhag.* **15**, 29.
Jones, J. G., Rizza, C. R., Hardisty, R. M., Dormandy, K. M., and MacPherson, J. C. (1962). *Brit. J. Haematol.* **8**, 120.
Kaneko, J. J., and Smith, R. (1967). *Calif. Vet.* **21**, 21.
Kaneko, J. J., Cordy, D. R., and Carlson, G. (1967). *J. Am. Med. Assoc.* **150**, 15.
Kinlough, R., Packham, M. A., and Mustard, J. F. (1969). *Federation Proc.* **28**, 509.
Kociba, G. J., Ratnoff, O. D., Loeb, W. F., Wall, R. L., and Heider, L. E. (1969). *J. Lab. Clin. Med.* **74**, 37.
Kroll, A. J., Alexander, B., Cochios, F., and Pechet, L. (1964). *New Engl. J. Med.* **270**, 6.

Langdell, R. D., Wagner, R. H., and Brinkhous, K. M. (1953). *J. Lab. Clin. Med.* **41**, 637.
Larrieu, M. J., Caen, J. P., Meyer, D. O., Vainer, H., Sultan, Y., and Bernard, J. (1968). *Am. J. Med.* **45**, 354.
Lewis, J. H. (1969). *Comp. Biochem. Physiol.* **31**, 667
Lorand, L., Konishi, K., and Jacobsen, A. (1962). *Nature* **194**, 1148.
MacFarlane, R. G. (1964). *Nature* **202**, 498.
McKenna, W. R. (1936). *Vet. J.* **92**, 370.
McKenzie, J. M., and Fowler, P. R. (1968). *Am. J. Physiol.* **214**, 786.
McMillan, C. W., and Roberts, H. R. (1966). *New Engl. J. Med.* **274**, 1313.
Marchioro, T. L., Hougie, C., Ragde, H., Epstein, R. B., and Thomas, E. D. (1969). *Science* **163**, 188.
Marcus, A. J., and Zucker, M. B. (1965). "Physiology and Blood Platelets." Grune & Stratton, New York.
Mayer, G., Selva, J., Mayer, S., and Waitz, R. (1965). *Pathol. Biol., Semaine Hop.* [N.S.] **13**, 1009.
Meier, H., Allen, R. C., and Hoag, W. C. (1962). *Blood* **19**, 501.
Merkens, J. (1938). *J. Ned. Ind, Bladen v. Diergeneesk. en Dierent.* **50**, 149.
Merskey, C., Johnson, A. J., Kleiner, G. J., and Wohl, H. (1967). *Brit. J. Haematol.* **13**, 528.
Miller, L. L., Hanavan, H. R., Titthasiri, N., and Chowdhury, A. (1964). *Advan. Chem. Ser.* **44**, 17.
Mustard, J. F., Secord, D., Hoeksema, T. D., Downie, H. G., and Rowsell, H. C. (1962). *Brit. J. Haematol.* **8**, 43.
Newcomb, T. F., and Hoshida, M. (1965). *Scand. J. Clin. & Lab. Invest.* **17**, Suppl. 84, 62.
Nilsson, I. M., Nilehn, J. E., Cronberg, S., and Norden, G. (1966). *Acta Med. Scand.* **180**, 65.
Norman, J. C., Lambillotti, G. P., Kojima, Y., and Sise, H. S. (1967). *Science* **158**, 1060.
Norman, J. C., Covelli, V. H., and Sise, H. S. (1968). *Surgery* **64**, 1.
Nossel, H. L. (1969). *Recent Advan. Blood Coag.* **1**, 39.
O'Brien, J. R. (1968). *Lancet* **I**, 894.
Oski, F. A., and Naiman, J. L. (1966). *New Engl. J. Med.* **275**, 352.
Owen, C. A., Jr., Amunden, M. A., Thompson, J. H., Jr., Spittell, J. A., Jr., Bowie, E. J. W., Stilwell, G. G., Hewlett, J. S., Mills, S. D., Sauer, W. G., and Gage, R. P. (1964). *Am. J. Med.* **37**, 71.
Pechet, L., Cochios, F., and Deykin, D. (1967). *Thromb. Diath. Haemorrhag.* **17**, 365.
Pilchard, E. I. (1966). *J. Am. Vet. Med. Assoc.* **148**, 48.
Pool, J. G., and Shannon, A. E. (1965). *New Engl. J. Med.* **273**, 1443.
Prydz, H. (1965). *Scand. J. Clin. & Lab. Invest.* **17**, Suppl. 84, 78.
Quick, A. J. (1966). *J. Am. Med. Assoc.* **197**, 418.
Ratnoff, O. D. (1966a). *In* "The Metabolic Basis of Inherited Disease" (J. B. Stanbury, J. B. Wyngaarden, and D. S. Fredrickson, eds.), 2nd ed., p. 1137. McGraw-Hill, New York.
Ratnoff, O. D. (1966b). *Progr. Hematol.* **5**, 204.
Rizza, C. R., and Biggs, R. (1969). *Recent Advan. Blood Coag.* **1**, 179.
Roberts, H. R., Scales, M. B., Madison, J. T., Webster, W. P., and Penick, G. D. (1965). *Blood* **26**, 805.
Roberts, H. R., Gross, G. P., Webster, W. P., Dejanov, I. I., and Penick, G. D. (1966). *Am. J. Med. Sci.* **251**, 81.
Robertson, J. H., and Trueman, R. G. (1964). *Blood* **24**, 281.
Rodman, N. F., Jr., Barrow, E. M., and Graham, J. B. (1958). *Am. J. Clin. Pathol.* **29**, 525.
Rosenthal, R. L. (1955). *J. Lab. Clin. Med.* **45**, 123.
Rosenthal, R. L., and Sloan, E. (1965). *J. Lab. Clin. Med.* **66**, 709.
Rowsell, H. C. (1963). *Gaines Vet. Symp.* **12**, 9.
Rowsell, H. C. (1969). *In* "Blood Coagulation and Hemorrhagic Disorders," p. 247. Williams & Wilkins, Baltimore, Maryland.
Rowsell, H. C., Downie, H. G., Mustard, J. F., Leeson, J. E., and Archibald, J. A. (1960). *J. Am. Vet. Med. Assoc.* **137**, 247.
Sanger, V. L., Moirs, R. E., and Trapp, A. L. (1964). *J. Am. Vet. Med. Assoc.* **144**, 259.
Shapiro, S. (1967). *J. Clin. Invest.* **46**, 147.
Shapiro, S. (1969). Personal communication.
Sharp. A. A., and Dike, G. W. R. (1963). *Thromb. Diath. Haemorrhag.* **10**, 494.
Spaet, T. H. (1964). *Blood* **23**, 839.
Stewart, J. H., and Castaldi, P. A. (1967). *Quart. J. Med.* **36**, 409.
Tasken, J. (1935). *Bull. Acad. Vet. France* **8**, 595.

Taylor, F. B., and Zucker, M. B. (1969). *Nature* **222**, 99.

Taylor, L. A., and Crawford, L. M. (1968). *J. Am. Vet. Med. Assoc.* **152**, 617.

Wall, R. L., McConnell, J., Moore, D., MacPherson, C. R., and Marson, A. (1967). *Am. J. Med.* **43**, 214.

Weaver, R. A., Price, R. E., and Langdell, R. D. (1964). *Am. J. Physiol.* **206**, 335.

Wurzel, H. A., and Lawrence, W. C. (1961). *Thromb. Diath. Haemorrhag.* **6**, 98.

6　　　　　　　　　Cerebrospinal Fluid

Embert H. Coles

I. INTRODUCTION

Diagnosis of diseases of the central nervous system in domesticated animals is often a problem to the clinician. Although much information relative to the lesion can be obtained from the history and by a careful systematic physical examination, confirmation of the diagnosis may be dependent upon the use of other techniques. Examination of cerebrospinal fluid (CSF) may provide clues as to the type of lesion present and be of assistance to the clinician in confirming a diagnosis and providing a more accurate prognosis.

This is presented as a brief review of the physiology of CSF, techniques for collection, and interpretation of CSF alterations in animals.

Although there is an abundance of information relative to the physiology of CSF, most of which has been determined in animals, there is a lack of definitive information concerning CSF alteration in diseases of the central nervous system in animals.

II. FORMATION AND DRAINAGE OF CSF

Basic to any discussion of CSF, is consideration of the site of formation.

A variety of techniques have been utilized in studying formation of CSF including: appearance of tracers in CSF; free drainage of fluid from the cerebral ventricles and subarachnoid spaces; steady-state studies of inulin dilution and clearance during perfusion of the CSF system; and the appearance of fluid on tissue surfaces. Perfusion of the CSF and studies of inulin dilution and clearance during perfusion, a method developed by Pappenheimer et al. (1961) and Heisey et al. (1962), has proven to be the most satisfactory and has provided the most reliable data. Bering (1957) reported that the values found from maximum free drainage rates agreed well with data obtained by the inulin-dilution technique.

The rate of total production of CSF, using the inulin-dilution technique, has been measured in man, monkey, goat (Heisey et al., 1962), dog (Bering and Sato, 1963), cat (Vates et al., 1964), and rabbit (Davson et al., 1962). The range of CSF formation was from 0.009 ml/min in the rabbit to 0.5 ml/min in a boy 12 years of age. These data are summarized in Table I.

More recently, Culter et al. (1968) studied the daily volume of CSF formation in twelve children. The mean rate of formation was 0.35 ml/min and was independent of short-term alterations in intraventricular pressure.

The chief site of CSF formation has been thought to be within the ventricular system. However, there is a considerable volume of literature suggesting and demonstrating the existence of an extraventricular formation of CSF (Bering, 1965; Bering and Sato, 1963; Boldrey, 1951; Hassin, 1924; Katzenelbogen, 1935).

In a series of experiments using the inulin-dilution technique in which they perfused from the lateral ventricle to the cisterna magna; from one lateral ventricle to the other after plugging the aqueduct of Sylvius; from the lateral ventricle to the fourth ventricle; and using subarachnoid–subarachnoid perfusions after occluding the outlets of the fourth ventricle; Bering and Sato (1963) quantitatively studied CSF production in dog. These experiments demonstrated that of the total CSF production (0.047 ml/min), 35% was derived from the lateral and third ventricles, 23% from the fourth ventricle, and 42% was formed in the subarachnoid space.

Estimates for ventricular and extraventricular formation of CSF in the cat were

TABLE I   RATE OF CSF PRODUCTION IN VARIOUS ANIMAL SPECIES USING
VENTRICULOCISTERNAL PERFUSION

	ml/min	Reference
Man (boy, age 12)	0.5	Heisey et al. (1962)
Dog	0.047	Bering and Sato (1963)
Cat	0.017	Vates et al. (1964)
	0.015	Hammerstad et al. (1968)
Monkey (Macaca mulatta)	0.097	Heisey et al. (1962)
Rabbit	0.009	Davson et al. (1962)
Goat	0.16	Heisey et al. (1962)
Calf	0.29	Calhoun et al. (1967)

59% intraventricular CSF formation, and 41% extraventricular formation (Bering, 1965).

Bering (1965) suggested that the source of extraventricular fluid was presumably from the brain as drugs and tracers applied to the cortex quickly penetrated the brain and a variety of substances were shown to enter the CSF from the cortex. He also remarked that the routes of entry and exit were not known.

Intraventricular formation of CSF is thought to be located in the choroid plexuses, although there is some experimental evidence demonstrating fluid from the brain (Bering and Sato, 1963; Bhattacharya and Feldberg, 1958; Davson, 1954). Curl and Pollay (1968) studied the transport of water and electrolytes between the brain and ventricular fluid in the rabbit. Their studies implied that the movement of CSF across the blood–brain–CSF barrier was an isotonic flow coupled to sodium transport and represented one-third of the total intraventricular formation of CSF.

In addition to the extrachoroidal formation of CSF, the choroid plexuses play a very important role in the production of CSF. Evidence favoring choroidal formation of CSF was presented by Welch (1963). The arteriovenous hematocrit differences and blood flow in the choroid plexus were measured. Using this technique it was confirmed that fluid was lost from blood on passage through the plexus. Direct evidence on the production of CSF by the choroid plexus was obtained in dogs by Bering (1957) and Bering and Sato (1963). They measured maximum CSF drainage prior to and following removal of the choroid plexuses from the lateral ventricles of a group of hydrocephalic dogs. Choroid plexectomy resulted in a drop in CSF production from 0.03 to 0.022 ml/min. However, plexectomy did not affect rates of entry of various isotopes into the CSF (Bering, 1955). It was admitted that the difference in rates of CSF formation was not of great statistical significance. However, if it were assumed to be a real difference, the choroid plexuses of the lateral ventricles could be assumed to have produced approximately 50% of the CSF arising from the lateral ventricles.

Additional evidence related to the secretory activity of the choroid plexuses was provided by a study of the exposed choroid plexus. This was described by Ames and his collaborators in four papers (De Rougemont et al., 1960; Ames et al., 1964, 1965a,b). These authors collected, under oil, freshly secreted fluid from the choroid plexus of an opened lateral ventricle of the cat. Fluid collected in this manner was submitted to chemical analysis. Concentrations of several ions in this fluid were compared with those in the CSF removed from the cisterna magna, and in plasma and plasma ultrafiltrate. Fluid from the choroid plexus did not differ from plasma ultrafiltrate in potassium and chloride concentration but did contain higher sodium, markedly higher magnesium, and lower calcium concentration than did the ultrafiltrate. Fluid from the cisterna magna differed from ultrafiltrate with respect to all five electrolytes that were measured. There was a higher concentration of chloride, sodium, and magnesium and a lower concentration of potassium and calcium in cisterna magna fluid than in the ultrafiltrate. Davson (1967) concluded that this work of Ames et al. (1964) which suggested that the choroid plexuses were continuously producing a characteristic fluid tended to support the view that these organs are one of the sources of CSF.

In summary, evidence would suggest that CSF is formed both in the ventricular system as well as in the subarachnoid space. Consequently, the fact that CSF formation may occur in many places must be considered in any study of mechanisms of formation and in any attempt to locate enzyme systems responsible for formation.

III. RELATIONSHIP BETWEEN CSF, BRAIN, AND CORD

According to Davson (1967) the simultaneous measurement of rates of penetration of nonelectrolytes into both CSF and brain tissue has led to the conclusion that gradients for diffusion from one compartment of the brain to the other are usually in favor of diffusion from brain tissue to CSF. In addition, quantitative comparisons between the blood–aqueous fluid and blood–CSF indicates that such a diffusion does occur.

Injection of material into the subarachnoid space has been used to study the blood–brain barrier. Among the first to do this was Goldman (1909) who injected trypan blue intravenously and found that the brain was unstained and the dye was not in the CSF even though the meninges and choroid plexuses were stained. In a second experiment (Goldman, 1913) trypan blue was injected in to the CSF. Following such an injection the entire brain was heavily stained and granular accumulations of the dye were present in all cell types. It was, therefore, concluded that there was a barrier between blood and nervous tissue that seemed to be almost absolute as trypan blue could not leave the vascular bed of the nervous tissue, although it could leave blood vessels of the choroid plexuses as the connective tissue of these bodies was stained. The barrier could be bypassed by direct injection into the CSF. These observations led to the view that the mode of entry of all substances into brain tissue was by way of the choroid plexuses.

Davson (1967) cautioned on the use of trypan blue as a technique for the demonstration of liquid flow within the CSF. He pointed out that trypan blue is phagocytosed and carried by wandering cells and furthermore is identified microscopically only when an accumulation has occurred in tissues. Therefore, failure to identify the dye in any particular location could have been the result of a failure of the cells in this region to take it up in sufficient quantity to be identified. He further cautioned that the use of such a dyestuff to establish the permeability of the meninges to colloidal matter had additional dangers. The principle of these was the fact that cells of the mesothelial linings of the subarachnoid space appeared to retain one of the more primitive characteristics shown by histiocytes as they are capable of phagocytizing particulate matter and may even leave the arachnoid membrane to become free mononuclear phagocytic cells.

Although dye studies provided a basis for the establishment of barriers within the central nervous system, Davson (1967) recommended that it was advisable to ignore such studies as a basis for the establishment of the interchange between CSF and nervous tissue.

The principle drainage route for the CSF appears to be the arachnoid villi. These arachnoid villi have been studied in detail in dogs and monkeys by Pollay and Welch (1962), Welch and Pollay (1963), and Welch and Friedman (1960). Welch and Friedman's study of the histological characteristics of the arachnoid villi indicated that they were composed of a porous tissue which they described as a series of interconnected tubes that, when opened, might allow for the passage of even microscopically visible particles. No attempt was made to determine the total area of the villi in animals studied by these workers but it is known that arachnoid villi are not evenly spread over the sinuses but occur mostly on the spinal nerves and around the veins.

As the escape of fluid by the route of the arachnoid villi probably constitutes an important factor in the consideration of the disappearance of substances injected into the ventricles or subarachnoid space, it must be considered in more detail.

It has been established that CSF pressure is greater than blood pressure in the dural sinuses (Weed and Flexner, 1933; Bedford, 1935; Shulman et al., 1964). Therefore, there is, under normal circumstances, a hydrostatic pressure which favors escape of CSF into blood.

Consideration has also been given to the effect of colloid osmotic pressure of the plasma (Weed, 1935). Weed found that when he withdrew CSF from cats and replaced it with a saline solution containing variable concentrations of gelatin that the rate of absorption was proportional to the effective filtration pressure. That is, it was proportional to the difference between hydrostatic pressure in the reservoir and the venous pressure in the sagittal sinus plus the difference in colloid osmotic pressure between CSF containing gelatin and the blood plasma. Using a high-concentration gelatin the rate was slower than with a lower concentration.

Davson (1967) indicated that this type of experiment was meaningless as exchanges of water between the nervous tissue and CSF were completely ignored. He further commented that although Weed's experiments were invalid, this did not prove that the outflow into dural sinuses was independent of colloid osmotic pressure of plasma protein and suggested that such osmotic pressure might be a factor of significance.

Consideration must also be given to the flow of fluid secreted by the choroid plexuses. Evidence suggests that fluid secreted by the choroid plexuses into the ventricles flows out into the cisterna magna and from this point through the intricate subarachnoid space to be absorbed through the arachnoid villi of serosinuses. Bering (1955) reported that fluid formed within the cerebral ventricles was actively pumped out of the ventricular system by the choroid plexuses. He contended that this was accomplished by volume changes of the plexuses that occurred with each heart beat. Filling of the choroid plexuses with blood caused an increase in the intraventricular contents; thus increasing the intraventricular pressure which could be relieved in two fashions, either by enlargement of the brain or by fluid flowing out of the ventricular system. He maintained that the latter factor was probably the greatest. Bering (1965), in summarizing the circulation of CSF, maintained that circulation was chiefly dependent on the pumping action of the choroid plexuses. Under these circumstances the plexuses acted as an unvalved pulse pump, resulting in a to-and-fro motion of the fluid. Any net flow of CSF varied with the site considered. He suggested that the flow of fluid seemed to be up over the hemispheres and anything that blocked the flow of CSF, prevented pulsation of the brain, or hampered venous drainage of great veins into the dura caused an increase in intraventricular pulse and an increase in the fluid tissue pressure gradient would result in ventricular enlargement. However, anything that decreased intraventricular pulse and fluid tissue gradient caused ventricles to decrease in size.

Bering further contended that CSF could not be regarded simply as a substance formed at a single site which flowed to another to be absorbed. Any attempt to interpret data based on such a concept could be misleading. Bering (1965) stated "the fluid is formed and absorbed throughout the ventricles and subarachnoid spaces, and is kept in constant motion by the pulsation of the choroid plexus, with a seeming progression to the surface of the cerebral hemispheres."

Phagocytosis is undoubtedly of great importance in determining the fate of particulate matter injected into the subarachnoid space. Essick (1920) reported that the mesothelial cells of the arachnoid characteristically reacted to foreign particulate matter. Injection of laked erythrocytes was followed by an aseptic meningitis, accompanied by an influx of neutrophils. Radovici et al. (1933) established that a similar reaction took place with other types of particulate matter. They injected thorotrast into the subarachnoid space and found that it was accumulated by macrophages in this space. Nine months following injection large aggregates of cells lining the pia were found to be stuffed with thorotrast granules. This resulted in an increased thickness of the pia mater and there was a ring of similarly stuffed cells in the perineural space surrounding the optic nerve. They were unable to demonstrate any of the material in the parenchyma of the central nervous system.

Stuck and Reeves (1938) also utilized thorotrast. Following intraventricular injection of thorotrast they were unable to demonstrate, using radiology, any spread of the material to the cervical lymph nodes. Following radiographs of the head of cats, dogs, and monkeys they studied the nervous system histologically and were unable to reveal any significant accumulation of thorotrast outside of the central nervous system and concluded that inanimate particulate matter could be retained in the central nervous system almost indefinitely with any small amount lost being most probably carried by macrophages.

Since results with colloidal suspensions indicated that very little escaped from the subarachnoid space, it is interesting to note that it has been established that whole blood can be eliminated from the arachnoid space quite rapidly. Sprong (1934) found that about 85% of erythrocytes injected into the subarachnoid space disappeared within 20 hours, whereas Meredith (1941) found that 75% of injected cells disappeared from the subarachnoid space of the dog within 2–4 hours. Simmonds (1953) injected ^{32}P-labeled erythrocytes and after 16 hours 12% of the injected cells were recovered in the general circulation. Bradford and Johnson (1962) conducted similar experiments by labeling erythrocytes with ^{59}Fe and injecting them into the subarachnoid space of dogs. Within 24 hours, 5–65% of the activity was found in the blood. They felt that since the ^{59}Fe label was more tightly bound than that of ^{32}P detection of this activity in the blood indicated unequivocally that there was an escape of erythrocytes from the subarachnoid space.

Courtice and Simmonds (1951) studied the fate of plasma proteins in the subarachnoid space. They injected plasma labeled with Evans blue into the cisterna magna of cats and rabbits and determined the plasma concentration of the dyed protein at repeated intervals. They found that the plasma concentration of the dyed protein rose to a peak within 3–5 hours and computed that at least 20% of the injected protein appeared in the circulation. They cannulated cervical and thoracic lymph ducts and demonstrated that the greatest proportion of the dyed protein entered the blood stream directly and not as a secondary feature following primary lymphatic absorption. Their results suggest that colloidal material can be absorbed directly into the blood stream from the subarachnoid space.

In addition to the escape route by means of arachnoid villi, direct passage into nervous tissue across ependyma and the pia glia may also be possible. Such an exchange might play an important role in the removal of protein from the tissue or alternatively a passage from CSF into tissue might be of significance in relation to immunological reaction and in the case of viral infection (Davson, 1967).

Radioautography and protein labeling by use of fluorescein have both been utilized for the study of passage of material out of CSF. Resolution by use of fluorescein-labeled material has been greatly superior to that obtained with autoradiography. Bowsher (1957) injected ^{35}S-labeled proteins into the subarachnoid space or ventricles of cats. Following this injection autoradiography showed a diffuse distribution in meningeal tissue and subarachnoid spaces. Not only were the sagittal sinus and spinal arachnoid villi filled with labeled material but also the sheaths of the emergent nerve routes, the cells of the pia mater and the cortex underlying the cerebral pia. These results indicated that the drainage route for bulk flow could be the arachnoid villi while passage into subpial and subependymal tissue could indicate either that the pia and the ependyma had pores permitting passage of these molecules between cells or that the cells lining the cavity actually took up the protein molecules.

Klatzo *et al.* (1962, 1964) utilized the fluorescent protein technique. Following ventriculocisternal perfusion, the cytoplasm of ependymal cells fluoresced indicating an intracellular absorption of protein. This protein was seen only in the gray matter lining the ventricles and not in the white matter. The blood vessels in the choroid plexuses had a bright green fluorescence and the epithelial cells and connective tissues were also fluorescent. The subpial tissue contained little protein and the authors concluded that, unlike the ependyma, the pia was completely impermeable to albumin.

The movement of colloidal particles has also been studied by Brightman (1965a) who injected ferritin into the ventricles of rats and examined the brains. Ferritin particles escaped into the brain along an intercellular route by moving through spaces between ependymal cells. There was also a pinocytotic mechanism in which particles were enveloped by an ependymal cell membrane and, after pinching off, collected in the cell where they eventually formed large aggregates. Ferritin within ependymal cells was contained in membrane-bound vesicles. Membranes of some vesicles remained continuous with the plasmalemma of the cell. The ferritin later became segregated in inclusions of three types identified as multivesicular bodies, dense bodies, and vacuoles. The dense bodies corresponded to lysosomes of the light microscope and were concentrated in the apical region of the cell.

In a second study, Brightman (1965b) injected ferritin into the subarachnoid space. These ferritin particles passed into the brain parenchyma and were taken up in pinocytotic vesicles by the glia and the neurons.

It would therefore appear that substances such as proteins may leave the ventricles across the ependyma by passing between the cells as well as into them. Although there is no direct evidence suggesting that it is true, it is possible that, having entered the cells, proteins may pass into the basal intercellular spaces by a process of reverse pinocytosis (Davson, 1967).

The evidence presented above would suggest that with large particles the main route of escape may be by the way of the arachnoid villi, although small amounts of material may be taken up by the nervous tissue. The fact that large molecules may leave the subarachnoid space or diffuse into the parenchyma of the brain and cord would suggest also that smaller molecules may be eliminated by the same routes (Davson, 1967). If the only route of escape is via the subarachnoid space, the materials are said to be carried by bulk flow and, consequently, the rate at which they disappear from CSF is a measure of bulk flow. However, as diffusion into the parenchyma of the brain and cord is possible, it may be expected that clearance of a great many substances may be greater than the rate of bulk flow. Consideration must also be given to the fact that the blood–brain barrier may operate as a mechanism affecting clearance by way of the brain. For example: If sucrose is present in the CSF, passage of this substance across the ependyma should be rapid, as this cellular sheet offers little resistance to diffusion (Rall et al., 1962). However, as sucrose passes into the brain it results in an increased concentration in the extracellular fluid of the tissue immediately adjacent to the ventricle. The concentration of sucrose soon becomes close to that in CSF and exchange stops as the concentration gradient becomes small. If sucrose is rapidly carried away by the blood, the concentration of sucrose in tissue will remain low and the concentration gradient sufficient to favor continuous escape of sucrose. According to Davson (1967), inulin and sucrose are not carried away by the blood to any great extent. Consequently, escape into the brain represents only a very small fraction of the total removal of these substances from the CSF. He also cautions that the choroid plexuses must not be forgotten as their area exposed to the fluid is quite large. Thus, if the epithelial cells of the choroid plexuses are permeable to the solute, they may also contribute appreciably to its clearance.

Strongly lipid-soluble substances, such as ethyl alcohol and ethylthiourea, escape into the blood by diffusion much more rapidly than do non-lipid-soluble substances (Davson, 1967). It was suggested that diffusion may represent the exclusive mode of exit from the ventricles by such strongly lipid-soluble substances.

The escape of substances from the cisterna magna was studied by Davson (1967). A given quantity of material, of known concentration, was injected into the cisterna magna and the needle left in place for 1 hour and the entire CSF withdrawn to determine the amount of solute lost. In order to relate the escape of the solutes, ^{24}Na was incorporated into all solutions injected and the loss of various substances expressed in terms of loss of ^{24}Na. Slow passage of inulin and sucrose was demonstrated as their escape was largely confined to bulk drainage with a larger rate of loss of ^{24}Na, urea, and thiourea, because of their measurable passage across the blood–CSF and blood–brain barriers, and finally a much more rapid loss of ethylthiourea. In order to establish that the escape of sucrose was by the way of bulk flow rather than diffusion, a high concentration of sucrose was maintained in the blood during the hour allowed for escape. In this experiment there was no significant difference in the rate of loss.

That an active transport system outward does exist was established by Pappenheimer et al. (1961). These authors studied ventriculocisternal perfusion in the goat and demonstrated that Diodrast, having a molecular weight of 405, and phenolsulfanophthalein, having a molecular weight of 346, were absorbed more rapidly than creatinine, having molecular weight of 113. They further established that there was absorption of Diodrast against a concentration gradient when concentration of Diodrast in plasma was held above that in the ventriculocisternal fluid. They were also able to demonstrate that Diodrast was actively absorbed almost exclusively by the choroid plexus of the 4th ventricle. In addition to Diodrast, the anions I^-, CNS^-, and probably Br^- are actively absorbed by the choroid plexuses in the rabbit (Pollay and Davson, 1963; Bito et al., 1966; Coben et al., 1965). Evidence for active cation transport between the blood and extracellular fluid of the brain was presented by Bito (1969). Using dogs and cats, it was found that the local environment of cells of mammalian cerebral cortex had a low potassium and high magnesium concentration when compared with the concentration of these cations in cisternal CSF. The author concluded, "Such concentration could not be maintained in the extracellular fluid of the brain by a simple combination of the known secretory activity of the choroid plexuses and a passive diffusional barrier at the blood–brain barrier. Rather, these results demonstrate the existence of an active transport function across the blood–brain barrier."

IV. COMPOSITION OF CSF

Cerebrospinal fluid has a different composition from that of blood plasma or plasma filtrate. This occurs, as previously indicated, as active transport mechanisms exist which have a tendency to accelerate certain molecules and ions while retarding others. The end result of these processes is to produce a fluid having a composition that is adapted to serve as an environment for the tissues which have a close relationship with the fluid. To some extent chemical composition of CSF is independent of chemical concentrations within the plasma, whereas with other chemical substances it appears to be directly related to plasma concentration. Any increase in total osmolarity of blood, as produced by intravenous injection of sodium chloride or mannitol, causes an abrupt withdrawal of water from CSF. This lowers the intracranial pressure and raises the osmolarity of the fluid. Many foreign substances injected into the blood find their way into CSF. Some solutions enter CSF easily and others with difficulty, indicating that there is a blood–CSF barrier.

The chemical composition of the CSF of animals is summarized in Table II. The significance and mechanisms for control of these concentrations will be discussed later.

Although cellular numbers are small in most animal species, knowledge concerning normal values must be considered in interpreting results of laboratory examinations. The normal cellular elements found in CSF of animals are summarized in Table III.

V. REMOVAL OF CSF

Cerebrospinal fluid examination is indicated when there is clinical evidence of pathology involving the central nervous system and occasionally as a prognostic method to determine the state of the disease and its response to therapy. Removal of CSF may also be of value for relief of abnormally high pressures and for drainage of blood or exudates from the subarachnoid space. Penetration of the subarachnoid space may also be used in initiating radiographic procedures and for the injection of medicaments into the spinal canal.

TABLE II   CHEMICAL COMPOSITION OF CEREBROSPINAL FLUID IN ANIMALS (AVERAGE VALUES)

Species	pH	Ca (mg/100 ml)	P (mg/100 ml)	Mg (mg/100 ml)	Cl (mg/100 ml)	K	Sugar (mg/100 ml)	Urea	Total protein (mg/100 ml)
Dog	7.42[a]	6.56[b]	3.09[b]	3.09[b]	808[b]	2.98 mEq/KgH$_2$O[c]	74[d] 64[b]	3.56 mEq/KgH$_2$O[c]	27.5[d]
Cat	Slightly alkaline[e]	5.2[f]	—	1.33 mEq/KgH$_2$O[g]	900[d]	2.98 mEq/KgH$_2$O[g]	85[d]	6.76 mEq/KgH$_2$O[c]	up to 20[d]
Horse	7.25[d]	6.26[d]	1.44[d]	1.98[d]	737[d]	12.66 mg/100 ml[d]	57.2[d]	3.28 mg/100 ml[h]	65.6 foal[d] 47.6 adult[d]
Cattle (adult)	7.4–7.6[i] 7.22[j]	4.1[k]	3.2[b] 1.9[j]	2.17[b]	650–725[d] 708[j]	41.2 mg/100 ml[k]	35–70[d] 68.1[j]	9.2 mg/100 ml[j]	20–33[d] 27.3[j]
Calves	7.26[j]	—	1.62[j]	—	722[j]	—	41.6[j]	8.2 mg/100 ml[j]	31.5[j]
Swine	—	—	—	—	—	—	48–87[d]	—	24–29[d]
Sheep	7.35[l]	5.77[d]	—	2.88[d]	832[d]	—	52–85[d]	—	29.42[d]
Goat	—	2.3	—	1.9	131	2.96	70[d]	—	12[d]
		mEq/KgH$_2$O[m]		mEq/KgH$_2$O[m]	mEq/KgH$_2$O[m]	mEq/KgH$_2$O[m]			

[a]Friedman et al. (1963)
[b]Fridman and Petrova (1935)
[c]Bito and Davson (1966)
[d]Fankhauser (1962)
[e]Kasahara and Fujisawa (1930)
[f]Katzenelbogen (1934)
[g]Ames et al. (1964)
[h]Adamsteau (1940)
[i]Fedotov (1947)
[j]Soliman et al. (1965)
[k]Josland (1934)
[l]Nikitin (1938)
[m]Held et al. (1964)

TABLE III   CELLULAR ELEMENTS IN CSF OF ANIMALS

Species	Lymphocytes		Other cells	Total cell count (cells/mm³)
	Large	Small		
Dog	5–40%[a]	15–95%[a]	0–40 degenerate	0–8[b]
Cat	all lymphocytes[b]			0–1[b]
				0–5[c]
Horse	50% lymphoid[b]		50 histiocytes[b]	1–7[b]
Cattle				
Adult	90–100%[d]		0–10% (endothelial)[d]	0–6[e]
			10–20[d]	0–3[b]
Calves	90–100%[d]		0–10% (endothelial)[d]	10–30[d]
Swine	—		—	0–7 up to 20[b]
Sheep	Small and large lymphocytes[b]		Mononuclears and endothelial cells[b]	0–5[b]
				1–11[f]
Goat	100%[b]			

[a] Bindrich and Schmidt (1952)
[b] Fankhauser (1962)
[c] Kasahara and Fujisawa (1930)
[d] Soliman et al. (1965)
[e] Fedotov (1960)
[f] Nikitin (1938)

Puncture of the spinal canal, either by lumbar or cisternal puncture, is a relatively safe and simple procedure, although it should not be performed unless there are definite indications for the procedure. In order to safely remove CSF from domestic animals, the clinician must be aware of the associated anatomy and the techniques for performing the puncture. These techniques were discussed in detail by Fankhauser (1962) and will not be repeated here.

Any procedure involving entering the subarachnoid space for the collection of fluid must be conducted using strict aseptic precautions. In all circumstances the area should be shaved, washed, and the skin disinfected prior to removal of the fluid. The cisternal approach is recommended for all species with the possible exception of the pig in which removal of fluid from the cisterna magna may be extremely difficult, being particularly difficult in swine weighing in excess of 180 pounds. In these animals the lumbosacral approach is preferred. The lumbosacral method may also be utilized in cattle and sheep. Although general anesthesia is not usually necessary for cattle or sheep, it is recommended for removal of fluid from all other animal species. The operator should remove only that amount of fluid necessary for analysis, and in small animals, should be limited to not over 1–2 ml in the dog and not over 10–50 drops in the cat.

VI. EXAMINATION OF CSF

Examination of CSF should include the following: physical examination, cytological examination, and chemical examination. The extent of chemical examination will be dependent upon the clinical observations and normally would include only protein determinations. However, under circumstances that suggest the presence of a bacterial infection or other lesion that might result in a high cell count, other chemical determinations such as glucose and chloride may be indicated. If there is some concern with respect to the acid–base balance in the body and its effect on the CSF, additional chemical examinations, including determinations for electrolytes, CO_2 combining power, and bicarbonate, might also be completed.

A. Physical Examination

Normal CSF is clear and colorless, although if hemorrhage occurred at the time of puncture blood will appear in the fluid. Additional discolorations include xanthochromia in which the fluid is yellow and clear. Xanthochromia may result from a previous hemorrhage into the arachnoid space and is probably due to the presence of free bilirubin which has resulted from the chemical breakdown of heme within the spinal canal. In advanced cases of icterus, varying amounts of bilirubin may be present in the CSF. Some of the more common causes of xanthochromia of CSF include subarachnoid hemorrhage, neoplasia, acute inflammation, abscesses, as well as spinal block.

In cases in which there is a recent hemorrhage into the subarachnoid space, or when blood has contaminated the specimen as a result of rupture of a blood vessel, such specimens may be centrifuged to detect alterations in color. If contamination with blood is the result of hemorrhage at the time of collection, the supernatant fluid is usually clear following centrifugation, in contrast to a yellow supernatant that will be present if an old hemorrhage exists.

Normal CSF has no turbidity, being completely transparent. Turbidity usually occurs as the result of the presence of cells. Turbidity does not, however, become grossly evident until there are 500 or more cells/mm³. In acute meningeal infections, the fluid may be slightly cloudy or frankly purulent.

Normal CSF does not coagulate. Coagulation occurs only if fibrinogen is present although occasionally a fibrin net containing blood cells may result from meningeal reactions. A heavy coagulation may occur in acute suppurative meningitis. Coagulation may occur if the CSF has been contamined with large quantities of blood, either as a result of a previous internal hemorrhage or from contamination at the time of collection.

B. Cytological Examination

Although the numbers and types of cells found in CSF are somewhat limited, detection of the total number and type of cell present may be of value in arriving at a diagnosis. The origin of these cells remains undetermined, although there are theories which would suggest meningeal, lymphogenous, hematogenous, or histogenous origins (Fedotov, 1960). The majority of the cells found in CSF are lymphocytes and rarely mononuclear phagocytes. As cells in CSF degenerate rapidly, total and differential counts should be completed as quickly as possible. If there is a delay in completing the differential count, the specimen may be preserved with an equal quantity of 50% ethanol and the smear prepared at a later time.

Techniques for completing total cell counts on CSF are described elsewhere (Coles, 1967; Cornelius, 1963) and will not be repeated here.

As contamination with peripheral blood is not uncommon in CSF samples obtained from domestic animals, it may be necessary to adjust the total count and total protein according to the following formula (Krieg, 1969):

$$WBC_{CSF} = WBC_0 - (WBC_b \times RBC_0)/RBC_b$$

WBC_{CSF}	=	leukocyte count (or total protein), presumably present in CSF prior to peripheral contamination
WBC_0	=	leukocyte count (or total protein) observed in CSF
WBC_b	=	leukocyte count (or total protein) of peripheral blood
RBC_0	=	erythrocyte count observed in CSF
RBC_b	=	erythrocyte count of peripheral blood

In utilizing the above formula, it is assumed that no erythrocytes were present in the CSF prior to collection. This formula is applicable only when it is impossible to obtain the needed information in any other fashion.

All CSF specimens, irrespective of their total count, should be examined to determine the cell types present. If the total cell number is under $500/mm^3$ or the specimen has been diluted with ethanol to preserve the cells, the sample should be centrifuged and smears prepared from the sediment. Smears are prepared in the usual fashion and an appropriate stain, such as Wright's, Geimsa, or new methylene blue, can be used. It has been suggested (Cornelius, 1963) that a wet mount coverslip method may be preferable as less cellular distortion, disintegration, and artifacts are observed with this technique than with the dried-film method. The preferred stain for a wet mount preparation is 0.5% new methylene blue in 0.9% saline.

If physical examination of the CSF suggests the presence of turbidity or other abnormality, direct smears for the identification of microorganisms should be made. Routine stains such as Gram's, Ziehl-Neelsen acid-fast stain or methylene blue may be utilized for tentative identification of the microorganisms. If bacteria are present, bacteriological cultures should be initiated as soon as possible.

C. CHEMICAL EXAMINATION

Protein determinations in CSF can be conducted by a variety of techniques. Qualitative procedures, such as the Pandy and Nonne-Apelt tests, are used for a preliminary examination and, if positive, indicate the presence of globulins. It must be remembered, however, that they are relatively insensitive tests and should be used only as a screening procedure to provide a rapid estimation. Quantitation of CSF protein may be based on ultraviolet absorption, micro-Kjeldahl reaction, the Folin-Ciocalteau reaction, the development of turbidity with trichloracetic acid or sulfosalicylic acid or by immunochemical methods.

There has recently been an increase in the study of cerebrospinal proteins using electrophoretic and immunoelectrophoretic techniques. Although the clinical use of cerebrospinal protein electrophoresis and immunoelectrophoresis has not yet been determined for animals, there is some evidence to suggest that it has a place in the diagnosis of diseases of the central nervous system in man.

Krieg (1969) suggests that immunoelectrophoretic demonstration of macroglobu-lins and lipoproteins may be a sensitive method for detection of injury to the blood–CSF barrier. He also reported that the majority of the CSF protein originates by diffusion from plasma across the blood–CSF barrier and that proteins larger than 9S do not readily diffuse from plasma unless there has been injury to the barrier. He also suggested that with a subarachnoid block there was an increase in CSF γ-globu-lin. However, a marked increase in serum γ-globulin may also result in an increase in CSF IgG γ-globulin.

Baltch *et al.* (1969) experimentally produced aseptic meningitis in dogs by intra-cisternal administration of streptokinase-streptodornase (SK-SD). The greatest pleocytosis and total protein increase were seen 48 hours following intracisternal injection of SK-SD. At the peak of pleocytosis and total protein increase, the greatest CSF protein increase was in the albumin fraction. A prompt return to normal albumin levels occurred within 4 weeks. The IgG was increased 14-fold during acute inflammation and remained elevated as long as 19 weeks. The total CSF protein returned to normal within 3–8 weeks. Antibodies to SK-SD first appeared and persist-ed longer and in higher titer in serum than in CSF. These data suggested that during an acute aseptic meningeal inflammation there is a significant change in the blood–CSF–brain barrier for protein which caused a marked albumin and later IgG increase without a concomitant change in the serum. The data also suggested that altered concentrations of CSF protein components can occur in the presence of a normal CSF total protein.

The mechanism of exchange of γ-globulins between blood CSF and brain was studied by Hochwald and Wallenstein (1967). They found that the clearance of ^{131}I labeled cat γ-globulin during steady-state ventriculocisternal perfusion was depend-ent on bulk absorptions of CSF but was independent of protein concentration. When ^{131}I γ-globulin was injected intravenously, the total amount of this protein that entered the ventricular system was 0.7 μg/min. The transfer of γ-globulin was similar to but did not exceed that of inulin clearance. Similar results were obtained on the study of the efflux of albumin from the CSF.

MacPherson (1967) studied the γ_c-globulin concentration in bovine CSF with-drawn from newly born, colostrum-deprived calves and older animals. She demon-strated that the average γ_c-globulin concentration in bovine CSF from new born calves was 1.4 mg/100 ml. This level decreased sharply for a few days after birth and the average value for 4-month-old animals was 0.44 mg/100 ml. The CSF of 3-year-old steers contained 0.22 mg/100 ml. The presence of γ_G-globulin was demonstrated in the CSF of newborn, colostrum-deprived calves but quantitation was not possible because of the small volume of available CSF and the low concentration of this globulin in the CSF. The level of γ_G-globulin increased with age so that the CSF of adult animals contained 2.22 mg/100 ml.

The significance of the presence of these various protein fractions in the CSF of domestic animals remains to be determined.

1. Glucose

Cerebrospinal fluid glucose levels are approximately 60–80% of the blood levels in most animal species. In man, it has been reported that with very high blood glucose levels (800 mg/100 ml and over) that the difference becomes more marked and CSF glucose is only about 30–40% of blood levels (Krieg, 1969). With an increase or decrease in blood glucose, CSF glucose will undergo a corresponding change within the next 1–3 hours. Such a time lag probably is a reflection of the slow transport of glucose across the CSF–blood barrier. Because of this relationship between blood glucose and CSF glucose levels, blood glucose should be estimated simultaneously with CSF glucose.

Hypoglycorrhachia is most commonly associated with bacterial meningitis, although it may also be seen in association with a marked hypoglycemia. The decreased level associated with bacterial meningitis is undoubtedly due to the glycolysis by the microorganisms present. There is some evidence to suggest that the glucose fall is the result of a synergism between the bacteria and leukocytes (Petersdorf et al., 1960a, b). There is also a suggestion that meningeal neoplasia may result in a decrease in CSF glucose (Krieg, 1969).

2. Chloride and Sodium

The fact that chloride and sodium concentrations in CSF are greater than that of the plasma suggests the presence of an active secretory mechanism for these substances into the CSF. Although the concentration difference is a realistic one, Davson (1967), in speaking of sodium and chloride, remarks "these ions constitute such an important fraction of the total osmolality of the cerebrospinal fluid in plasma that it seems unlikely that their concentrations in the cerebrospinal fluid could be held at levels that were independent of the plasma levels." Thus, it is impossible to separate the serum and plasma levels of these two substances from levels which may occur in CSF.

Alterations in chloride levels undoubtedly do occur but other than the hypochloremia associated with meningitis and that which may occur as a result of protracted vomiting and in advanced pneumonia are probably of little diagnostic significance.

3. Calcium and Magnesium

The normal concentration of CSF calcium is much lower than in plasma. The principle reason for the discrepancy is the great degree of protein binding with calcium. When a comparison is made between plasma dialysate and CSF, the discrepancy is not large but the concentration of ionized calcium in plasma is greater than that in CSF. According to Davson (1967), studies on man and experimental animals, in which plasma calcium was lowered or raised, demonstrated the virtual independence of CSF concentration of calcium to that in plasma.

In contrast, the concentration of magnesium in CSF of most species is greater than in plasma dialysate and is virtually independent of plasma concentration.

Alterations in CSF calcium and magnesium in disease states have not been extensively studied and probably have little clinical significance, although in man a slight increase in calcium and decrease in magnesium has been recorded in patients with tubercular meningitis (Hunter and Smith, 1960).

4. Cholesterol

Cholesterol concentration in CSF of animals is small, varying from none to minute traces. Normal values have been reported as high as 0.65 mg/100 ml in the horse (Fankhauser, 1962); and in goats, cholesterol values have been reported as high as 0.51 mg/100 ml (Mould and Dawson, 1965).

According to Cornelius (1963) increased values of CSF cholesterol occur in association with brain abscesses, tumors, meningitis, and hemorrhages involving the central nervous system.

5. Potassium

The concentration of potassium in CSF is considerably less than that of a plasma dialysate. Increases in plasma potassium do not produce a significant increase in the concentration of potassium in CSF.

Bekaert and Demeester (1951a,b, 1952) stated that lowering of plasma potassium, following injection of insulin or glucose or by treatment with DOCA, likewise had a small or negligible effect on CSF potassium. It has been suggested (Cornelius, 1963) that potassium alterations in CSF would be most likely to occur when there is an escape of whole plasma or blood into CSF.

6. Acid–Base Balance

Cerebrospinal fluid is slightly more acid than arterial plasma. It has been suggested that CSF is more likely to be in equilibrium with venous than with arterial plasma, and as venous blood is more acid than arterial, may be the explanation for the difference between CSF pH and that of arterial plasma. Davson (1967) suggested that this is only a partial explanation of the variation.

Response of CSF pH to changes in the blood are of considerable physiological interest. It has been established (Davson, 1967) that pH of CSF does not accurately follow that of blood. In the case of metabolic acidosis, the pH of the two fluids may move in opposite directions (Cestan et al., 1925). They injected HCl into dogs and found that although the blood became more acid, CSF became more alkaline. The difference in pH was thought to be due to the fact that although the bicarbonate concentration of plasma fell rapidly, bicarbonate concentration of CSF fell more slowly. That there is a low permeability of the blood (CSF barrier to HCO_3^-) was demonstrated in 1920 by Collip and Backus. They reported that injection of $NaHCO_3$ had no measurable effect on concentration in the CSF until 1 hour after injection. In contrast to the slow movement of HCO_3^-, there was a very rapid transport of CO_2 between blood, brain, and CSF. Coxon and Swanson (1965) studied the passage of this labeled CO_2 from blood to CSF and concluded that passage of this labeled material into CSF was quite rapid, with the maximum peak occurring approximately 15 minutes following injection of $^{14}CO_2$ into the blood stream.

The effects of respiratory alkalosis and acidosis in dogs have been studied by Leusen (1954, 1965; Leusen and Demeester, 1960). There was a shift of blood and CSF pH in the same direction without an appreciable alteration in the concentration of HCO_3^- in the fluids.

Posner *et al.* (1965) studied arterial and CSF, pH, PCO_2, and HCO_3^- in 35 control. and 48 human patients with an acid–base disorder. They found that metabolic acidosis was associated with only a slight shift in CSF pH, as the concentration of bicarbonate in CSF did not fall proportionately to that in blood. They also found that the difference in PCO_2 of venous blood, with which the CSF apparently was in approximate equilibrium, had become closer to that of arterial blood. They suggested that this might have been due to an increased blood flow following the fall in blood pH.

Such parameters have not been extensively measured in animals and consequently, no definite conclusion can be reached although the mechanisms would appear to be similar in man and animals.

7. Urea

The concentration of urea in CSF apparently occurs in a purely passive manner in response to concentration gradient differences between blood and CSF. Thus, we might expect that in any animal having an increase in blood–urea nitrogen would have a corresponding increase in the concentration of urea nitrogen in the CSF. Cockrill (1931) found in experimental uremia in cats that a concentration of urea in blood and CSF increased at about the same rate with the urea of CSF always slightly lower than that in the blood.

8. Enzymes

As enzymes are relatively large molecules of proteins, usually of the globulin type, the concentration of enzymes found in the blood will be small if their entry and exit are controlled in a fashion similar to those of the main protein constituents. Some enzymes, however, may be derived from the central nervous system and under certain conditions may be present in higher proportions in CSF (Davson, 1967).

Cerebrospinal fluid levels of glutamic oxalacetic transaminase (GOT) and glutamic pyruvic transaminase (GPT) were studied by Hibbs and Coles (1965). In a series of 37 dogs, the mean CSF–GOT was 20.1 units with a range of 9–46 units. In the same animals the CSF–GPT was 13.7 units with a range of 2–32 units. Hibbs (1962) also estimated the CSF levels of GOT and GPT in a series of dogs with distemper. Eleven of fourteen dogs had increased enzymic activity in the CSF. The mean CSF–GOT was 81.5 units and mean CSF–GPT was 30.7 units.

Belsey (1966) produced purulent meningitis in a series of dogs by intracisternal and intravenous inoculation of *Diplococcus pneumoniae* type III. In six of seven dogs that died as a result of meningitis, the CSF–GOT was significantly elevated. In animals that developed meningitis but recovered, the CSF–GOT was normal or rose slightly, followed by a return to normal. No elevation in CSF–GOT was noted in animals without meningitis. He assumed that the increased CSF–GOT activity during meningitis was the result of brain injury.

Wakim and Fleisher (1956) produced cerebral infarctions in dogs by intracarotid injection of vinyl acetate and found that following infarction there was an increase in both serum GOT activity, which doubled, and in the CSF–GOT which rose severalfold. At the same time, the brain tissue lost more than 80% of its activity. This suggested that the CSF-GOT was derived from the brain tissue. When the serum level of GOT was raised as a result of liver damage, following poisoning with carbon tetrachloride, the rise in activity in CSF was negligible (Fleisher and Wakim, 1956).

Increased levels of CSF lactate dehydrogenase (LDH), with a normal serum LDH, has been described in man in association with bacterial meningitis, metastatic carcinoma, subarachnoid hemorrhage, and cerebral infarction (Krieg, 1969).

There are indications in man that the use of isocitric dehydrogenase (ICD) levels in the CSF of man may be of some value. Van Rymenant et al. (1966) found a marked increase of ICD in meningitis and a transient elevation in seven cases in which there were cerebrovascular lesions. They also felt that ICD was promising in the diagnosis of the presence of tumors of the CNS, as in a group of individuals having CNS tumors the increase in ICD often preceded alterations in either the CSF leukocyte count or protein content.

VII. CSF IN DISEASE

A. Dog

Knowledge concerning CSF alterations in diseases of the dog are somewhat limited. As a result, accurate interpretation of CSF alterations and their direct relationship to diseases of the central nervous system remain to be determined.

Fankhauser (1962) divided CSF findings into three distinct groups:

1. Cerebrospinal fluids having slight alterations or which are almost normal. Such fluid can be found in intoxications, acute serous meningoencephalitis (acute distemper, infectious canine hepatitis, leptospirosis, posttraumatic encephalopathy, tetanies, congenital hydrocephalus, as well as traumatic, neoplastic, and inflammatory lesions concerning only the spinal cord, and in disc herniation). Changes noted include pleocytosis (up to 30 cells/cu mm) and a slightly elevated protein concentration.

2. Cerebrospinal fluids with xanthochromia, erythrocytes, protein levels from 90 to 500 mg/100 ml, and with the Nonne-Apelt and Pandy tests strongly positive. This type of fluid was usually associated with inflammatory processes, such as toxic encephalopathies and in acute meningoencephalitides accompanied by severe vascular lesions and hemorrhages.

3. Cerebrospinal fluid which was clear or slightly turbid (when the total cell count reaches 200/mm³ or more), sometimes having either white flakes or a fibrinous network, with cell numbers ranging from 10 to 1000/mm³.

Canine Distemper

In experimental canine distemper, Bindrich and Schmidt (1952) found that the cell types in CSF of these animals were small lymphocytes, large lymphocytes, and degenerate forms. Fankhauser (1962) reported that in spontaneous nonpurulent encephalitides the cellular elements consisted of erythrocytes, small lymphocytes and naked nuclei of small lymphocytes, medium-sized and large lymphocytes, mononuclear cells and monocytes, plasma cells, endothelial cells, gitter cells, neutrophils, and degenerating cells. The most common and numerous cell types were lymphocytes and mononuclear cells. Markiewicz (1965) studied the CSF of 47 dogs with a nervous form of distemper and found that the cellular increase was mainly in lymphoid cells.

In canine distemper there also is an increase in CSF protein (Fankhauser, 1962; Markiewicz, 1965). According to Fankhauser the increase is not great and usually parallels the increase in cells. The total protein CSF values ranged from 40 to 150 mg/100 ml and the Nonne-Apelt and Pandy reactions were usually positive, although they occasionally were negative. The glucose concentration was usually within normal range (Fankhauser, 1962) but may be either decreased or increased. Markiewicz (1965) reported that the cerebrospinal glucose in dogs with a nervous form of distemper was decreased. The CSF chlorides have been reported to be increased (Markiewicz) or normal (Fankhauser). Croft (1955) reported only slightly lower glucose levels in the CSF of 17 dogs with distemper. These dogs also had an elevated CSF total protein (130 to 15,000 mg/100 ml) and uric acid.

In general, diseases of the meninges produce greater alterations in CSF than do lesions of the parenchyma of the central nervous system. Thus, if neutrophil counts, protein values, and total cell counts are greatly increased, involvement of the meninges should be suspected.

Belsey (1966) experimentally produced meningitis in dogs by the injection of *Diplococcus pneumoniae* type III. A significant pleocytosis with cell counts up to 2500 were recorded in these animals. In addition, he reported a significant increase in CSF–GOT activity in infected animals and suggested the possibility that CSF–GOT might be useful in clinical studies of meningitis.

Cornelius (1958) reported the following alterations in CSF in various clinical conditions in dogs in California:

1. Lymphosarcoma. Marked pleocytosis with 1250 cells/mm^3. These cells were distributed as 81% large mononuclear, 8% small mononuclear, and 11% neutrophils. The total protein was 57 mg/100 ml.

2. Brain tumor with spondylitis. Xanthochromia was evident, total cell count was 55/mm^3 of which 78% were neutrophils and 22% small and large mononuclears. Erythrocytes were present at a concentration of 4800/mm^3 and the total protein was 200 mg/100 ml.

3. Chronic encephalomyelitis. CSF was clear, colorless, had 100 cells/mm^3 of which 3% were neutrophils and 95% small mononuclears, and the total protein was 320 mg/100 ml.

4. Distemper. The CSF in distemper was slightly turbid, leukocytes numbered 17/mm^3 composed of 13% neutrophils and 87% small mononuclears. Erythrocytes numbered 480/mm^3, the Pandy test was 2+ and total protein 51.3 mg/100 ml.

5. Hypertrophic spondylitis. This fluid was pink, cloudy, and xanthochromic. Neutrophils were present at a concentration of 32 cells/mm^3, erythrocytes numbered 12,000/mm^3 and total protein was 79.8 mg/100 ml.

6. Chronic disseminated nonsuppurative meningoencephalitis. Cerebrospinal fluid from this animal was clear and colorless, had 30 cells/mm^3 of which 9% were neutrophils and 91% large mononuclear cells. The erythrocyte count was 24/mm^3 and total protein 51 mg/100 ml.

Monlux (1948) studied CSF in experimental leptospirosis of the dog. He found xanthochromia present in CSF from dogs with icterus. In most experimental cases, the fluid was free from pleocytosis and an elevation in protein. He was unable, however, to find erythrocytes in the CSF even though there were gross and microscopic lesions indicating hemorrhage. In naturally occurring cases of leptospirosis, however, erythrocytes were found.

Infection with rabies virus produced a severe meningial reaction in animals with total cell counts ranging from 30 to 1200 cells/mm^3, of which 60 to 98% were lymphocytes (Durand, 1951).

B. Cat

Although much experimental work on the physiology of CSF has been reported in the cat, there is little information concerning alterations in CSF in diseases of the central nervous system.

In cerebellar ataxia due to encephalitis of the cerebellum and marked atrophy, there was a positive Pandy reaction, increased protein, and a pleocytosis with a cell count of 900/mm^3. The cells were small and large lymphocytes, mononuclears, and endothelial cells (Fankhauser, 1962). In a case of head injury with hemorrhage and softening in the hypothalmus, Fankhauser (1962) found a positive Pandy test, a blood-stained fluid with 10,000 erythrocytes and approximately 120 lymphocytes/mm^3. He also reported the presence of some granulocytes and gitter cells. Two Siamese cats with congenital tremor and a cat experimentally infected with *Leptospira pomona* had normal CSF (Fankhauser, 1962).

C. Horse

Although CSF is somewhat difficult to obtain from the horse, there are several reports concerning CSF alterations in diseases of this animal.

In equine encephalomyelitis, Meyer *et al.* (1931, 1934) found that there was a greater pleocytosis (600–25,000) in infection with the eastern strain than with the western strain of encephalomyelitis virus (12–30/cells/mm^3). In horses affected with Russian equine encephalomyelitis, abnormal quantities of albumin and globulin, an increase in sugar and a decrease in alkali reserve were noted. The pH and calcium content were both high (Fridman *et al.*, 1935). In a later study (Fridman, 1938) a considerable decrease in vitamin C content was reported in horses experimentally infected with the virus of Russian meningoencephalitis.

Müller and Schulze (1953) studied CSF alterations in horses affected with Borna disease. The total cell numbers increased after the fourth day reaching 10–33/mm^3. The Nonne-Apelt reaction was markedly positive in 20 of 30 horses studied and the Pandy reaction was nearly always positive, ranging from slight to marked. Cerebrospinal fluid glucose was increased in eight cases and decreased in six. Fankhauser (1962) concluded that CSF alterations in Borna disease were of inconstant nature and therefore should not be considered diagnostic.

A case of purulent leptomeningitis from which *Spherophorus necrophorus*, *Staphyloccus albus*, and *Staphyloccus aureus* were isolated was reported by Schulze (1953). Cerebrospinal fluid in this animal was turbid, viscous, and yellow. The cell count was greater than 350/mm^3 and almost all cells observed were neutrophils. The CSF glucose was 27 as compared to a blood glucose of 123 mg. Both the Pandy and Nonne-Apelt reactions were strongly positive. Fankhauser (1962) reported opacity and rapid coagulation of CSF from a horse with severe purulent leptomeningitis. Bacteriological examination of the fluid revealed the presence of *Staphyloccus albus*.

In horses with clinical signs of immobility resulting from a chronic swelling or edema of the brain, Fankhauser (1962) reported that there were no gross alterations in CSF. Cerebrospinal fluid was colorless, the total cell count from 0 to 2/mm^3 with the Pandy test markedly positive, a total protein of 40–75 mg/100 ml and a glucose of 50–87 mg/100 ml. In horses with clinical signs of liver disease, Fankhauser (1962) reported the presence of xanthochromia, heavy quantities of protein (100–400 mg/100 ml) and a tendency for the formation of a fibrin clot.

D. CATTLE

The most exhaustive study of CSF alterations in diseases involving the central nervous system was reported by Fankhauser (1962). As a result of his studies he was able by examination of the CSF, to differentiate various clinical syndromes involving the central nervous system. In tuberculosis of the central nervous system he distinguished two groups:

1. The typical alterations of the CSF in acute tuberculous leptomeningitis or meningoencephalitis included the presence of a fibrinous clot, a high content of cells and protein, low sugar, and markedly pathological colloidal tests. He concluded, however, that a positive diagnosis could be provided only by a positive bacteriological test.

2. Atypical alterations occurred in CSF in intracerebral tuberculosis with only a slight meningeal reaction or in space-occupying tuberculous growths originating from the surrounding tissues. In these cases, CSF alterations were less pronounced but seldom absent. In two cases of this type involving what was termed "tuberculoma of the cerebellum" the CSF was clear and colorless with 5 and 23 cells/mm^3 with protein 40 and 70 mg/100 ml, the Nonne-Apelt and Pandy reactions were slightly positive to negative, the CSF glucose was 47 and 59 mg/100 ml, respectively.

In purulent meningoencephalitis (Fankhauser, 1962) CSF was opaque, whitish, or yellowish, with fibrinous filaments or flakes, often coagulating. The total cell count ranged from 75 to several thousand per mm^3 and was mostly neutrophils. The total protein was increased and both the Pandy and Nonne-Apelt tests were distinctly positive. In these cases, the CSF sugar ranged from 50 to 78 mg/100 ml.

In nonpurulent meningoencephalitis and -myelitis, CSF was usually clear, colorless, occasionally had a slight opalescence with fine fibrinous filaments. The total cells, most of which were lymphocytes and mononuclears, ranged from 10 to 140/mm^3. Total protein was up to 300 mg/100 ml with an average of 88 mg/100 ml. Protein content and cell count generally were parallel although this was not always true. The Pandy was negative to 3+ and Nonne-Apelt was 1+ to 2+.

Fankhauser also reported the CSF findings in a steer with traumatic encephalopathy. In this animal the CSF was clear and colorless; the pressure was noticeably increased; the cell count was 70/mm³, predominantly lymphocytes and histiocytes; the total protein was 42 mg/100 ml of which 6.6 mg was globulin and 35.4 mg albumin; the Pandy and Nonne-Apelt reactions were negative. In a second case of a cow with endogenous intoxication and edema of the brain, the total cell count was not increased; the total protein was 50 mg/100 ml; the Pandy reaction was 1+; the Nonne-Apelt reaction was negative; the CSF sugar was 55 mg/100 ml. In a cow with extensive brain abscesses in the left cerebral hemisphere, Fankhauser (1962) found the CSF formed a fibrinous clot after a few minutes; the fluid was slightly turbid containing 20 cells/mm³; total protein was 500 mg/100 ml; the Nonne-Apelt and Pandy reactions were positive; the sugar was 70 mg/100 ml. The presence of a high protein concentration in the absence of a high cell count enabled him to exclude the presence of a purulent leptomeningitis.

Howard (1969) summarized methods for neurological disease differentiation in cattle and pointed out that examination of CSF provides information concerning the type and degree of inflammatory or degenerative process present.

Howard emphasized that diseases causing severe inflammatory reactions in tissue contacting CSF (i.e., thromboembolic meningoencephalitis and other bacterial infections) result in escape of blood proteins into the fluid and strong Pandy's tests. In contrast, bacterial infections limited to deep brain tissues are also exudative, but the proteins are filtered by the surrounding tissues so that the intensity of the Pandy reaction is reduced or negative. This, he reported, is true of listeriosis and may also occur in other focal bacterial encephalitides. Lesions that do not affect blood vessel contiguity may not result in a positive Pandy test (polioencephalomalacia, coccidial encephalopathy, idiopathic myelopathy, and viral infections).

He reported that total cell counts in viral degenerative and toxic conditions ranged from less than 25 to 100/mm³. Cell counts in listeriosis and streptococcosis ranged between 100 and 200/mm³. Cell types were also characteristic as mononuclear cells accompany viral infections, polioencephalomalacia, idiopathic myelopathy, coccidial encephalopathy, and listeriosis. Neutrophils accompany purulent diseases such as thromboembolic meningoencephalitis, and staphylococcal, *Corynebacterium*, and *Pseudomonas* encephalitis and meningitis.

E. SWINE

In experimental Teschen disease (Fankhauser, 1962) the total cell count ranged from 16 to 70/mm³ and consisted predominantly of small and large lymphocytes and mononuclear cells. The total protein was not over 50 mg/100 ml and Pandy and Nonne-Apelt reactions not always positive. Lax (1961) studied the CSF in 74 pigs that were either experimentally or spontaneously infected with Teschen's disease. In about half the cases, the CSF developed a fibrinous precipitation within 24 hours. Globulin tests ranged from negative to positive and there was generally an increase in the number of lymphocytes and in albumin content. Similar findings were reported by Fischer and Starke (1951) as they found the fluid to be clear and colorless, slightly turbid when the pleocytosis reached 170/mm³, and sometimes the presence of fibrinous filaments forming a fine "spider web".

Rauch (1961) studied CSF from pigs prior to and following subcutaneous injections of crystal violent vaccine. Inoculation of the vaccine was followed by a moderate to average lymphocytosis and an increase in protein content of the CSF reaching its highest concentration 3 to 9 days following the second dose of vaccine.

Fankhauser (1962) reported on the CSF findings in a boar with paraplegia of some days duration. A lumbosacral puncture revealed a turbid yellowish CSF which coagulated after a few minutes. The fibrinous clot retracted and the supernatant fluid was xanthochromic, had 1 cell/mm^3; a protein concentration of 2500 mg/100 ml with very strong Nonne-Apelt and Pandy reactions.

F. Sheep

Data concerning pathological alterations in the CSF of sheep are scarce. This occurs in spite of the fact that neurological disorders of sheep occur which are of considerable economic importance.

Sigurdsson (1954) and Sigurdsson et al. (1957) reported some data on the CSF in rida, a chronic encephalitis, and visna, a subacute demyelinating encephalomyelitis and meningitis of sheep in Iceland. A long-lasting pleocytosis was said to be characteristic of visna and often began months before onset of clinical signs. The increase in protein varied in experimental cases from 31 to 295 mg/100 ml. Sigurdsson believed that presence of pleocytosis permitted differentiation of visna from rida.

Buck (1964) induced convulsions in sheep by inhalation of carbon dioxide, subcutaneous injection of insulin, and oral administration of heptachlor. He found a twofold increase in CSF protein, glutamic oxalacetic transaminase, and lactate dehydrogenase following insertion of a catheter into the cisterna magna. During CO_2 inhalation induced seizures were very acute. Both blood and CSF glucose levels doubled during seizures and there were definite elevations in serum and, to a lesser extent, CSF potassium values within 6 minutes that returned to near normal within 1 hour. Both blood and CSF pH decreased by 0.5–0.7 units within 1 minute and returned to normal within 1 hour. GOT activities were elevated in both blood and CSF of the two sheep from which analyses were made. He also found that the CSF calcium and magnesium increased inconsistently during carbon dioxide seizures.

Convulsive seizures were induced in five sheep by injecting insulin and in four sheep by giving heptachlor orally. Physiological and biochemical changes were much less acute than during CO_2 induced seizures. Blood and CSF glucose decreased to below 10 mg/100 ml during insulin shock seizures but after treatment with glucose or DL-glutamic acid, returned to above control levels. Blood and CSF glucose levels increased markedly in sheep given heptachlor prior to the time that clinical signs of toxicity were evident. Slight elevations in blood serum GOT were noted in the sheep given insulin and both blood and CSF elevations were noted in those given heptachlor.

G. Goat

Little work has been done on CSF alterations in diseases of this animal, although a great deal of research has been conducted concerning the physiological relationship between CSF and respiration.

Mould and Dawson (1965) studied the free and esterified cholesterol in CSF of goats affected with experimental scrapie. They found that the total cholesterol in CSF remained relatively constant but a small increase occurrred in clinically affected animals. The proportions of free cholesterol increased in all goats when only slight histological damage to brain tissue was present. The mean value for total cholesterol was 4.0 mg/liter in experimental animals and of this 48% was free cholesterol when the terminal elevations were ignored.

Millson *et al.* (1960) reported that the concentration of total protein, glucose, chloride and urea in CSF of goats affected with scrapie showed no deviation from normal.

REFERENCES

Adamesteau, I. (1940) *Rev. Vet. Milit. (Bucarest)* **11**, 217.

Ames, A., Sakanoue, M., and Endo, S. (1964), *J. Neurophysiol.* **27**, 672.

Ames, A., Higashi, K., and Nesbett, F. B. (1965a). *J. Physiol. (London)* **181**, 506.

Ames, A., Higashi, K., and Nesbett, F. B. (1965b). *J. Physiol. (London)* **181**, 516.

Baltch, A. L., Fuller, T., and Osborne, W. (1969). *J. Lab. Clin. Med.* **73**, 883.

Bedford, T. H. B. (1935). *Brain* **58**, 427.

Bekaert, J., and Demeester, G. (1951a). *Arch. Intern. Physiol.* **59**, 262.

Bekaert, J., and Demeester, G. (1951b). *Arch. Intern. Physiol.* **59**, 393.

Bekaert, J., and Demeester, G. (1952). *Arch. Intern. Physiol.* **60**, 172.

Belsey, M. A. (1966). *Antimicrobial Agents Chemotherapy* pp. 19–23.

Bering, E. A., Jr. (1955). *J. Neurosurg.* **12**, 385.

Bering, E. A., Jr. (1957). *Clin. Neurosurg.* **5**, 77.

Bering, E. A., Jr. (1965). *In* "Cerebrospinal Fluid and the Regulation of Ventilation" (C. McC. Brooks *et al.*, eds.) p. 395. Davis, Philadelphia, Pennsylvania.

Bering, E. A., Jr., and Sato, O. (1963). *J. Neurosurg.* **20**, 1050.

Bhattacharya, B. K., and Feldberg, W. (1958). *Brit. J. Pharmacol.* **13**, 156.

Bindrich, H., and Schmidt, D. (1952). *Arch. Exptl. Veterinaermed.* **6**, 162.

Bito, L. Z. (1969). *Science* **165**, 81.

Bito, L. Z., and Davson, H. (1966). *Exp. Neurol.* **14**, 264.

Bito, L. Z., Bradbury, M. W. B., and Davson, H. (1966). *J. Physiol. (London)* **185**, 323.

Boldrey, E. B. (1951). *Bull. Los Angeles Neurol. Soc.* **16**, 225.

Bowsher, D. (1957). *Anat. Record* **128**, 23.

Bradford, F. K., and Johnson, P. C. (1962). *J. Neurosurg.* **19**, 332.

Brightman, M. W. (1965a). *J. Cell Biol.* **26**, 99.

Brightman, M. W. (1965b). *Am. J. Anat.* **117**, 193.

Buck, W. B. (1964). *Ann. N. Y. Acad. Sci.* **3**, 751.

Calhoun, M. C., Hurt, H. D., Eaton, H. D., Rousseau, J. E., Jr., and Hall, R. C., Jr. (1967) *Univ. Conn., Coll. Agr. Expt. Sta. Bull.* **401**.

Cestan, R., Sandrail, M. and Lassalle H. (1925). *Compt. Rend. Soc. Biol.* **93**, 475.

Coben, L. A., Gottesman, L., and Jacobs, M. (1965) *Neurology* **15**, 951.

Cockrill, J. R. (1931). *A. M. A. Arch. Neurol. Psychiat.* **25**, 1297.

Coles, E. H. (1967). "Veterinary Clinical Pathology" Saunders, Philadelphia, Pennsylvania.

Collip, J. B., and Backus, P. L. (1920). *Am. J. Physiol.* **51**, 551.

Cornelius, C. E. (1958). *Calif. Vet.* **12**, No. 2, 18.

Cornelius, C. E. (1963). *In* "Clinical Biochemistry of Domestic Animals" (C. E. Cornelius and J. J. Kaneko, eds.), p. 385. Academic Press, New York.

Courtice, F. C., and Simmonds, W. J. (1951). *Australian J. Exptl. Biol. Med. Sci.* **29**, 255.

Coxon, R. V., and Swanson, A. G. (1965). *J. Physiol. (London)* **181**, 712.

Croft, P. G. (1955). *Vet. Record* **67**, 872.

Curl, F. D., and Pollay, M. (1968). *Exptl. Neurol.* **20**, 558.

Cutler, R. W. P., Page, L., Galicich, J., and Watters, G. V. (1968). *Brain* **91**, 707.

Davson, H. (1954). *Acta Physiol. Pharmacol. Neerl.* **3**, 553.

Davson, H. (1956). "Physiology of the Ocular and Cerebrospinal Fluids." Little, Brown, Boston, Massachusetts.

Davson, H. (1966). *In* "The Scientific Basis of Medicine Annual Reviews," p. 238. Brit. Med. Federation.

Davson, H. (1967). "Physiology of the Cerebrospinal Fluid." Churchill, London.

Davson, H., Kleeman, C. R., and Levin, E. (1962). *J. Physiol. (London)* **161**, 126.

De Rougemont, J., Ames, A., Nesbett, F. B., and Hofmann, H. F. (1960). *J. Neurophysiol.* **23**, 485.

Durand, P. (1951). *Arch. Inst. Pasteur Tunis* **30**, 55.

Essick, C. R. (1920). *Contrib. Embryol. Carnegie. Inst.* **9**, 377.

Fedotov, A. I. (1947). *Veterinariya* **24**, No. 6, 19.

Fedotov, A. I. (1960). "Cerebrospinal Fluid of Domestic Animals." Nat. Inst. Health, Bethesda, Maryland.

Fischer, K., and Starke, G. (1951). *Exptl. Veterinaermed.* **5**, 38.

Fleisher, G. A., and Wakim, K. G. (1956). *Proc. Staff Meetings Mayo Clinic* **31**, 640.

Fankhauser, R. (1962) *In* "Comparative Neuropathology" (J. R. M. Innes and L. Z. Saunders, eds.), p. 21–54, Academic Press, New York.

Fridman, A. P. (1938). *Sovet. Vet.* **15**, No. 1, 20.

Fridman, A. P., and Petrova, V. V. (1935). *Arkh. Biol. Nauk.* **39**, 209.

Fridman, A. P., Shokhor, N. I., Glinka-Cernorucka, E. L., Petrova, V. V., and Arkina, R. (1935). *Sovet. Vet.* **12**, No. 12, 39.

Friedman, S. B., Austin, W. G., Rieselbach, R. E., Block, J. B., and Rall, D. P. (1963). *Proc. Soc. Exptl. Biol. Med.* **114**, 801.

Goldman, E. E. (1909). *Bruns Beitr. Klin. Chir.* **64**, 192.

Goldman, E. E. (1913). *Abhandl. Preuss. Akad. Wiss., Phys.-Math. Kl.* No. 1, 1–60.

Hammerstad, J. P., Lorenzo, A. V., and Cutler, R. W. P. (1968). *Neurology* **18**, 296.

Hassin, G. B. (1924). *J. Nervous Mental Disease* **59**, 113.

Hassin, G. B. (1933). *J. Am. Med. Assoc.* **101**, 821.

Heisey, S. R., Held, D., and Pappenheimer, J. R. (1962). *Am. J. Physiol.* **203**, 775.

Held, D., Fencl, V., and Pappenheimer, J. R. (1964). *J. Neurophysiol.* **27**, 942.

Hibbs, C. M. (1962). M. S. Thesis, Kansas State University Manhattan, Kansas.

Hibbs, C. M., and Coles, E. H. (1965). *Proc. Soc. Exptl. Biol. Med.* **118**, 1059.

Hochwald, G. M., and Wallenstein, M. C. (1967). *Exptl. Neurol.* **19**, 115.

Howard, J. R. (1969). *J. Am. Vet. Med. Assoc.* **154**, 1174.

Hunter, G., and Smith, H. V. (1960). *Nature* **186**, 161.

Josland, S. W. (1934). *New Zealand Dept. Agr., Ann. Rept.* pp. 25–26.

Kasahara, M., and Fujisawa, Y. (1930). *Z. Ges. Exptl. Med.* **73**, 11–13 and 14–18.

Katzenelbogen, S. (1934). *J. Pharmacol. Exptl. Therap.* **51**, 435.

Katzenelbogen, S. (1935). "The CSF and its Relation to the Blood." Johns Hopkins Press, Baltimore. Maryland.

Klatzo, I., Miquel, J., and Otensasek, R. (1962). *Acta Neuropathol.* **2**, 144.

Klatzo, I., Miquel, J., Ferris, P. J., Prokop, J. D., and Smith, D. E. (1964). *J. Neuropathol.* **23**, 18.

Krieg, A. F. (1969). *In* "Clinical Diagnosis by Laboratory Methods" (I. Davidsohn and J. B. Henry, eds.), pp. 1161–1169. Saunders, Philadelphia, Pennsylvania.

Lax, T. (1961). *Sb. Cesk. Akad. Zemedel. Ved, Vet. Med.* **6**, 147.

Leusen, I. (1954). *Am. J. Physiol.* **176**, 513.

Leusen, I. (1965). *In* "Cerebrospinal Fluid and the Regulation of Respiration" (C. McC. Brooks *et al.*, eds.), pp. 55–89. Davies, Philadelphia, Pennsylvania.

Leusen, I., and Demeester, G. (1960). *Arch. Ges. Physiol.* **270**, 390.

MacPherson, C. F. G. (1967). *J. Immunol.* **98**, 1039.

Markiewicz, K. (1965). *Med. Welt.* **21**, 528.

Meredith, J. M. (1941). *Surgery* **9**, 524.

Meyer, K. F., Wood, F., Harding, C. M., and Howitt, B. (1931). *Science* **74**, 227.

Meyer, K. F., Harding, C. M., and Howitt, B. (1934). *Proc. Soc. Exptl. Biol. Med.* **32**, 56.

Millson, G. C., West, L. C., and Dew, S. M. (1960). *J. Comp. Pathol. Therap.* **70**, 194.

Monlux, W. S. (1948). *Cornell Vet.* **38**, 109–121; **38**, 199.

Mould, D. L., and Dawson, A. McL. (1965). *Res. Vet. Sci.* **6**, 274.

Müller, L. F., and Schulze, J. (1953). *Berlin. Muench. Tieraerztl. Wochschr.* **66**, 117.

Nikitin, N. A. (1938). *Tr. Vet. Fak. Vologodskogs Sel'skokhoz. Inst.* **2**, 113; abstract in *Vet. Bull.* (*Commonwealth Agr. Bur.*) **12**, 473 (1942).

Pappenheimer, J. R., Heisey, S. R., and Jordan, E. F. (1961). *Am. J. Physiol.* **200**, 1.

Pappenheimer, J. R., Heisey, S. R., Jordan, E. F., and Downer, J. deC. (1962). *Am. J. Physiol.* **203**, 763.

Petersdorf, R. G., Swarner, D. R., and Garcia, M. (1960a). *Proc. Soc. Exptl. Biol. Med.* **103**, 380.

Petersdorf, R. G., Swarner, D. R., and Garcia, M. (1960b). *Proc. Soc. Exptl. Biol. Med.* **104**, 65.

Pollay, M., and Davson, H. (1963). *Brain* **86**, 137.

Pollay, M., and Welch, K. (1962). *J. Surg. Res.* **2**, 307.

Posner, J. B., Swanson, A. G., and Plum, F. (1965). *Arch. Neurol.* **12**, 479.

Radovici, A., Bazgan, I., and Meller, O. (1933). *Compt. Rend. Soc. Biol.* **114**, 207.

Rall, D. P., Oppelt, W. W., and Patlak, C. S. (1962). *Life Sci.* **2**, 43.

Rauch, H. (1961). *Arch. Exptl. Veterinaermed.* **15**, 1147.

Schulze, J. (1953). *Monatsh. Veterinaermed.* **8**, 165.

Shulman, K., Yarnell, P., and Ranshoff, J. (1964). *Arch. Neurol.* **10**, 575.

Sigurdsson, B. (1954). *Brit. Vet. J.* **110**, 341.

Sigurdsson, B., Pálsson, P., and Grímsson, P. (1957). *J. Neuropath. Exptl. Neurol.* **16**, 389.

Simmonds, W. J. (1953). *Australian J. Exptl. Biol. Med. Sci.* **31**, 77.

Soliman, M. K., Amrousi, S. E., and Youssef, L. B. (1965). *Zentr. Veterinaermed.* **A12**, 769.

Sprong, W. (1934), *Surg., Gynecol Obstet.* **58**, 705.

Stuck, R. M., and Reeves, D. L. (1938). *A. M. A. Arch. Neurol. Psychiat.* **40**, 86.

Van Rymenant, M., Robert, J., and Otten, J. (1966). *Neurology* **16**, 351.

Vates, T. S., Jr., Bonting, S. L., and Oppelt, W. W. (1964). *Am. J. Physiol.* **206**, 1165.

Wakim, K. G., and Fleisher, G. A. (1956). *Proc. Staff Meetings Mayo Clinic* **31**, 391.

Weed, L. H. (1935). *Brain* **58**, 383.

Weed, L. H., and Flexner, L. B. (1933). *Am. J. Physiol.* **105**, 266.

Welch, K. (1963). *Am. J. Physiol.* **205**, 617.

Welch, K., and Friedman, V. (1960). *Brain* **83**, 454.

Welch, K., and Pollay, M. (1963). *Anat. Record* **145**, 43.

7   Synovial Fluid

Victor Perman and Charles E. Cornelius

I. INTRODUCTION

Articular diseases rank high among the crippling diseases of domestic animals. The study of the origin and nature of joint fluids has allowed for a more accurate interpretation of abnormalities encountered in pathological synovial effusions. In recent years, more attention has been focused on the cellular and chemical analysis of such pathological joint fluids in veterinary medicine. The characteristic of normal synovial fluids of the dog (Bennett *et al.*, 1932; Sawyer, 1963), horse (Davies, 1945; Andreev, 1948; Van Pelt, 1962, 1967d), cow (Bauer *et al.*, 1930, 1933, 1940; Blair *et al.*, 1961; Van Pelt, 1965; Van Pelt and Conner, 1963a,b,c; Preston *et al.*, 1965; Smith and Frame, 1965; Dabich and Neuhaus, 1966a,b), pig (Crimmins and Sikes, 1965), and man (Labor and von Balogh, 1919; Key, 1929; Forkner, 1930; McEwen, 1935; Blair *et al.*, 1961; Shaw and Martin, 1962; Tanner, 1966) provide substantial data on normal mammalian synovial fluid. The availability of large quantities of synovial fluid from cattle for physicochemical studies has extended our knowledge on basic properties of these fluids.

The distribution of electrolytes and nonelectrolytes between plasma and the synovial fluid is in accord with its origin as a protein containing dialyzate of blood plasma (Ropes *et al.*, 1939). Early investigators suggested that the origin of synovial fluid occurred as follows: (1) from synovial membrane glands (Havers, 1691); (2) as the result of disintegration of the synovial membrane and transudation (Freichs, 1850); (3) destruction of the cartilage from constant use (Ogston, 1876); (4) gland secretion and transudation from capillaries and lymphatics (Mayeda, 1920); and (5) synovial fluid is a fluid matrix with a specialized connective tissue lining a large tissue space (Hueck, 1920). Most early theories were based primarily upon histological studies prior to the time physiological studies indicated the synovial fluid to be a modified dialyzate of plasma.

The concept of a modified dialyzate is in keeping with the resemblance of synovial fluid to other body transudates. The major differences between synovial fluid and other body fluids derived primarily from plasma is the high mucin content resulting in exceptionally high colloid osmotic pressure and elevated ionic calcium levels due to the high base-combining power of mucin. Mucin appears to be derived from auricular cartilage rather than the synovial membrane (Shaw and Martin, 1962) and provides an elastohydrodynamic film in lubrication of joints (Tanner, 1966) and plays a role in the exchange of water and metabolites between the vascular pool and joint cavity. Protein is present in synovial fluid in small amounts, approximately one-seventh to one-third as much as serum (Neuhaus, 1962). Albumin forms 60 to 70% of the protein with complete absences of proteins whose molecular weights are greater than 160,000. Synovial fluid is free of all blood-clotting factors (Neuhaus, 1962). The alkaline phosphatase level of synovial fluid is generally higher than serum and with exceptionally high activity in synovial fluid of cattle (Bauer *et al.*, 1940; Dabich and Neuhaus, 1966b). The synovial alkaline phosphatase migrates differently than serum but similar to the enzyme of cartilage and bone extraction (Dabich and Neuhaus, 1966b).

Anatomically, a typical diarthrosis consists of opposing articular cartilages, a connecting capsule, and a variable amount of synovial fluid. In human fetal embryos, the anlage is completely formed by the third month. The two chondrogenous plates are separated by mesenchymal tissue, which becomes liquid and develops into the articular cavity. The synovial membrane, within the joint, lines the fibrous capsule, covers intraarticular ligaments and tendons, and is reflected onto intracapsular bone. It consists of an inner surface layer (intima) and a subsynovial layer. At the articular margins the intimal layer thins to become nonexistent and the subsynovial layer blends with the intraarticular periosteum. Thus, the synovial membrane only partially encloses the synovial space, a logical explanation for various physiochemical properties, similar to a dialyzate of plasma, but modified by local production of mucin and other substances. The articular cartilage obtains its nutrition via the synovial fluid. The intimal layer has an abundance of capillaries, lymphatics, and nervous tissue. The cells of the intimal layer form a compact interlacing layer one to three cells thick; however, not in a continuous unbroken layer (Barland *et al.*, 1962). The lining cells have long cytoplasmic processes that interlace with other cells, such as mast cells, the ground substance, capillaries, lymphatics, and nerves. There is no basement membrane (Barland *et al.*, 1962). Articular cartilage lacks regenerative ability. In contrast, the joint capsule and lining structures can be completely replaced in 8 weeks after its surgical removal.

Theories concerning the lubrication of mammalian joints require a concept of an articular "sponge" not only soaking up fluid and thus insuring its adhesion to bearing surfaces, but also permitting it to be squeezed out, thus insuring an instantaneous formation of a lubricant film with the ability of self-movement. Recently, Crook (1961) applied elastohydrodynamic principles to explain lubrication of synovial joints. It appears that as long as synovial fluid is normal (thixotropic and elastic) and the articular cartilage remains elastic, the articular surfaces do not contact (Dintenfass, 1963). The large molecules of hyaluronic acid maintain the low friction wear of the thin synovial film (Tanner, 1966). The high rate of blood flow (Cobbald and Lewis, 1956), the marked response to temperature changes, and the intraarticular movement of fluid appear to be essential to rapid joint movement.

II. EXAMINATION OF SYNOVIAL FLUID

Routine laboratory examination of synovial fluid may include the following.
1. Physical characteristics: quantity, turbidity, color, specific gravity, clot formation, and viscosity.
2. Cell counts and types: total leukocyte count, red blood cell count, and differential cell count.
3. Chemical examination: total protein concentration, sugar concentration, and the quality of mucin following precipitation with acetic acid.
4. Bacteriological examination: aeorbic and anaeorbic culture, mycoplasma culture, and stains.

A. Physical Characteristics

Studies on the physical and chemical characterization of synovial fluid indicate a close similarity between mammals with minor notable exceptions. The cow and man have been studied extensively, the former in part because of availability of synovial fluid and the latter with emphasis on pathogenesis of joint diseases.

Normal bovine synovial tarsal joint fluid is a clear, colorless to straw-colored, viscous liquid which does not clot after standing (Ropes et al., 1939; Van Pelt and Conner, 1963b). According to Van Pelt and Conner (1963a) the volume of synovial fluid obtained from tibiotarsal joints of 77 adult cattle was 12.6 ml (4–20).* Amrousi and associates (1966) found an average of 15 ml (12–30) of synovial fluid in the tibiotarsal joint on 50 cattle 1 to 2 years old, and 20 ml (10–29) for 60 bulls over 7 years of age. The specific gravity of bovine synovial fluid averages 1.010 with a range of 1.008–1.015. The average content of solids is 2.084% with a range of 1.672–3.886%. The freezing point of the fluid is between −0.509 and −0.556 C. According to Ropes and associates (1939) the average relative viscosity of fluid from the hock joint of cattle at 25°C is 3.72 (2.84–4.15) and is chiefly due to the presence of mucin, a macromolecular acido-glycoprotein which contains hyaluronic acid. Van Pelt and Conner (1963b) obtained an average relative viscosity of 3.79 (1.57–13.01) with an inverse-relationship between relative viscosity and volume of fluid, i.e., the highest relative viscosity occurs with the lowest volume. Further, the relative viscosity increased

---

*The numbers in parentheses refer to the range of valves obtained.

significantly with age of animal. The relative viscosity of human and horse synovial fluid is higher than for cattle. The average osmotic pressure for bovine synovial fluid against Ringer-Locke's solution is 150 mm water. Albumin and globulin, according to Ropes et al. (1939), accounts for only 57 mm water pressure with the remainder of the osmotic pressure due to the mucin. Mucin has a calculated value of nine times the osmotic pressure of albumin. The average pH of cattle fluid is 7.31 (Bauer et al., 1940) and 7.4 (Amrousi et al., 1966), compared to 7.4 for postmortem human synovial fluid (Bauer et al., 1940). The mucin clot quality after precipitation with acetic acid was normal for 92–95% of cattle and fair for remaining animals (Van Pelt and Conner, 1963b; Amrousi et al., 1966).

Horse synovial fluid is a clear, straw-coloured, viscous, tenacious and adhesive liquid, which becomes gelatinous (thixotropism) in 2–3 hours after its removal, but returns to normal consistency on agitation (Müller, 1929; Wheat, 1955; Van Pelt, 1962, 1967d). Van Pelt (1962) examined synovial fluid from radiocarpal, intercarpal metacarpophalangeal, tibiotarsal, and metatarsophalangeal joints of 29 horses. The total volume obtained averaged 4.2, 6.2, 3.3, 10.3, and 4.6 ml and the relative viscosity at 37°C averaged 12.4, 16.8, 21.6, 4.4, and 46.7 for the respective joints The quality of the mucin clot was normal for the majority of specimens (88.5–100%). The liquid did not clot for 48 hours; however, thixotropism occurred occasionally in fluids left unagitated.

Sawyer (1963) studied various joints on 46 normal dogs. The volume of synovial fluid obtained from normal articulations averaged 0.24 ml (0.01 to 1.0). The pH range was 7.0 to 7.8 and the mucin clot quality was normal for most subjects. McCarty et al. (1966) found normal synovial fluid pH from the dog stifle was identical to that of blood. Olson et al. (1967) compared the osmotic activity of dog synovial fluid to arterial plasma and found no significant differences between means of total osmotic activity. Müller (1929) found a slightly negative pressure in normal human and dog joint cavities, ranging from −2 to −12 cm of water pressure and varying with muscle tone and position. Investigation concerning the viscosity of sheep synovial fluid as well as sedimentation measurements of the hyaluronic acids from various fluids have been made (Fessler et al., 1954). Particle weights for hyaluronic acid from the synovial fluid of sheep were 5 to 6 $\times$ 10⁶ as compared to 10⁷ for the ox and 1 to 4 $\times$ 10⁶ in human fluids. Preston et al. (1965) found molecular weight estimates of hyaluronic acid to vary from 8 $\times$ 10⁶ to 10 $\times$ 10⁶ based on sedimentation and viscosity to 12 $\times$ 10⁶ to 14 $\times$ 10⁶ by light scattering methods. The authors suggested the existence of inter- and intraspecies differences in specific biochemical properties of synovial hyaluronic acid. Crimmins and Sikes (1965), on limited numbers of adult swine, found a volume of 4.0 ml (1.3–9.2) for stifle joints. The pH was 7.069 (7.0–7.2), specific gravity 1.015 (1.010–1.018), and normal mucin clot tests were recorded. Normal joints of smaller animals such as the cat and small dogs, contain small quantities of fluid and rarely can more than a drop or two be aspirated (Rhinelander et al., 1939; Warren et al., 1935).

B. Cytological Examination

Aseptic technique must be used in withdrawal of synovial fluid to guard against contamination of the joint cavity. The skin, subcutaneous tissues, and joint capsule should first be infiltrated with a local anesthetic. The use of at least an 18-gauge short-beveled needle with stylet is advised. A needle with a larger bore will plug less readily with thick exudates. A 20-ml syringe can be used to remove the joint fluid by suction. Synovial fluid should always be collected in an anticoagulant appropriate for the determination. For cytological examination 1 mg/ml of EDTA is preferable to oxalates and citrates, since the latter induce marked morphological changes in cells on contact.

1. Total Cell Counts

Synovial fluid is counted for cells, undiluted or diluted with physiological saline. An acid diluent precipitates mucin in the field. The cells are best counted under high power magnification and the number of fields counted should be sufficient to insure accurate counts. In obvious exudative conditions, prior examination of a stained smear will usually indicate whether cell counts are practical based on excessive numbers, clumping, clots, and degenerative cellular changes.

Normal cell counts for synovial fluids on animals (Table I) are variable between species, and within species will tend to vary considerably between joints. In general, low counts are the order and higher counts probably should be log transformed to account for skewness, thus giving more realistic values for comparison.

Normal cell counts for bovine synovial fluid (Ropes et al., 1939; Warren et al., 1935; Van Pelt and Conner, 1963a; Amrousi et al., 1966) are similar considering that variation between fluids from different joints exist. Six series of studies of bovine tarsal fluids contained an average 112, 131, 182, 224, 316, and 103 nucleated cells per mm^3 and in two series of carpal fluids, 213 and 222 nucleated cells per mm^3 were observed on average. The range for nucleated cell counts varies between series, particularly at the higher end. Highest counts reported were 575 and 725 cells per mm^3. Erythrocyte counts on bovine synovial fluid (Ropes et al., 1939) were 194 (0–1540/mm^3). Average total cell counts in the horse vary greatly from joint to joint (Davies, 1945; Van Pelt, 1962, 1967d). Davies (1945) reports average cell counts (per mm^3) on atlantooccipital, 594 (348–1162); elbow, 207 (107–336); knee, 671 (390–1638); radiocarpal, 234 (40–453); and temporomandibular, 983 (412–2350). Van Pelt (1962, 1967d) lists average leukocyte counts for equine synovial fluid (per mm^3) as radiocarpal, 124 (25–300); intercarpal, 91 (9–555); metacarpophalangeal, 226 (44–1350); tibiotarsal, 167 (25–464); metatarsophalangeal, 164 (66–611); and tibiotarsal, 79 (11–178). The mean red blood cell count for horse tibiotarsal fluid was 1314/mm^3 (0–16,500), the high value probably as a result of contamination. For dogs (Warren et al., 1935; Sawyer, 1963; McCarty et al., 1966) average cell counts of 963 (327–1450), 430 (0–2900), and 633 (50–2725) per mm^3 for different joints indicates greater variability for this species. Total cell counts in sheep vary considerably from joint to joint. Average values have been reported (cells per mm^3), for atlantooccipital, 200, and elbow joints, 1100 (Davies, 1945). Crimmins and Sikes (1965) record nucleated cell counts for swine as 220 (50–450) cell/mm^3. Explanation for the apparent differences between nucleated cell counts of synovial fluid taken from various anatomic locations if lacking. However, since the cells involved participate in the inflammatory process, variation between sites may be anticipated even in apparent by normal animals.

TABLE I   TOTAL CELL COUNTS AND DIFFERENTIAL CELL COUNTS ON SYNOVIAL FLUID FROM DOMESTIC ANIMALS

Animal	No. of spec.	Cell count/mm³		No. of spec.	Differential (%)[a]							Reference
		Total cells	Range		N	L	M	E	Macro	Clasm	Other	
Cattle												
Tibiotarsal	21	90		21	1	1.3	87.0			3.7	7.0	Bauer et al., 1930
	25	181.8	55–575	25	2.2	40.1	36.4			15.0	6.1	Warren et al., 1935
	15	131	65–250									Ropes et al., 1939
	21	194.2	50–316									Davies, 1945
—[b]	50	224.0	—	50	7.2	47.8	38.4	0.6	6.0			Amrousi et al., 1966
—[c]	60	316.0	—	60	6.8	46.8	39.8	0.8	5.8			Amrousi et al., 1966
Tarsal	76	103.5	0–725	60	6.0	49.1	38.2	0.8	5.9			Van Pelt and Conner, 1963a
Caropmetacarpal	5	170.4	—	5	0.6	1.6	79.8			6.4	6.8	Bauer et al., 1930
	12	213.3	100–555	12	2.2	40.1	36.4			15.0	6.1	Warren et al., 1935
Radiocarpal	20	246.2	130–530									Davies, 1945
Atlantooccipital	22	783.9	542–1208									Davies, 1945
Atlantoepistrophial	21	888.4	549–1604									Davies, 1945
Temporomandibular	21	1337.5	800–1756									Davies, 1945
Stifle	41	246.6	86–483									Davies, 1945
Elbow	15	197.3	53–500									Davies, 1945
Horses												
Tibiotarsal	18	192	72–368	18								Davies, 1945
	34	166.8	25–466	23	7.2	32.2	48.1	0.6	4.6			Van Pelt, 1962
Tarsal	14	79	11–178	79	3.0	66.9	27.5	0.2	2.4			Van Pelt, 1967d
Radiocarpal	17	234	50–453									Davies, 1945
	17	123.8	25–300	11	7.6	48.5	33.2	0.7	9.3			Van Pelt, 1962
Intercarpal	26	91.2	9–555	18	7.6	56.5	31.4	1.0	4.1			Van Pelt, 1962

Metacarpophalangeal	11	266.0	44–1350	7	4.1	33.9	56.9	0.3	4.9	Van Pelt, 1962
Metatarsophalangeal	4	163.8	66–411	4	0.0	54.0	40.5	0.0	5.5	Van Pelt, 1962
Atlantoöccipital	5	594	358–1162							Davies, 1945
Atlantoepistrophial	10	534	346–678							Davies, 1945
Temporomandibular	14	983	412–2350							Davies, 1945
Stifle	16	671	390–1638							Davies, 1945
Elbow	12	207	107–336							Davies, 1945
Dogs										
Stifle	14	963.8	327–1450	14	1.7	15.7	68.5	6.5	8.2	Warren et al., 1935
	58	716	50–2725	42	32.4	28.7	17.7		20.2	McCarty et al., 1966
Average of six[d]	55	430	0–2900	64	1.4	44.2	39.7	4.2		Sawyer, 1963
Swine										
Unspecified	5	220	50–450	5	32	49	17	0	2	Crimmins and Sikes, 1965
Sheep										
Tibiotarsal	24	207.3	81–405							Davies, 1945
Radiocarpal	15	157.5	73–298							Davies, 1945
Atlantoöccipital	49	926.9	228–1974							Davies, 1945
Atlantoepistrophial	14	1060.7	728–1960							Davies, 1945
Temporomandibular	13	993.5	347–1478							Davies, 1945
Stifle	16	254.7	113–519							Davies, 1945
Elbow	19	200.1	73–411							Davies, 1945

[a] N = neutrophils; L = lymphocytes; M = monocytes; E = eosinophils; Macro = macrophages; Clasm = clasmatocytes; Other = synovial cells, histiocytes, unclassified cells.
[b] Tibiotarsal of male calves.
[c] Tibiotarsal of bulls.
[d] Carpal, elbow, shoulder, hip, stifle, and hock.

2. Differential Counts

Cover glass smears are preferred to glass slides since the fluid films are thinner. Wright's or Giemsa stains are practical; however, Schalm's use of new methylene blue on dried films (1961), gives excellent tinctorial properties to the cells and does not induce additional fixation artifact, so common to alcohol-fixed specimens. Supravital stains (Sabin, 1923) are needed in order to differentiate the various types of mononuclear cells (monocytes, lymphocytes, and mononuclear phagocytes). It is not important, however, to differentiate the specific type of mononuclear cells in routine clinical studies, since the differences may be in stages of transition and, furthermore, the greatest diagnostic significance is attached to numbers of polymorphonuclear leukocytes. There is considerable variation in terminology concerning cell types among various investigators. For purposes of discussion, clasmatocytes will be classified as mononuclear cells other than lymphocytes, monocytes, and macrophages. Bauer and co-workers (1930) used graphite suspension for differentiation studies on the basis of phagocytosis. Eggers (1959) examined synovial fluid on 20 healthy horses and reports on many specific cell types other than those coming exclusively from the blood stream. Andreev (1948) reported the presence of lymphocytes, monocytes, histiocytes, and epithelioid cells of the synovial membrane in a study concerning the joint fluid of 50 stabled horses. Differential cell counts for synovial fluid for several species of animals are summarized (Table I).

Normal synovial fluids from domestic animals should have less than 10% polymorphonuclear leukocytes present; however, the absolute number must also be considered. Studies have revealed that much variation in the total numbers of cells normally occurs in the mononuclear cell counts. Erythrocytes have been reported as absent or in low number. It is probable that red blood cells are introduced into synovial fluid during the process of aspiration.

C. CHEMICAL CHARACTERISTICS

1. Normal Synovial Mucin

The lubricating synovial mucin is an acido-glycoprotein, the acid polysaccharide portion of which is hyaluronic acid. Mucin was first prepared by Freichs (1850) by the addition of acetic acid to synovial fluid. By this procedure, the mucin normally separates into a tough ropey mass. Mucin is precipitated by the common protein precipitants, but denaturation results in the polysaccharide moiety becoming partly depolymerized. Mucin can also be salted out with 60% ammonium sulfate. In most methods of serum protein fractionation, it appears in the globulin fraction. Mucin concentrations vary greatly among the joints in the same animal. Van Pelt and Conner (1963b) report the highest viscosity of synovial fluid in cattle with the smallest volume of fluid. Average concentrations of tarsal and carpal joint mucin have been reported to be 140 and 600 mg/100 ml, respectively. Human fluids have been found to contain on an average over 10 times as much mucin as in synovial fluid from cattle (Fisher, 1929). Ropes et al. (1939) reported that only one-eighth of the fluid protein (0.138 gm/100 ml) is mucin. Friechs (1850) found higher levels (0.326 gm/100 ml) of mucin in the fluid of newborn calves. Cows maintained in stalls for long periods of time had mucin levels of 0.24 gm/100 ml; white cattle free to graze on pastures had levels of 0.5 gm/100 ml mucin in their fluid. Von Holst (1904) determined the level of mucin in normal cattle to be 0.5 gm/100 ml. Mucin nitrogen levels in the bovine astrogalotibial joint (Ropes et al., 1939) bovine carpometacarpal joint (Bauer et al., 1940), and canine carpal joint (Bauer et al., 1930) were 22 (5–40), 96 (63–202), and 43–58 mg/100 ml, respectively. Carpal fluid from cattle and horses have been reported to contain 200 ± 57 mg/100 ml and 136 ± 77 mg/100 ml of hyaluronic acid, respectively (Levine and Kling, 1956). Others have reported levels in cattle tarsal joints as low as 20–25 mg/100 ml (Meyer, 1947). Hyaluronic acid levels in the tempomandibular joint of the horse and knee joint of the rabbit (Sundblad, 1953) have been reported to be 56 and 389 mg/100 ml, respectively. The carpal synovial fluid of the horse exhibits a lower degree of polymerization of the hyaluronic acid, as evidenced by its lower intrinsic viscosity. The lower viscosity of horse synovial fluid as compared to that of cattle may be due to both the lower concentration of hyaluronic acid and the lesser degree of its polymerization. Differences in the concentration and polymerization of hyaluronic acid of synovial fluid and hence viscosity, vary according to age, species, and the specific joint examined. Fessler et al. (1954) suggested that hyaluronic acid differs chemically within species (sheep, man) as well as between species.

Recent studies upon the physical and chemical properties of hyaluronic acid in bovine synovial fluid have been quite interesting (Blumberg and Ogston, 1956; Curtain, 1955; Platt et al., 1956; Blair et al., 1961; Smith and Frame, 1965; Preston et al., 1965). Bovine fluids, in addition to containing one-third of the nitrogen concentration of human synovial fluids, also show differing hyaluronic acid components (P_1, P_2, and P_3) which migrate faster electrophoretically than serum albumin. Seven of eleven bovine synovial fluids had only the P_1 component. The other fluids contained P_2 and P_3 components with an absence of the P_1 component (Platt et al., 1956). Preston and associates (1965) describe measurements of refractive properties, osmotic pressure, light-scattering, viscosity, sedimentation, and optical rotatory dispersion. Ox synovial fluid hyaluronic acid, prepared by filtration and deproteinized, contained 21% of protein in the ultrafilter residue. Measurements of light-scattering and viscosity suggest that the structure of hyaluronic acid may be some degree of branching and of crosslinkage. Optical rotatory dispersion measurements support a structure less simple than a linear random coil. Preston et al. (1965) found hyaluronic acid to contain glucosamine 1.51–190 mEq/gm, total acetyl 1.76–2.31 mEq/gm, O-acetyl 0.04–0.05 mEq/gm, sialic acid 0.049–0.052 mEq/gm, glucuronic acid 1.98–2.59 mEq/gm, total nitrogen 3.74–5.91%, and ash 3.2–12.9%. A comparison of data on hyaluronic acids has been compiled by Preston et al. (1965). Synovial fluid hyaluronic acid from cattle is composed as follows: (1) recovery % 95.7–97.5, (2) acetylglucosaminyl 36.4–46.9%, (3) glucuronyl 36.6–45.5%, (4) protein 3.0–21.9%, and about 1.4–2.1% based on gm/100 gm dry weight.

Whether polysaccharides and proteins exist combined as mucin or as independent substances is not entirely clear. Electron microscopic studies of Smith and Frame (1965) suggest that the washed mucin clot contains no appreciable amount of free protein and is regarded as a hyaluronate–protein complex. The protein of synovial fluid is of vascular origin (Curtain, 1955), whereas hyaluronic acid most likely arises from the articular cartilage (Shaw and Martin, 1962). Studies concerning synovial tissue in tissue culture indicate a continual elaboration of this viscous material (Kling *et al.*, 1955).

2. Proteins

Bovine synovial fluid has been reported to have an albumin:globulin ratio of 1.21 ± 0.02 with the presences of albumin, α_{-1}-, β-, and γ_{-2}-globulins. A few fluids contained α_{-1} and α_{-2}-globulins (Platt *et al.*, 1956). Eggers (1959) reported averages in the synovial fluid of 10 normal horses (%): albumin, 39.5 ± 4.47; α-globulins, 10.5 ± 2.3; β-globulins, 21.3 ± 4.2; and γ-globulins, 28.7 ± 4.0. Prior to the separation of proteins electrophoretically, albumin:globulin ratios as high as 3.9:1 were reported (Butler and Montgomery, 1932). Van Pelt (1967d) records total synovial fluid protein for the horse as 1.37 gm/100 ml (0.83–2.17), and albumin:globulin ratio 3.9 (0.31–8.06), by a modified biuret procedure. Amrousi *et al.* (1966) found bovine synovial protein (0.9 gm/ml) to be less than that for horses and considerably less than for man. Average protein concentration excluding mucoproteins in cattle fluid was reported to be 0.88 gm/100 ml (Bauer *et al.*, 1940). Fisher (1929) indicated non-mucin protein levels in cattle were on an average 0.92 gm/100 ml. Total protein levels for equine carpal fluid (Bywaters, 1937) and knee joint fluid in the rabbit (Sundblad, 1953) have been reported to be 1.4 (0.88–1.95) and 3.6 gm/100 ml, respectively. Synovial fluid protein for swine is recorded as 3.9 (3.1–5.4) gm/100 ml (Crimmins and Sikes, 1965) higher than the normal for man (Neuhaus, 1962).

The protein in synovial fluid is distributed as free protein and in complex with hyaluronate, the mucopolysaccharide of mucin. Smith and Frame (1965) studied the two major constituents of bovine synovial fluid mucin by electron microscopy of the acidified mucin clot. They conclude that free protein was not included, rather a hyaluronate protein complex exists.

Synovial fluid enzymes have not been extensively studied except for alkaline phosphatase. The enzymes of synovial fluid studied by West *et al.* (1963) are lactic dehydrogenase, aldolase, phosphohexase, isomerase, malic dehydrogenase, isocitric dehydrogenase, glutothione reductase, glutamic pyruvic transaminase. In addition, diatase, lipase, and protease have been detected in synovial fluid (Podkaminsky, 1931). The enzyme levels are lower than corresponding serum levels and correlate with leukocyte number, suggesting origin from the latter. However, enzymes of small molecular weight may enter directly from plasma or be produced locally. Van Pelt (1967d) reports on horse tibiotarsal synovial fluid, enzymes as alkaline phosphatase 1.02 (0.28–2.05) Sigma units/ml, acid phosphatase 0.09 (0.00–0.27) Sigma units/ml, lactic dehydrogenase 44 (0–94) LDH units/ml, aldolase activity 9 (1–29) Sibley-Lehninger units/ml, glutamic oxalacetic transaminase 26 (8–60) Sigma-Frankel units/ml, and glutamic pyruvic transaminase activity 10 (0–23) Sigma Frankel units/ml. Comparison with serum levels reveals significantly lower values for all enzymes except for aldolase.

Alkaline phosphatase has been reported to be high in human synovial fluid (C. H. Barnett *et al.*, 1961). Van Pelt (1967d) reports lower than serum levels of alkaline phosphatase for the horse synovial fluid, while Dabich and Neuhaus (1966a,b) studied the origin of alkaline phosphatase in bovine synovial fluid since the specific activity is often 100 times higher than the serum value (Bauer *et al.*, 1940). Dabich and Neuhaus (1966a,b) conclude that the synovial enzyme differs from the serum enzyme in electrophoretic motility and is similar to the enzyme of cartilage and bone extracts.

3. Electrocytes

The concentration and distribution of synovial fluid electrolytes agree with that expected from the Gibbs-Donnan theory of membrane equilibrium. The values obtained from cattle fluid agree, in general, with studies of "*in vivo* dialysates" (Greene and Power, 1931) and also with values reported for lymph, edema, and ascitic fluid.

Values for synovial fluid chloride and bicarbonate are slightly higher than in the serum while the concentrations of magnesium, sodium, calcium, and potassium are slightly lower in the synovial fluid. Total inorganic phosphate is equal in both fluids. Distribution ratios for cattle synovial fluid are as follows: (fluid:serum) Cl, 1.01; HCO_3 1.065; PO_4, 1.00; Na, 0.93; K, 0.75; Ca, 0.83; and Mg, 0.88. Theoretical ratios for Donnan's equilibrium would be near 0.93 for electrolytes. The average ratio for total anions of serum to total anions of synovial fluid is 0.99 (Bauer *et al.*, 1940). Calculations concerned with the ratios of ionic calcium in the synovial fluid to that in the serum give values on an average of 1.18. This ratio is obviously higher than would be expected from membrane equilibration phenomena and is most likely due to the high base-combining power of the synovial mucin.

The theory that synovial fluid is a dialyzate of blood plasma can explain many of its physical and chemical properties. The presence of serum albumin and globulins which are derived from capillary permeability to protein, and mucin which is produced most likely from adjacent connective tissue, in no way invalidates this concept.

4. Nonelectrolytes

The distribution of nonelectrolytes has been found to be similar to that found in a dialyzate of blood plasma. Urea concentrations in cattle fluid (8.2 mg/100 ml) are on an average the same as in serum (8.5 mg/100 ml). This would be expected if the membrane of separation were permeable to urea (Bauer *et al.*, 1940). Distribution ratios of the total non-protein nitrogen (0.87) and uric acid (0.84) between the synovial fluid and serum of cattle are somewhat lower but are still of the same general magnitude. Similar distribution ratios have been found in the synovial fluid of horses (Hare and Cohen, 1929). It can be assumed that the average distribution ratios for most nonelectrolytes are only slightly under 1.00, since in individual cases their concentration in serum and synovial fluid has been found to be nearly equal.

Average glucose concentrations of bovine synovial fluid have been found to be slightly lower than the serum glucose levels. Occasionally, however, samples will approach a distribution ratio of 1.00. Bauer *et al.* (1940) have suggested that the struggling prior to sampling could easily elevate the blood glucose concentration from hepatic glycogenolysis and insufficient time would elapse for its equilibration between plasma and the synovial fluid. Nonfasting conditions could also account in part for any differences in the blood and synovial glucose concentration.

Van Pelt and Conner (1963c) studied the blood sugar level of tarsal fluid from cattle on full feed and slaughtered cattle from which feed had been withheld for 18 hours. With cattle on full feed, no significant differences between blood, plasma, or synovial fluid sugar levels were noted, nor between bulls, cows, and steers. However, with the slaughtered fasted cattle, blood plasma, and synovial sugar levels were greater than the nonfasted group. In addition, plasma sugar levels were significantly greater for plasma and all sugar values for cows were significantly greater than bulls and steers. Van Pelt (1967d) reports horse synovial fluid levels similar to that of blood; however, the range in synovial fluid sugar levels 70 (33–105) mg/100 ml is great. Bacterial joint infections and increased cell counts are responsible for low concentrations of monosaccharides in the joint fluid from their glycolytic activities. The absence of such reducing substances in infectious joint effusions is a common finding.

III. PATHOLOGICAL CHANGES IN SYNOVIAL FLUID

A. Classification

Human pathological synovial fluids have been divided into differing groups. Information concerning pathological animal fluids appear to agree generally with such a classification (Bauer *et al.*, 1940; Van Pelt, 1965).

Group I.   Fluids Produced by Effusion from Traumatic Origin

The fluid is usually clear, does not clot, and contains no great increase in leukocytes, which are of the mononuclear type. Mucin precipitated by acetic acid is ropey as in normal fluid and the resulting supernatant solution is clear. The reduction in viscosity is minimal and glucose levels are not greatly lowered. Degenerative joint disease (osteoarthritis) and trauma are the main etiological causes. Van Pelt (1967 a–c, 1968a) studied tarsal hydrarthrosis of cattle and horses and synovial fluid of cattle with leukemia. The fluids were classed as group I with no major deviation from normal.

Group II.   Intermediate Fluids

Some fluids will exhibit some characteristics of both groups I and III. These may be from arthritis or hydroarthrosis, which at first may show a great inflammatory reaction, and later return gradually to the consistency of normal fluid. Rheumatoid arthritis is a well-documented disease of man with fluids frequently of the group II type. Ankylosing, spondylitis (Archibald and Cawley, 1959), and the polyarthritis of systemic lupus erythematous (Lewis and Hathaway, 1967) may have group II-type changes.

Group III.   Septic Fluids (Infectious Arthritides)

These show evidence of exudation with marked elevations in the total protein and polymorphonuclear leukocytes. The mucin may not precipitate upon addition of

TABLE II   LABORATORY FINDINGS ON SEVERAL SYNOVIAL FLUIDS[a]

Animal	Fluid	Diagnosis	Laboratory findings
Horse	Stifle	Polyarthritis (joint Ill)	Turbid, yellow fluid; clots; TP 5.5 gm/100 ml; cell count, too numerous to count; lymphocyte, 1%; total neutrophils, 96%; monocyte, 1%; macrophages, 1%; tart cell, 1%. *Corynebacterium equi* and hemolytic staphlococcus.
		Traumatic synovitis	Cloudy, straw-colored; TP 3.7 gm/100 ml; WBC, 1925/mm³; RBC, 1150/mm³; lymphocyte, 22%, total neutrophils, 71%; monocytes, 1%; clasmatocytes, 6%. No bacteria on culture.
	Carpus	Aseptic arthritis	Turbid fluid; clots; TP 5.5 gm/100 ml; cells, numerous; total neutrophils, 96%; eosinophils, 2%; clasmatocytes, 1%; macrophages, 1%. No bacteria on culture.
	Tibiotarsal	Polyarthritis (joint Ill)	Yellow, turbid fluid; TP 5.0 gm/100 ml; WBC, too numerous to count; lymphocytes, 6%; total neutrophils, 90%; clasmatocytes, 3%; macrophages, 1%. No bacteria on culture.
Cow	Stifle	Traumatic synovitis	Clear, viscous fluid; AP gr 1.011; TP 0.7 gm/100 ml; WBC, 60/mm³; RBC, 470/mm³. Too few cells for differential count. Majority clasmatocytes and few lymphocytes.
Pig	Stifle	Arthritis–synovitis	Whitish, turbid fluid; WBC 60,000/mm³; lymphocyte, 9%; total neutrophils, 90%; monocytes, 1%. Hypersegmentation of neutrophils prominent. No bacteria on culture.
Dog	Radioulnar	Septic arthritis	Pinkish, turbid fluid; clot; WBC, packed field; lymphocyte, 8%; total neutrophils, 83%; clasmatocytes, 8%; monocytes, 1%. *Escherichia coli*; hemolytic staphalococcus.
—[b]	Radioulnar	Fibrinopurulent polyarthritis	Pinkish, turbid fluid; clots; LE test negative, WBC 35,000/mm³; lymphocyte, 2%; total neutrophils, 97%; clasmatocytes, 1%. Fibrin strands present. No bacteria on culture.
—[b]	Stifle	Rheumatoid arthritis, canine systemic lupus Erythematosus	Pinkish fluid; LE test, positive; Rheumatoid factor, positive; WBC, 30,000/mm³; lymphocytes, 17%; total neutrophils, 72%; LE cells, 11%. Classical LE cells observed on direct smear of synovial fluid. No bacteria on culture.

[a]Medical Records, Department of University Veterinary Hospitals, University of Minnesota, St. Paul, Minnesota.
[b]Lupus erythematosus (LE) cell test.

acetic acid, and the supernatant solution will be cloudy. The viscosity and glucose levels are greatly reduced.

Table II gives synovial fluid findings from animals with various diseases. Figure 1 illustrates cytological features.

B. PATHOLOGICAL CHANGES IN MUCIN

Mucin becomes denatured and hyaluronic acid undergoes depolymerization in infective arthritides from bacterial enzyme action. This causes the fluid to be of

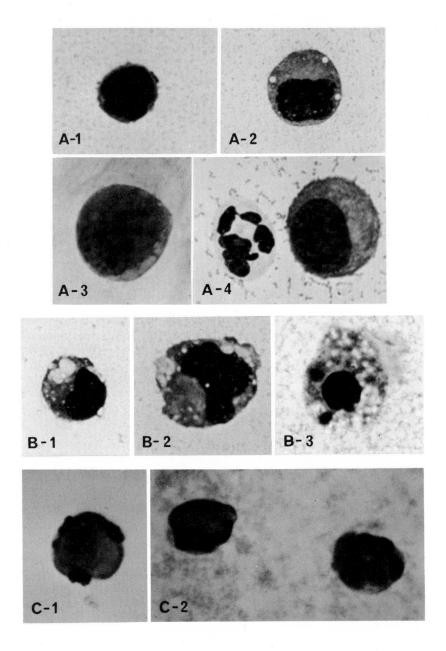

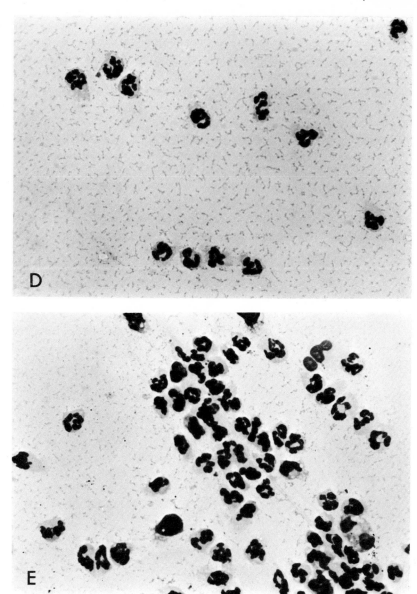

Fig. 1. Synovial fluid cytology. (A) Equine synovial fluid from stifle joint (Wright's stain). This normal appearing fluid of low cellularity contained predominantly mononuclear cells. (1) small lymphocyte; (2) and (3) large mononuclear cells; and (4) segmented neutrophil and large mononuclear. (B) Equine traumatic carpitis (Wright's stain). This cloudy, straw-colored fluid contained 400 leukocytes/ mm³. The mononuclear cells are (1) and (2) phagocytic and (3) phagocytic and degenerate.   (C) Canine polyarthritis associated with canine systemic lupus erythematosus, stifle fluid (Wright's stain). The pinkish fluid contained 30,000 leukocytes/mm³ with 17% lymphocytes, 72% neutrophils and 11% LE cells. Classical LE cells (1) and (2) present on direct smear.   (D) Bovine suppurative synovial fluid (Wright's stain). This whitish, turbid fluid contained 10,200 leukocytes/mm³ with predominantly neutrophils present.   (E) Porcine arthritis–synovitis, stifle (Wright's stain). This whitish, turbid fluid contained 60,000 leukocytes/mm³ with predominantly neutrophils. No bacteria on culture.

a lower viscosity. Infected fluids show an increase in turbidity and/or no precipitation upon the addition of acetic acid. Traumatic joint fluids, however, may maintain their normal mucin concentration despite an increase in the volume of the joint fluid (Ropes *et al.*, 1947). In myxedema and osteoarthritis, the mucin level and hence viscosity may increase. Rheumatoid arthritis is characterized by a loose clot (Johansen and Sylvest, 1961) or tends toward a flocculent precipitate (Thrift, 1966). Curtiss (1964) emphasizes that spontaneously formed clots in pathological fluid from fibrin formation should not be confused with the mucin clot. Ropes *et al.* (1941, 1947) and Ropes and Bauer (1953) reported that physical changes in the mucin may be of great value in the differential diagnosis of joint disease as follows.

1. Traumatic or degenerative joint lesions: The mucin concentration is normal, the viscosity is within normal limits usually, and the acetic acid test is normal.

2. Infectious arthritides: The mucin concentration and viscosity are lowered due to bacterial degeneration of the mucin. An abnormal acetic acid test is present.

C. Changes in Cytological Characteristics

Information concerning cytological changes in joint disease in veterinary medicine is increasing, however, still scantly in relation to diseases affecting joints. Wheat (1955) found sterile, clear, and viscous synovial fluids containing usually less than 100 mononuclear cells/mm³ in traumatic equine joint effusions. Less viscous and cloudy fluids, which contained flocculent particles and polymorphonuclear cell counts over 5000/mm³, were observed in bacterial joint infections. Van Pelt and Riley (1967) and Van Pelt (1968a) noted minor leukocyte increases in tarsal hydroarthrosis of horses. Van Pelt (1967a,c) observed increases in leukocyte counts of synovial fluid in bovine leukemia and tarsal hydroarthrosis, although the fluid was classified as group I.

Nonseptic polyarthritis of dogs (Table II) is characterized by greatly elevated leukocyte counts. The synovial fluid clotted immediately, however, no observation of mucin clot quality was made. A cellular reaction seen in rheumatoid arthritis in which peculiar cytoplasmic inclusions "R.A. cell" ("ragocytes") were found was described by Hollander *et al.* (1965). The inclusions are best seen in unstained leukocytes under high power or under phase constrast microscopy. Under ordinary light microscopy the granules are 0.5–1.5 μ in diameter and from 1 to 20 in number. Although frequently (95% of cases) encountered in rheumatoid arthritis, Hollander *et al.* (1965), Sones *et al.* (1968), and Astorga and Bollet (1965) discuss their presences in other forms of arthritis. The presence of L.E. cells in synovial fluid in polyarthritis of canine systemic lupus is evident (Table II and Fig. 1).

Andreev (1948) observed that synovial fluid from horses with septicemia contained many desquamated mesothelial cells, tissue histiocytes, monocytes, small lymphocytes, and plasma cells. He indicated that the lymphoid reaction in the joints was associated with a neutrophilia in the peripheral blood. Warren *et al.* (1935) on the other hand, reported that synovial cellular components were not affected by variations in the blood cytology of dogs and cows in experimental leukocytosis. In this regard, inflammation of joints characterized by high number of neutrophils has been induced by injection of synovial space with monosodium urate (McCarty and Hollander, 1961), calcium pyrophosphate (McCarty *et al.*, 1962), and esters of adrenocorticosteroid (McCarty and Hagan, 1964). In further studies, Phelps *et al.* (1966) and Phelps and McCarty (1966) conclude the influx of neutrophils is necessary for the inflammatory response suggesting greater importance to interpretation of neutrophil number as indication of great clinical importance. Recent reports by E. V. Barnett (1968) and Barnhart (1968) on the pathogenesis of the inflammation indicate the complexity of the inflammatory response and illustrate the importance of blood constituents to the development of lesions in arthritis.

Septic synovial infections are well recognized. Joint ill in foals has long been known to be associated with naval infections (Magnusson, 1919; Snyder, 1925; Dimock *et al.*, 1928). Similar infections occur in cattle and other animals. Probably the first advance on record in clarifying the etiology of purulent polyarthritis in foals was made by Bollinger (1873) in which joints and umbilical abscesses were associated. The most complete descriptions of these fluids were those produced by *Actinobacillus equuli (Shigella equirulis, Bacterium viscosum equi)*. Additional cytological studies on suppurative arthritis in the horse have been made by Berezhkov (1955).

Emmel (1945) described a suppurative polyarthritis of Florida range cattle caused by streptococcal infections introduced into infected navels by the eggs of screwworm flies. Discolored synovial fluids, containing degenerative tissue and many leukocytes, have been reported in cows in experimental avian tuberculosis synovitis following joint inoculation (Crawford and Frank, 1940). Vaughan (1960) studied thirteen cases of osteoarthritis of the bovine stifle joint and found a slight increase of turbid synovial fluid. Fluid collected from six stifle joints was found to be sterile. Bauer *et al.* (1930) had previously observed constant differences in the synovial fluid of the carpometocarpal and astragalotibial articulations in aging cows, and later (Bennett and Bauer, 1931) explained these differences by finding areas of degeneration in the articular cartilages of the articulations.

Van Pelt (1965, 1967a,c) and Van Pelt and Langham (1968) studied several causes of synovial fluid alteration of cattle. They classified infectious arthritis with respect to duration and dependent on its pathogenesis, as primary, secondary, or tertiary. Infectious arthritis synovial effusions were primarily exudative and classed under group III, septic synovial effusions. Excessive volume of fluid with reduced viscosity and poor quality mucin clots were characteristic. The synovial fluid sugar level is approximately one-half the blood level. The alkaline phosphatase levels were reported to exceed the blood level. The synovial fluid leukocyte counts were variable with generally markedly increased values. *Corynebacterium pyogenes*, whether singly or in combination with *Escherichia coli, Streptococcus fecalis*, or an α-hemolytic *Streptococcus* sp. were not necessarily the most common isolate, however, were associated with the most severe reaction. Van Pelt (1967b) described the use of punch biopsy of the synovial membrane as an added means of study of joint disease associated with synovial effusions.

Synovial disease is common in swine and of varied etiology (Switzer, 1964). Crimmins and Sikes (1965) (Sikes, 1960, 1968) described synovial fluid in a rheumatoidlike arthritis caused by *Erysipelothrix rhusiopathiae*. The synovial fluid was described as less viscous than normal with mucin clot formation thick, white, and ropey, or weblike, white, and friable. The nucleated cell counts were greatly elevated with neutrophils in preponderance. Roberts *et al.* (1968) described synovial membrane changes in *Streptococcus equisimilis* infection of swine; however, no qualitative or quantitative change in synovial fluid are recorded.

D. BIOCHEMICAL CHANGES

The lack of large protein molecules (160,000 MW) in normal synovial fluid is changed in disease and reflects primarily the exudation of plasma constituents. Eggers (1959) has investigated by electrophoresis, alterations in the serum protein fraction of the synovial fluid in various diseases. He reported averages on the synovial fluid of ten normal horses (%): albumin, 39.5 $\pm$ 4.47; α-globulin, 10.5 $\pm$ 2.3; β-globulins, 21.03 $\pm$ 4.2; and γ-globulins, 28.7 $\pm$ 4.0. From a large series of various clinical joint diseases in the horse, he concluded that in acute noninfectious inflammations, there is eventually a decrease in the percent of albumin and an increase in the globulins. In acute purulent joint infections, a decreased albumin and increased globulin percentage was consistently observed. Chronic noninfectious joint involvement produced synovial fluids with an increase in percentage of β-globulins.

In tarsal hydrarthrosis of the horse (Van Pelt and Riley, 1967; Van Pelt, 1967c) the total protein levels found were 1.66 (1.28–2.14) and 1.79 (0.81–5.34) gm/100 ml, respectively. Albumin:globulin ratio of the horse tarsal hydrarthrosis fluid was 3.85 (1.28–15.44) (Van Pelt, 1968a) compared to cattle 1.23 (0.94–2.03) (Van Pelt, 1967c). In addition, synovial fluid of cattle with malignant lymphoma contained protein (gm/100 ml) 1.29 (0.54–3.17) with an albumin:globulin ratio of 2.93 (0.48–9.13) (Van Pelt, 1967a).

It is quite apparent that many environmental and disease factors may effect the mucin and nonmucin protein concentrations quite differently. In all pathological joint conditions, the nonmucin protein concentration will increase owing to changes in the permeability or degeneration of blood vessels immediately adjacent to the joint cavity. The proteins elevated and present in infection will be those also found elevated in the serum. Fibrinogen is present in variable amounts. Nonmucin protein levels may double their concentration in traumatic and degenerative joint conditions, while the mucin levels are slightly lowered. In severe infectious arthritides, nonmucin protein levels may increase threefold, whereas the mucin concentrations are halved. Total protein levels will, therefore, be established from the summation of the changes of the various proteins involved, i.e., mucoproteins, nonmucoprotein, including fibrinogen.

The enzymes of synovial fluid (West *et al.*, 1963) are probably derived from cells, since the enzyme level correlates with leukocyte number. Van Pelt (1968a) studied equine tarsal hydrarthrosis and found that the mean alkaline phosphatase, acid phosphatase, lactic dehydrogenase and glutamic oxalacetic transaminase activity levels were higher than for control horses. The mean activity of aldolase was the same while the glutamic pyruvic transaminase was not significantly altered.

The electrolytes and nonelectrolytes of synovial effusions are not remarkable except for the serum–synovial sugar ratio. Bacterial joint infections and increased cells counts are responsible for low concentrations of monosaccharides in the joint fluid from their glycolytic activities. The absence of such reducing substances in infectious joint effusions is a common finding. Van Pelt (1967c, 1968a,b) studied tarsal hydrarthrosis of cattle and horses and found no significant deviation from a synovial–serum ratio of 1:1. Van Pelt and Langham (1968) observed an average synovial–serum sugar ratio of 0.5–1.0 for various infections arthritides.

Cholesterol and fatty acids are not normally present since the capillary membrane is impermeable to such molecules. These determinations are, however, rarely made. In a report on a chylous synovial fluid in a patient with rheumatoid arthritis (Newcombe and Cohen, 1965) the authors review additional reports that indicate cholesterol (as crystals), chylomicrons, lipoproteins, phospholipids, and triglycerides to be elevated.

IV. SUMMARY

Biochemical changes in the composition of synovial fluid produced by disease depend upon two fundamental functional alterations (Bauer *et al.*, 1940) altered permeability of adjacent tissues and disturbances in intra-articular metabolism. Experimental studies have indicated that bacteria gain entrance to joint fluid more readily than to spinal fluid, aqueous humor, and urine. The great permeability of the synovial tissue as compared to "true" membranes is quite apparent. Changes in permeability of the adjacent joint tissues allows for the entrance of water, fibrinogen, leukocytes, antibody globulin, and some enzymes. Alterations in joint tissue and synovial lymphatics leads to diminished removal of colloidal and particulate materials from the cavity. The inability to remove these colloids, which gain entrance in inflammation, increases the osmotic pressure and hence the quantity of joint effusion. Seifter *et al.* (1949) measured the permeability of "synovial membranes" by the speed of absorption and excretion into the urine of phenolsulfonphthalein (PSP) instilled into joints of rabbits. Hyaluronidase increased the permeability while adrenal cortical extract (Sharp, 1963a,b) and estrone decreased it. Deoxycorticosterone increased maximally its permeability.

The possibility of increased permeability of the joint capsule in relation to pathogenesis of the arthritic response is part of the complexity of the biochemistry of inflammation. The role of blood coagulation factors (Barnhart, 1968) in inciting the inflammatory process becomes of greater significance because of chemotaxis of polymorphonuclear cells into the synovial fluid, the latter (Phelps and McCarty, 1966) apparently necessary for the inflammatory response. The extension of infectious osteomyelitis is apparently a major factor in the pathogenesis of synovitis in turkeys (Nairn, 1969). In man, the principal features of rheumatoid arthritis, have been produced by a variety of agents and it is possible that the initial inflammatory agent may not be responsible for perpetuation or extension of the disease. In other words, the chronic inflammatory process may be the result of an immunological reaction to altered somatic tissue.

Altered joint metabolism is quite obvious following the examination of synovial glucose and mucin concentrations. Low serum levels from glycolysis and a decreased mucin concentration with a low viscosity are quite common in infections. Such fluids show an elevated difference between the concentration of total glucosamines and the mucin glucosamine and, therefore, indicate that an accelerated breakdown of synovial mucoproteins is occurring.

Ropes *et al.* (1941) have recommended the tests shown in Table III to aid in the

TABLE III   LABORATORY FINDINGS ON SYNOVIAL FLUID FROM INFECTIVE AND TRAUMATIC ARTHRITIS[a]

Characteristic	Infective arthritis	Traumatic arthritis
1. Physical appearance	Clear to turbid	Clear
2. Coagulation	Usually	None
3. Leukocytes/mm^3	< 3000	< 1000
4. Neutrophils/mm^3	< 1000	< 500
5. Protein, gm %	3–9	< 5
6. Mucin precipitate with acetic acid	Friable precipitate and cloudy supernatant	Ropey with clear supernatant
7. Drop in the synovial fluid sugar concentration (from serium concentration)	< 20	< 10

[a]Ropes et al. (1941)

differential diagnosis of joint involvement. These tests must be interpreted in light of a complete history, physical examination and other clinical findings. In addition, surgical biopsy to determine the nature and extent of the inflammatory process (Van Pelt, 1967b) may be useful.

REFERENCES

Amrousi, S. E., Soliman, M. K., and Youssef, L. B. (1966). Can. J. Comp. Med. Vet. Sci. 30, 251.
Andreev, P. P. (1948). Veterinariya 25, 20.
Archibald, J. A., and Cawley, A. J. (1959). Vet. Scope 4, 3.
Astorga, G., and Bollet, A. J. (1965). Arthritis Rheumat. 8, 511.
Barland, P., Novikoff, A. B., and Hamerman, D. (1962). J. Cell Biol. 14, 207.
Barnett, C. H., Davies, D. V., and MacConnaill, M. A. (1961). "Synovial Joints; Their Structure and Mechanics." Thomas, Springfield, Illinois.
Barnett, E. V. (1968). Biochem. Pharmacol. Suppl., 77.
Barnhart, M. I. (1968). Biochem. Pharmacol. Suppl., 205.
Bauer, W., Bennett, G. A., Marble, A., and Claflin, D. (1930). J. Exptl. Med. 52, 835.
Bauer, W., Short, C. L., and Bennett, G. A. (1933). J. Exptl. Med. 57, 419.
Bauer, W., Ropes, M. W., and Waine, H. (1940). Physiol. Rev. 20, 272.
Bennett, G. A., and Bauer, W. (1931). Am. J. Pathol. 7, 399.
Bennett, G. A., Bauer, W., and Maddock, S. J. (1932). Am. J. Pathol. 8, 499.
Berezhkov, N. K. (1955). Tr. Buryat-Mongol-Zootech.-Vet. Inst. No. 9, 125; cited from Vet. Bull. (Commonwealth Bur. Animal Health) 27, 3684 (1957).
Blair, M. G., Pigman, W., and Holly, H. L. (1961). Arthritis Rheumat. 4, 612.
Blumberg, B. S., and Ogston, A. G. (1956). Biochem. J. 63, 715.
Bollinger, O. (1873). Arch. Pathol. Anat. Physiol. 58, 329.
Butler, A. M., and Montgomery, H. (1932). J. Biol. Chem. 99, 173.
Bywaters, E. G. L. (1937). J. Pathol. Bacteriol. 44, 247.
Cobbald, A. G., and Lewis, O. J. (1956). J. Physiol. (London) 133, 467.
Crawford, A. B., and Frank, A. H. (1940). J. Am. Vet. Med. Assoc. 96, 459.
Crimmins, L. T., and Sikes, D. (1965). Can. J. Comp. Med. Vet. Sci. 29, 312.
Crook, A. W. (1961). Nature 190, 1182.
Curtain, C. C. (1955). Biochem. J. 61, 688.
Curtiss, P. H. (1964). J. Bone Joint Surg. 46, 873.
Dabich, D., and Neuhaus, O. W. (1966a). J. Biol. Chem. 241, 415.
Dabich, D., and Neuhaus, O. W. (1966b). Proc. Soc. Exptl. Biol. Med. 123, 584.

Davies, D. V. (1945). *J. Anat.* **79**, 66.

Dimock, W. W., Edwards, P. R., and Bullard, J. F. (1928). *J. Am. Vet. Med. Assoc.* **73**, 163.

Dintenfass, L. (1963). *Nature* **197**, 496.

Eggers, H. (1959). *Wien. Tieraerztl. Monatsschr.* **46**, 24.

Emmel, M. W. (1945). *Florida, Univ., Agr. Expt. Sta. (Gainesville), Bull.* **407**, 1.

Fessler, J. H., Ogston, A. G., and Stanier, J. E. (1954). *Biochem. J.* **58**, 656.

Fisher, A. G. T. (1929). "Chronic (Non-Tuberculous) Arthritis, Pathology and Principles of Modern Treatment." Macmillan, New York.

Forkner, C. E. (1930). *J. Lab. Clin. Med.* **15**, 1187.

Freichs, D. D. (1850). *In* "Handwörterbuch der Physiologie," Vol. 3, p. 463.

Greene, C. H., and Power, M. H. (1931). *J. Biol. Chem.* **91**, 183.

Hare, T., and Cohen, H. (1929). *Proc. Roy. Soc. Med.* **22**, 1121.

Havers, C. (1691). "Osteologia Nova, or Some New Observations on the Bones and the Parts Belonging to Them, with the Manner of Their Accretion and Nutrition," communicated to the Royal Society in several discourses. S. Smith, London.

Hollander, J. L., McCarty, D. J., Jr., Astorga, G., and Castro-Murillo, E. (1965). *Ann. Internal Med.* [N.S.] **62**, 271.

Hueck, W. (1920). *Beitr. Pathol. Anat. Allgem. Pathol.* **66**, 330.

Johansen, P. E., and Sylvest, O. (1961). *Acta Rheumatol. Scand.* **7**, 240.

Key, J. A. (1929). *J. Bone Joint Surg.* **11**, 705.

Kling, D. H., Levine, M. G., and Wise, S. (1955). *Proc. Soc. Exptl. Biol. Med.* **89**, 261.

Labor, M., and von Balogh, E. (1919). *Wien. Klin. Wochschr.* **32**, 535.

Levine, M. G., and Kling, D. H. (1956). *J. Clin. Invest.* **35**, 1419.

Lewis, R. M., and Hathaway, J. E. (1967). *J. Small Animal Pract.* **8**, 273.

McCarty, D. J., Jr., and Hagan, J. M. (1964). *Arthritis Rheumat.* **7**, 359.

McCarty, D. J., Jr., and Hollander, J. L. (1961). *Ann. Internal Med.* [N.S.] **54**, 452.

McCarty, D. J., Jr., Kohn, N. N., and Faires, J. S. (1962). *Ann. Internal Med.* [N.S.] **56**, 738.

McCarty, D. J., Jr., Phelps, P., and Pyenson, J. (1966). *J. Exptl. Med.* **124**, 99.

McEwen, C. (1935). *J. Clin. Invest.* **14**, 190.

Magnusson, H. (1919). *J. Comp. Pathol. Therap.* **32**, 143.

Mayeda, T. (1920). *Mitt. Med. Fak. Tokio* **23**, 393.

Meyer, K. (1947). *Physiol. Rev.* **27**, 335.

Müller, W. (1929). *Deut. Z. Chir.* **218**, 395.

Nairn, M. E. (1969). Thesis, University of Minnesota, St. Paul, Minnesota.

Neuhaus, O. W. (1962). *Mich. State Med. Soc.* **61**, 458.

Newcombe, D. S., and Cohen, A. S. (1965), *Am. J. Med.* **38**, 156.

Ogston, A. (1876). *J. Anat. Physiol.* **10**, 49.

Olson, M. E., Kubicek, W. C., Sampson, G. R., Bilka, P. J., and Kottke, F. J. (1967). *Arthritis Rheumat.* **10**, 180.

Phelps, P., and McCarty, D. J., Jr. (1966). *J. Exptl. Med.* **124**, 115.

Phelps, P., Prockop, D. J., and McCarty, D. J. (1966). *J. Lab. Clin. Med.* **68**, 433.

Platt, D., Pigman, W., Holly, H. L., and Patton, F. M. (1956). *Arch. Biochem. Biophys.* **64**, 152.

Podkaminsky, N. A. (1931). *Langenbecks Arch. Klin. Chir.* **165**, 383.

Preston, B. N., Davies, M., and Ogston, A. G. (1965). *Biochem. J.* **96**, 449.

Rhinelander, F. W., Jr., Bennett, G. A., and Bauer, W. (1939). *J. Clin. Invest.* **18**, 1.

Roberts, E. D., Ramsey, F. K., Switzer, W. P., and Layton, J. M. (1968). *Am. J. Vet. Res.* **29**, 253.

Ropes, M. W., and Bauer, W. (1953). "Synovial Fluid Changes in Joint Diseases." Harvard Univ. Press, Cambridge, Massachusetts.

Ropes, M. W., Bennett, G. A., and Bauer, W. (1939). *J. Clin. Invest.* **18**, 351.

Ropes, M. W., Coggeshall, H. C., and Bauer, W. (1941). *J. Clin. Invest.* **20**, 455.

Ropes, M. W., Robertson, W. van B., Rossmeisl, E. C., Peabody, R. B., and Bauer, W. (1947). *Acta Med. Scand.* Suppl. **196**, 700.

Sabin, F. R. (1923). *Bull. Johns Hopkins Hosp.* **34**, 277.

Sawyer, D. C. (1963). *J. Am. Vet. Med. Assoc.* **143**, 609.

Schalm, O. W. (1961). *Calif. Vet.* **15**, 28.

Seifter, J., Baeder, D. H., and Begany, A. J. (1949). *Proc. Soc. Exptl. Biol. Med.* **72**, 277.

Sharp, G. W. G. (1963a). *Ann. Rheumatic Diseases* **22**, 50.

Sharp, G. W. G. (1963b). *J. Endocrinol.* **25**, 443.

Shaw, N. E., and Martin, B. F. (1962). *J. Anat.* **96**, 359.

Sikes, D. (1960). *Can. J. Comp. Med. Vet. Sci.* **24**, 347.

Sikes, D. (1968). *Am. J. Vet. Res.* **29**, 1719.

Smith, J. B., and Frame, J. (1965). *Nature* **208**, 867.

Snyder, E. M. (1925). *J. Am. Vet. Med. Assoc.* **66**, 481.

Sones, D. A., McDuffie, F. C., and Hunder, G. G. (1968). *Arthritis Rheumat.* **11**, 400.

Sundblad, L. (1953). *Acta Soc. Med. Upsalien.* **58**, 113.

Switzer, W. P. (1964). *In* "Diseases of Swine" (H. W. Dunne, ed.), p. 498. Iowa State Univ. Press, Ames, Iowa.

Tanner, R. I. (1966). *Phys. Med. Biol.* **2**, 119.

Thrift, E. G. (1966). *Ann. Phys. Med.* **8**, 292.

Van Pelt, R. W. (1962). *J. Am. Vet. Med. Assoc.* **141**, 1051.

Van Pelt, R. W. (1965). *Dissertation Abstr.* **26**, 3258.

Van Pelt, R. W. (1967a). *Am. J. Vet. Res.* **28**, 421.

Van Pelt, R. W. (1967b). *J. Am. Vet. Med. Assoc.* **150**, 1121.

Van Pelt, R. W. (1967c). *J. Am. Vet. Med. Assoc.* **151**, 590.

Van Pelt, R. W. (1967d). *Can. J. Comp. Med. Vet. Sci.* **31**, 342.

Van Pelt, R. W. (1968a). *Am. J. Vet. Res.* **29**, 569.

Van Pelt, R. W. (1968b). *J. Am. Vet. Med. Assoc.* **153**, 446.

Van Pelt, R. W., and Conner, G. H. (1963a). *Am. J. Vet. Res.* **24**, 112.

Van Pelt, R. W., and Conner, G. H. (1963b). *Am. J. Vet. Res.* **24**, 537.

Van Pelt, R. W., and Conner, G. H. (1963c). *Am. J. Vet. Res.* **24**, 735.

Van Pelt, R. W., and Langham, R. F. (1968). *Am. J. Vet. Res.* **29**, 507.

Van Pelt, R. W., and Riley, W. F. (1967). *J. Am. Vet. Med. Assoc.* **151**, 328.

Vaughan, L. C. (1960). *Vet. Record* **72**, 534.

von Holst, G. (1904). *Z. Physiol. Chem.* **43**, 145.

Warren, C. F., Bennett, G. A., and Bauer, W. (1935). *Am. J. Pathol.* **11**, 953.

West, M., Poske, R. M., Black, A. B., Pilz, C. G., and Zimmerman, H. J. (1963). *J. Lab. Clin. Med.* **62**, 175.

Wheat, J. D. (1955). *J. Am. Vet. Med. Assoc.* **127**, 64.

8   Transudates and Exudates

Victor Perman

I. INTRODUCTION

The occurrence of fluids in the serous body cavities is a dynamic process. The interchange of substance between blood plasma, interstitial tissue space, and the serous body spaces involves the processes of filtration, absorption, and lymph transport. The accumulation of excessive amounts of fluid of normal or altered composition is influenced by many factors. The transudation of fluid in right heart failure, and chronic liver disease is of great significance to the clinician of today, since management of these diseases is demanded with increasing frequency. Frequently, the fluid accumulation is exudative in nature, associated with inflammatory processes of diverse etiology in various species of animals.

This chapter will deal with the physical, chemical, and cellular characteristics of transudates and exudates. It will be readily apparent that only scanty information is available on the chemical aspects of these fluids, whereas the primary emphasis relates to the cellular aspects, particularly in diseases of neoplastic and inflammatory nature. Although it is recognized that anatomic and physiological differences exist between various species of animals, including man, it will be apparent that many observations cited relate to the latter, since adequate data on animals is not available.

II. NORMAL SEROUS FLUIDS

A. FORMATION

Under normal physiological conditions, transudation of small quantities of serous fluids into pericardial, pleural, and peritoneal spaces occurs. The origin of the serous fluid is considered to be a dialyzate of blood plasma; however, the flow of fluid may be regulated by the lining mesothelial cells (Kloss, 1968).

The physical and chemical composition of serous fluids depends on the concentration of blood constituents, membrane permeability of the constituent, the charge of the ion, and the concentration of nondiffusible ions in the blood plasma and interstitial fluid. For electrolytes, the concentration in the serous fluid (transudate) will differ from blood plasma in accordance with the Gibbs-Donnan law for heterogeneous solutions.

Nonelectrolytes readily pass through membranes from blood plasma into interstitial fluid and serous body fluids, providing a steady state is present. Nondiffusible ions (proteins) are governed by the microanatomy of various portions of the vascular and interstitial compartments. Semipermeability to the protein is relative to molecular size. That proteins do leave the vascular compartment under normal conditions is readily determined by the examination of lymph from various organs or portions of the body (Courtice, 1968). The protein content of efferent lymph is usually about one-half the blood plasma concentration, with hepatic lymph five-sixths of the plasma concentration. The high amount of protein in hepatic lymph is mainly of vascular origin (Mayerson et al., 1960). The passage of macromolecules from the vascular space through interstitial fluid into lymphatic channels is possible because of the loose bonding of endothelial cells of capillaries and lymphatics. It appears that endothelial cells of lymphatics are not closely adhesed together (Casley-Smith, 1965). The supporting basement membrane is discontinuous allowing the free interchange of large particles. This concept would tend to suggest that little difference is expected between lymph protein content and interstitial fluid protein content.

A similar exchange of lipoprotein macromolecules occurs between vascular tissue and lymphatic spaces probably on the same order as the larger globulin proteins (Courtice, 1968). The exchange of free fatty acids is like that of other highly diffusible substances; although, in interstitial fluid it binds to albumin in equilibrium. Chylomicrons are carried by intestinal lymphatics and are observed in serous fluids in pathological states.

It appears that the serous body spaces are in essence comparable to the extracellular interstitial tissue compartment. The passage of constituents into this space is governed by similar factors. In addition, the peritoneal cavity is in communication with lymphatics, particularly the space bounded by the diaphragm. Particulate substances, intact leukocytes, and red blood cells readily pass from the peritoneal cavity by means of lymphatics, mainly the right lymphatic duct (Courtice *et al.*, 1953). The route and extent of absorption of particulate material from the pleural cavity is similar (Wilson *et al.*, 1960). However, little is known about the pericardial fluid transport (Rusznyak *et al.*, 1967). The passage of diffusible substances from the serous cavities into the vascular compartment is continuous, as is the removal of serous fluids from these cavities via the lymphatics.

The relation of the serous cavities to the lymphatic system both morphologically and physiologically has resulted in regarding serous fluid and lymph as it drains the area to be analogous. Serous fluids cannot be regarded as protein-free serum filtrates since it has been adequately demonstrated to contain significant protein in a variety of animals (Maurer *et al.*, 1940).

B. COMPOSITION

The examination of normal serous fluids is not without problems because of the difficulty in collection and the small quantities available for study. Yamada (1933) obtained pleural fluid from less than one-third of healthy people studied. Quantities of fluid collected ranged from a few drops to 20 ml. Maurer and associates (1940) obtained significant data on pericardial fluid from 34 dogs, lesser numbers of other mammals and birds, and on 12 humans, the latter at autopsy. Peritoneal fluids were obtained from some of these animals. The pericardial fluids were obtained by aspiration on direct exposure of the pericardial sac in anesthesized animals. The volume of fluid collected from the pericardial sac of dogs ranged from 0.5 to 2.5 ml. The fluids clotted readily; however, no measurement of fibrinogen level was made. The protein content ranged from 0.83 to 2.88 gm/100 ml with an average of 1.70 gm/100 ml. Peritoneal fluid collected on eleven dogs ranged in volume from 0 to 75 ml. Clots were found invariably after collection. The protein level ranged from 1.63 to 3.71 gm/100 ml with an average of 2.56 gm/100 ml, levels slightly higher than for pericardial fluid. Serum levels of protein were reported, a factor necessary for interpretation, since data on animals suggests a relationship between lymph and serum protein levels. Biochemical data on serous fluids from Maurer et al. (1940) are summarized in Table I. Cellular constituents of normal serous fluids (Maurer *et al.*, 1940) ranged from 0 to 100 red blood cells per mm^3 of fluid and similar numbers of leukocytes. Stewart and Burger (1958) report data on pleural fluid obtained from six normal dogs. The volume of fluid collected ranged from 0.2 to 15.0 ml (1.3 ml average) while total protein ranged from 0.5 to 3.5 gm/100 ml (1.39 gm/100 ml average). The average red blood cells were 6300 per mm^3 and leukocytes were 2820 per mm^3. Additional but limited data on other animals on the composition of normal serous fluid has been compiled by Altman (1961).

C. MECHANISMS OF INCREASE

The accumulation of excessive fluid in a serous body cavity is usually a sign of serious clinical disease. The mechanism of accumulation and the composition may vary with the disease process; however, several factors are common to the occurrence of transudates. By definition, a transudate is a liquid or substance produced by transudation, the passing of fluid through a membrane. Normal serous body

TABLE I   PROTEIN AND CHLORIDE VALUES ON PERICARDIAL AND PERITONEAL FLUIDS AND SERUM FROM NORMAL DOGS[a]

	No. of dogs	Mean	Range
Serum			
Protein content (gm %)	11	5.93	4.38–7.00
Albumin/globulin ratio	5	1.19	0.94–1.88
Chloride (mg %)	11	4.12	3.68–4.42
Pericardial			
Protein content (%)	34	1.70	0.83–2.88
Albumin/globulin ratio	5	1.58	1.07–2.62
Chloride (mg %)	11	4.40	4.10–5.10
Peritoneal			
Protein content (%)	11	2.56	1.63–3.38
Albumin/globulin ratio	3	1.46	1.36–1.62
Chloride (mg %)	5	4.48	4.23–4.86

[a]Adapted from Maurer et al. (1940).

cavity fluids are transudates by definition, yet are seldom recognized until the quantity of fluid is increased.

The permeability of blood capillaries was first described by Starling (1894, 1896). In these studies, Starling describes free permeability of capillaries to crystalloids and water and relative permeability to colloids or large molecules. Landis (1927) measured the hydrostatic pressure and rate of fluid movement across membranes in individual capillaries. These observations greatly advanced knowledge concerning movement of fluid across membranes, or transudation. The four major factors that determine the direction of movement between blood and interstitial tissues are: (1) the capillary pressure, (2) the interstitial fluid pressure, (3) the plasma colloid osmotic pressure, and (4) the interstitial fluid oncotic pressure. The causes of transudation arising from abnormal capillary and interstitial fluid dynamics are varied and indeed complex. Since the composition of the fluid accumulated depends on the mechanism of transudation, a brief discussion of important considerations is germane to the subject.

1. Increased Capillary Pressure

Increased capillary pressure may result from venous obstructions, hypervolemia, and arterial dilation. Principal clinical cause to be considered is myocardial failure.

2. Increased Interstitial Fluid Pressure

Increased interstitial fluid pressure can be explained in local tissue areas; however, in relation to serous transudation, it is poorly understood. Interference with lymphatic drainage is a factor. However, the lymphatic system, so adequately reviewed by Rusznyak and his associates (1967) is complex and the extent of involvement is difficult to determine. The thoracic duct is greatly distended and the flow after cannulation is increased six to eight times in ascitic conditions caused by cardiac failure or cirrhosis (Dumont and Mulhollond, 1960; Dumont, 1968). It is postulated that failure of the lymphatic–venous junction to accommodate to increase lymph flow is the cause of the obstruction, rather than increased venous pressure, since thoracic duct distension occurs regardless of the venous pressure. Mechanical block-age of the thoracic ducts in itself does not cause ascites; however, in malignancy and inflammation, occlusion of collateral ducts may also occur (Howard, 1968). This type of transudation, since it may be of liver origin is frequently high in pro-tein content. The affect of thoracic duct lymph drainage on ascites accumulation is most likely mediated through removal of hepatic lymph, since the latter accounts for 50% of thoracic duct lymph in dogs (Nix et al., 1951). The drainage of the peritoneal space is primarily through the right thoracic duct (Wasserman and Mayer-son, 1951).

3. Plasma Colloid Osmotic Pressure

Lowering the oncotic pressure of plasma will allow for increased accumulation of fluid in tissues. A severe drop in the oncotic pressure must occur to initiate excessive transudation. Since albumin has a much greater influence on the oncotic pressure than the globulins, a measurement of albumin and total protein is a more reliable assessment of the deficiency. Hypoalbuminemic and hypoproteinemic con-ditions do occur in severe blood loss, nutritional edema, malabsorption, severe liver disease, and the nephrotic syndrome. Plasma albumin values of less than 1 gm/100 ml are generally necessary before appreciable transudation occurs. It is this mechanism associated with sodium retention that leads to the classical description of a tran-sudate, a fluid that is cell poor and low in protein.

4. Interstitial Oncotic Pressure

A rise in interstitial oncotic pressure occurs when the integrity of the capillary membrane is altered, causing increased filtration into the area. These mechanisms may effect the steroid regulation of sodium allowing for its retention and thus markedly influencing the dynamics of fluid transudation. The role of aldosterone in the formation of transudates associated with different diseases is of great significance (Kojima, 1966; Wolff et al., 1966). The control of aldosterone secretion by the adrenal is influenced to a great extent by the concentration of ACTH, the concentra-tion of angiotensin and the Na^+/K^+ ratio at the production site (Wolff et al., 1966). It is generally agreed that aldosterone acts primarily on sodium transport at or distal to the ascending limb of the loop of Henle. The liver is concerned in aldosterone metabolism and in activation, a major factor in transudations of liver disease. The metabolites and some unchanged steroid are excreted by the kidney. Vorburger (1968) reviewed the role of hemodynamic influence on release of angiotensin. It has been shown in dogs with experimental heart failures that blood flow to the outer cortical region of the kidney is reduced, while blood flow through the outer medulla is increased. This difference in flow may influence Na^+ retention since it is postulated that superficial cortical glomeruli are associated with short loops of Henle, a factor that may account for increased Na^+ retention (Vorburger, 1968).

The formation of transudates is in delicate balance between these several factors. This was illustrated by Osborne *et al.* (1969) by the disappearance of ascites and edema in a dog with an amyloid nephrotic syndrome following a minor increase in serum protein levels. Clinical treatment of the uremic condition with sodium chloride was associated with reoccurrence of transudation.

The cellular composition of transudates is subject to variation associated somewhat with the mechanism of fluid accumulation. In the dog, chronic passive congestion associated with heart failure, and cirrhosis is characterized frequently by sanguineous effusions. The mechanism of the sanguineous effusion may be related to the formation of bloody lymph, the major source of the effusion in these conditions or to capillary hemorrhage. As a result, the composition of this type transudate is modified and of itself may provoke a mild inflammatory response. Hence, the separation of transudates and exudates, the subject for this chapter, becomes exceedingly difficult.

The formation of ascites may at times be associated with pleural and pericardial effusions. The mechanism of pleural effusion following ascites has been explained on the basis of small defects in the diaphragm (Lieberman *et al.*, 1966). Separation of the pleural and peritoneal fluids by the diaphragm is the usual finding, and it can be postulated that the flow from one cavity to the other would be associated with such defects or possibly peculiar lymphatic pathways.

The mechanism of exudative serous accumulations is generally associated with the effect of the high protein level of the fluid from the inflammatory site, increasing the oncotic pressure of the interstitial fluid space. The same explanation is offered for the ascites associated with neoplasms (McDermott and Brown, 1964). An alternate mechanism of greater probable importance is the obstruction of lymphatics by tumor emboli and growth (Howard, 1968). A similar mechanism of mechanical blockade of lymph flow associated with inflammation may be as important in the exudative processes as the change in interstitial oncotic pressure.

III. TRANSUDATES

The composition of serous fluids may be altered when excessive quantities are formed. In previous discussion, the impression that serous fluids are simple filtrates of plasma should have been corrected. The passage of macromolecular substances into interstitial fluid, lymph, and serous fluid has been reviewed by Courtice (1968). Since several factors may effect the transudative process in disease, it is not surprising that the composition of the fluid may vary considerably. This is more apparent when hepatic lymph and intestinal lymph are compared for macro-molecular content, and it is recognized that transudates and lymph are indeed similar.

A. Occurrence

The mechanism of formation of the transudate does affect the physicochemical properties of the fluid. When the macromolecular composition approaches that of plasma, it gives rise to a so-called modified transudate (Shafer *et al.*, 1962). The typical low protein and cell poor transudate associated with hypoproteinemic conditions such as malnutrition, malabsorption, nephrotic syndrome, and certain liver diseases are usually very similar in composition. The fluid is generally clear, transparent, and of low specific gravity as reflected by the low protein content, the latter consistent with the hypoproteinemic state. Transudates associated with changes in blood circulation are of serious consequence. Various causes of heart failure may result in hepatic congestion. Impairement of the liver outflow through the vena cava of the dog as a cause of ascites was recorded nearly three hundred years ago by Lower (cited by McDermott and Brown, 1964). Cirrhosis of the liver results in obstruction to hepatic flow, a frequent cause of ascites in several species of animals. Obstructing flow through the liver results in excessive hepatic lymph flow, the latter escaping through the capsule into the peritoneal cavity. The transudates formed are especially high in protein content since hepatic lymph is nearly five-sixths that of plasma (Smith and Hamlin, 1965). The exudative fluid frequently contains many of the formed blood elements, to the extent that at times it is impossible to distinguish the cellular response from inflammatory exudate. Both mechanisms are complicated by sodium retention as a result of increased aldosterone levels.

Obstruction of lymphatic flow draining the body cavities may result in serous fluid accumulations. Neoplasms arising from the mesothelium or other tissues may exfoliate sufficient cells, which enter and grow in lymphatics causing obstruction. Although typical transudates may result, the fluid is frequently sanguineous from extravasation of blood. Chylothorax associated with thoracic duct rupture is essentially a transudate. Because the major source of thoracic duct lymph is hepatic lymph, the protein content is usually high (3–5 gm/100 ml). Chylomicrons from intestinal lacteals and other lipids are present in variable amount, consistent with the intestinal content of lipid material and the state of absorption.

Lymphatic obstruction may occur in neoplasia of lymphoreticular tissue (Leukemia). In the cervical–mediastinal form of leukemia, a pleural effusion is of frequent occurrence. The physicochemical properties of the fluid are that of lymph and the cellularity is variable, but frequently high in lymphocyte number and of the type involved in the neoplastic process.

B. PHYSICOCHEMICAL PROPERTIES

Transudates from peritoneal, pericardial, and pleural serous spaces are similar in composition. The volume of fluid is variable, dependent on the distensibility of the space. The unmodified transudate is a clear, transparent fluid, with color characteristics similar to the plasma from which it is derived. The specific gravity is stated to be under 1.018 with 1.010 as an average value (Benjamin, 1961; Biberstein, 1963; Medway, 1969; Coles, 1967). The protein content of these fluids is under 3.0 gm/100 ml with values of 0.5 gm/100 ml. Transudates with greater specific gravity and protein levels are termed modified transudates. Albumin is the principle protein of transudates. The globulin proteins present are in proportion to molecular size and to some extent to relative proportions in plasma. Fibrinogen is present in transudates, although the levels may be exceedingly low. The transudative fluid does not clot, but on standing small fibrin clots will be found in the sediment. Fibrinogen is reported to occur in serous fluids of all body cavities of man and in lymph in quantities consistent with the permeability factors for macromolecules (Courtice, 1968). The concentration of lipids is low in transudates and are similar to those discussed for serous fluids. Only scanty data is available for animals, unless the data for lipids and lipoproteins of lymph is considered (Courtice, 1968). The clinical value of chemical analysis of ascitic fluid of man has been studied by Spak (1960). This monograph contains data of extensive chemical analysis including electrophoretic protein patterns, determination of mucoproteins, and several enzymes. Similar data on studies of animals are not available.

C. CELLULAR COMPOSITION

The body cavities are lined by a single layer of flattened mesothelial cells, that have a low brush border. The visceral and parietal layers are held in close apposition, except for the small amount of serous fluid present. Excessive transudation is accompanied by changes in the mesothelial lining cells. The flat cells become cuboidal and may increase in number to form a multilayer lining of cells. Small papillary projections are not uncommon in the case of long-standing effusions. Exfoliation of a few mesothelial cells occurs into normal serous accumulations and an increased number of mesothelial cells are present in excessive accumulations of fluid. These cells are large, 15–25 μ with highly basophilic cytoplasms, a low brush border, hyperchromatic nucleus, and single or multiple large nucleoli. It has been suggested that the fluid may act as a cell culture for exfoliate cells, a factor in clustering of cells and the frequency of mitotic figures. Although the cell clusters are usually small, at times large clusters originating from papillary outgrowth of mesothelium are found. Figure 1 illustrates some of the mesothelial cell formations observed in transudates.

The occurrence of hyperchromatophilic basophilic mesothelial cells in clusters and the presence of mitotic cells prompted the term "black sheep" of cancer diagnosis (Soderstrom, 1966) because of frequent misdiagnosis. This error can be avoided by a conservative approach in interpretation and the assistance of cytologist and pathologists on appropriate specimens (Roszel, 1967).

Large pale-staining mesothelial cells, 15–20 μ, occur in transudates in low number. These cells usually show evidence of phagocytic activity. Pale-staining mesothelial cells have a loosely structured nucleus with pale blue vacuolated cytoplasm. These cells are difficult to separate from phagocytic cells of lymphoreticular origin. Pale mesothelial cells are thought to be degenerate, however, may be transformed mesothelial cells that have become phagocytic.

Blood leukocytes are present in transudates, however, in very low number except for modified transudates. The number of leukocytes and red blood cells in transudates of hepatic origin, frequently approach that found in active exudative processes. In chylothorax, lymphocyte number may range from a few thousand to 10,000 or more per mm³. The lymphocytes are predominantly of the small type, with some large lymphocytes, and a few lymphoblasts. Mitotic figures may be present, a feature of normal efferent lymph draining stimulated lymph nodes. In fluids associated with leukemia, the lymphocyte number may be compatible with that of thoracic duct lymph, but on cytological examination, the distinctive appearance of neoplastic cells (lymphoblasts) allows for separation of these conditions (Squire, 1965). Figures 1 and 2 illustrate characteristics of fluids associated with physical injury and neoplasia.

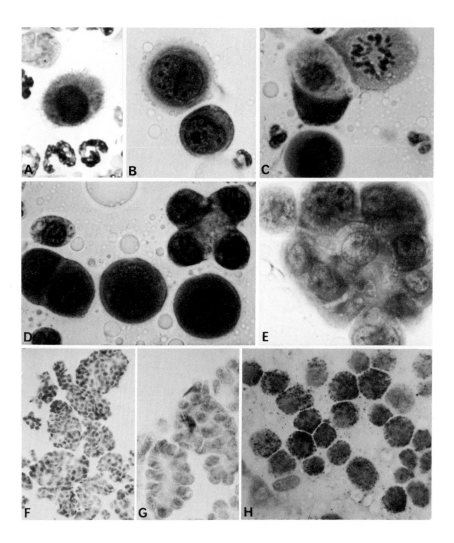

Fig. 1 Transudate and exudate cytology. (A) Pleural effusion. Basophilic mesothelial cell with hyperchromatophilic nucleus and low brush border on cytoplasmic membrane. (Wright's stain.) (b) Peritoneal fluid, transudate. Basophilic mesothelial cells, one binucleate form. (New methylene blue stain.)   (C) Peritoneal fluid, transudate. Basophilic mesothelial cells, one mitotic figure. (New methylene blue stain.)   (D) Peritoneal fluid, transudate. Bosophilic mesothelial cells. Single, multi-nucleate and cluster form. (New methylene blue stain.)   (E) Peritoneal fluid, transudate. Morula clusters of basophilic mesothelial cells. (New methylene blue stain.)   (F) Peritoneal fluid, dog. Clusters of neoplastic cells of an ovarian adenocarcinoma. (New methylene blue stain.)   (G) Peritoneal fluid, dog. Same fluid as (F), however, a thicker portion of the smear. Glandular origin of neoplastic cells suggested by rosette formation. (New methylene blue stain.)   (H) Peritoneal fluid, dog. Disseminated mast cell sarcoma. (New methylene blue stain.)

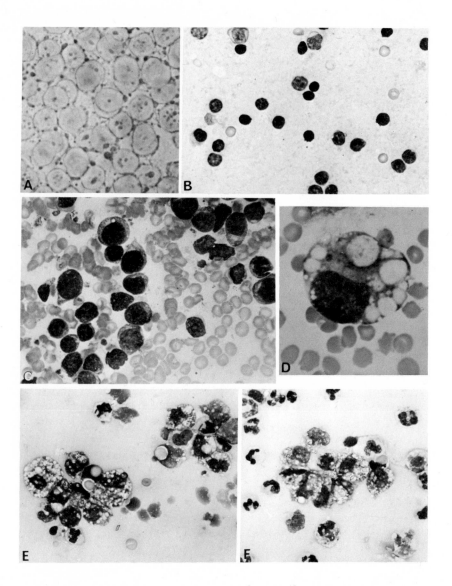

Fig. 2. Transudate and exudate cytology. (A) Pleural effusion, dog. Chlyothorax. Note lipid droplets ringing red blood cells as outlined with a water-based stain. (New methylene blue.) (B) Pleural effusion, dog, Chlyothorax. Note normal small and large lymphocytes. (Wright's stain.) (C) Pleural effusion, dog. Lymphocytic leukemia. Pleomorphic lymphoblasts predominate. (Wright's stain.) (D, E, F) Peritoneal fluid. Hemoperitonium associated with disseminated hemangiosarcoma. (D) Erythrophagia. (Wright's stain.) (E) Erythrophagia and blood pigment-filled macrophages. (F) Blood pigment-filled macrophages including crystalline bilirubin-type pigment. (Wright's stain.)

IV. EXUDATES

The line of division between transudates and exudates as judged from the previous discussion is in reality, nonexistent. Since modified transudates are the most frequent type of the former, the usual separation of the two fluids on accepted criteria becomes extremely difficult, if not impossible in many cases (Pillay, 1963). The mechanism of the exudative process gives rise to larger quantities of macromolecules in these fluids, but at times may also induce a transudative process that tends to alter the composition of the fluid expected.

A. Occurrence

The occurrence of inflammatory exudates into serous body cavities varies between animal species, dependent on the nature and type of disease common to the animal in question. For instance, the cat is frequently affected with pyothorax, a complication of many infectious and parasitic respiratory diseases (Wilkinson, 1966). Feline leukemia may result in pleural or peritoneal effusions (Gilmore, 1962, 1966) that may be classified transudative and at times exudative. Feline infectious peritonitis, a newly described disease of cats (Wolfe and Griesemer, 1966), is associated with fluids of high protein content and low cellularity.

Exudative fluid accumulations are not uncommon in dogs. Several infectious agents mycotic and bacterial, may result in fluid accumulations in pleural and or the peritoneal cavity. Systemic actinomyces infections, which include nocardiosis, occurs in both dogs and cats. If the presence of large quantities of blood in body cavities may be termed exudation, trauma and neoplasia are causes for exudation into all serous cavities. Hemoperitoneum is particularly perplexing clinically, since auto-transfusion may occur rapidly (Clark, 1959). The ascitic fluid associated with ruptured bladder is high in urea nitrogen, a useful diagnostic determination. Of similar importance is the determination of amylase or lipase levels in ascitic fluid obtained in acute pancreatitis of dogs.

In dairy cattle, a common cause of exudative fluids in body cavities is so-called "hardware disease." Traumatic perforations of various abdominal organs, the diaphragm, the pericardial sac, and the pleura results in both diffuse and focal accumulations of exudates. The value of examination of peritoneal fluids, to distinguish between noninflammatory and inflammatory lesions of the abdomen of cattle is recognized. Similarly, the analysis of abdominal fluid in colic of horses is frequently an aid to differential diagnosis.

B. Physicochemical Properties

Physical characteristics of exudates are variable, from that of transudates to obvious purulent exudates. The consistency of exudative fluid ranges from watery to thick creamy pus, many times altered with variable quantities of blood. On aspiration, the fluid may clot rapidly or contain clots and aggregates of inflammatory debris of macroscopic proportions. The viscosity of exudates may be increased by the presence of mucopolysaccharides. In addition, the viscosity induced by release of cell nucleoprotein is frequently overlooked.

A specific exudate may contain virtually no cells because of the highly necrotic effect of the inflammatory process and bacterial toxins. Such fluids when poured, may show increased viscosity because of the high content of nucleoprotein. In contrast, a fluid of marked cellular content may be of low viscosity. The high leukocyte content is probably the result of a more favorable environment for longer cell life rather than indicative of the severity of the exudative process. Inflammatory exudates usually clot, but at times fibrinolysis or mechanical defibrination may affect the clotting mechanism. The color of exudates tends to vary depending on the composition of the fluid. The presence of red blood cells gives rise to a sanguineous appearance. The milky appearance of chyle may be associated with intestinal perforation and escape of lipids. On occasion bile pigments in jaundiced animals or injury to the biliary tract will impart distinctive yellow-orange to greenish discoloration of the fluid.

The protein content of exudates varies considerably, however, is usually less than that of plasma. Increased vascular permeability allows the macromolecular content to approach the relative quantities found in the plasma. Sufficient data on protein types in exudative fluids are not available. Limited data on man indicate that in exudative fluids of high protein content, the proteins are distributed similarly to those of plasma. With marked necrosis of leukocytes, certain enzymes may be increased over that of plasma. Exudates associated with acute pancreatitis may for instance, be high in serum amylase or lipase.

The lipid content of fluids is variable. Lipid values for lymph draining the intestinal tract are higher than from other areas of the body (Courtice, 1968). Intestinal perforation or thoracic duct rupture may be a cause of grossly apparent chylous lymph. The presence of lipid as lipoprotein is usually of blood plasma origin.

C. CELLULAR COMPOSITION

Exudates are unusually high in leukocytes. Accurate cell counts are frequently not possible because of the fragile nature of the cells and tendency to clump in aggregates of various sizes. At times, purulent exudates are composed of cellular debris rather than intact cells and in other instances, the leukocytes will undergo hypersegmentation, a normal aging phenomena, to the extent that Arneth counts would be significant (Riis and Wulff, 1960). Karyolysis, karyorrhexis, and pyknosis, all signs of cell death, are more common in septic disease and as such are frequently a clue to the presence of microorganisms. Macrophages of lymphoreticular origin and to some extent from the mesothelium are variable in number (Goodman, 1964; Volkman, 1966). Frequently, the macrophages are laden with lipid, degenerate cells, and even pigment from red blood cell destruction. Basophilic and pale-staining mesothelial cells are usually present in increased number, the latter frequently phagocytic. The occurrence of mesothelial cells in clumps, however, is variable.

In chronic infection, lymphoreticular cells, including plasma cells, are present in variable number. The presence of plasma cells is indicative of chronicity. Eosinophils and basophils are not of frequent occurrence, unless the exudative process is associated with these cells as part of the cellular response in the disease. Such is the case frequently in the ascites of heart failure associated with dirofilariasis. Mononuclear cell aggregates or giant cells are found in some granulomatous diseases.

At times, exfoliate cells of organs involved in the inflammatory process may be observed. In the process of aspiration of fluid, it is possible to penetrate organs adhesed to the peritoneum or pleura; hence, liver cells or other somatic cells may be introduced.

Tumor cells are not infrequent in body fluids especially those associated with leukemia. Although the fluid associated with neoplasms may have features of inflammatory exudates, the blood components generally arise from extravasation in areas of tissue degeneration. Mesotheliomas and adenocarcinomas of the ovary are, in our experience, frequently associated with massive fluid accumulations. In both instances, difficulty distinguishing between neoplastic cells and mesothelial reaction is encountered by cytological methods. Histological examination of the sediment proves to be extremely useful, particularly with the adenocarcinomas.

D. OTHER CONSTITUENTS

The etiological causes of exudative fluids in body cavities are numerous. Marked degenerative changes in leukocytes and the presence of plasma cells, epithelioid, and giant cells are usually indicative of microbial causes. Protozoa, microfilaria, nematodes, viruses, mycoplasma, and other forms of pathogens may be encountered (Fig. 3). Positive identification is possible in some instances, whereas with many, cultural procedures are necessary. The examination of smears of these fluids stained with Wright's or other stains is recommended. It has been experienced that most microorganisms in these inflammatory exudates are readily observed by direct examination of appropriately stained specimens. In the case of certain pathogenic yeasts, positive identification from smears may eliminate the hazards encountered by growing an organism in culture.

V. TRANSUDATES VERSUS EXUDATES

It is readily apparent that transudates are distinguished from exudates with difficulty, and that in some instances, both processes are involved. Traditionally, several parameters are used in the clinical evaluation of fluids. Great importance is attached to the specific gravity or protein concentration. This approach is not without problems since the values for transudates and exudates overlap to a considerable extent in many cases. Understanding the mechanism of effusion of fluid is necessary to laboratory evaluation and eventual correlation of results with other findings on the patient. It may at times be academic to determine whether the fluid is transudative or exudative when evaluation of the fluid for specific constituents may substantiate the clinical findings.

Routine laboratory examination of body fluids may include the following:
1. Physical Characteristics: quantity, turbidity, color, specific gravity, and viscosity.
2. Cell Counts: total nucleated cell count and red cell count.
3. Chemical Determination: total protein concentration, A/G ratio, electro-

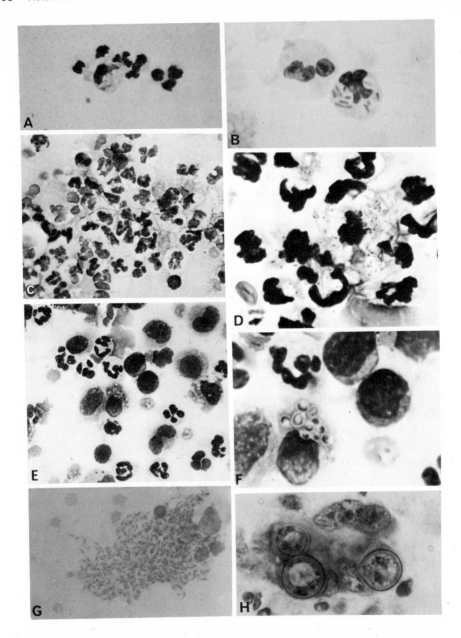

Fig. 3. Exudate cytology. (A) Feline infectious peritonitis. The fluid is typically cell poor and high in protein. Occasional clusters of neutrophils and macrophages are present on a granular background of proteinaceous material. (Wright's stain.) (B) Thromboembolic colic. Peritonitis associated with intestinal infarction. (Wright's stain.) (c) Pyothorax, cat. Actinomycosis. Slender, filamentous, branching organism surrounded by degenerate neutrophils.   (D) Peritonitis, dog. Actinomycosis. Slender pleomorphic organism surrounded by neutrophils. (Wright's stain.)   (E, F) Peritoneal fluid, dog. Histoplasmosis. Mixed inflammatory cell response. Macrophages contain numerous yeast. (G) Pleural effusion, piglet. Toxoplasmosis. Numerous toxoplasma clustered as released from cyst. (Wright's stain.)   (H) Pleural effusion, dog. Blastomycosis. Note budding, thick wall yeast associated with a multinucleated giant cell. (New methylene blue.)

phoretic pattern of protein, lipids, specific enzymes, urea nitrogen, and others.
4. Smears: differential cell count, presence of microorganisms, or neoplastic cells.
5. Microbiological Examination: aerobic and anaerobic culture, cell culture, and special stains.

REFERENCES

Altman, P. L. (1961). *In* "Blood and Other Body Fluids" (D. S. Dittmer, ed.), p. 337. Fed. Am. Soc. Exptl. Biol., Washington, D.C.
Benjamin, M. M. (1961). "Outline of Veterinary Clinical Pathology." Iowa State Univ. Press, Ames, Iowa.
Biberstein, E. L. (1963). *In* "Clinical Biochemistry of Domestic Animals" (C. E. Cornelius and J. J. Kaneko, eds.) pp. 419–439. Academic Press, New York.
Casley-Smith, J. R. (1965). *Brit. J. Exptl. Pathol.* **46**, 35.
Clark, C. H. (1959). *Am. J. Vet. Res.* **20**, 1062.
Coles, E. H. (1967). "Veterinary Clinical Pathology," p. 241. Saunders, Philadelphia, Pennsylvania.
Courtice, F. C. (1968). *In* "Lymph and the Lymphatic System" (H. S. Mayerson, ed.), pp. 89–126. Thomas, Springfield, Illinois.
Courtice, F. C., Harding, J., and Steinbeck, A. W. (1953). *Australian J. Exptl. Biol. Med. Sci.* **31**, 215.
Dumont, A. E. (1968). *In* "Lymph and the Lymphatic System" (H. E. Mayerson, ed.), pp. 232–256. Thomas, Springfield, Illinois.
Dumont, A. E., and Mulholland, J. H. (1960). *New Engl. J. Med.* **263**, 471.
Gilmore, C. E. (1962). *Small Animal Clinician* **2**, 234
Gilmore, C. E. (1966). *J. Am. Vet. Med. Assoc.* **149**, 1769.
Goodman, J. W. (1964). *Blood* **23**, 18.
Howard, J. M. (1968). *In* "Lymph and the Lymphatic System" (H. S. Mayerson, ed.), pp. 153–168. Thomas, Springfield, Illinois.
Kloss, L. G. (1968). "Diagnostic Cytology and its Histopathologic Bases." Lippincott, Philadelphia, Pennsylvania.
Kojima, M. (1966). *Japan. Circulation J.* [*English Ed.*] **30**, 525.
Landis, E. M. (1927). *Am. J. Physiol.* **82**, 217.
Lieberman, F. L., Hidemura, R., Peters, R. L., and Reynolds, T. B. (1966). *Ann. Internal Med.* [N.S.] **64**, 341.
McDermott, W. V., Jr., and Brown, H. (1964). *Ann. Rev. Med.* **15**, 79.
Maurer, F. W., Warren, C. F., and Drinker, C. K. (1940). *Am. J. Physiol.* **129**, 635.
Mayerson, H. S., Wolfram, C. G., Shirley, H. H., Jr., and Wasserman, K. (1960). *Am. J. Physiol.* **198**, 155.
Medway, W. (1969). *In* "A Textbook of Veterinary Clinical Pathology" (W. Medway *et al.*, eds.), pp. 473–475. Williams & Wilkins, Baltimore, Maryland.
Nix, J. T., Mann, F. C., Bollman, J. L., Grindlay, J. H., and Flocks, E. V. (1951). *Am. J. Physiol.* **164**, 119.
Osborne, C. A., Johnson, K. H., and Perman, V. (1969). *J. Am. Vet. Med. Assoc.* **154**, 1545.
Pillay, V. K. G. (1963). *S. African Med. J.* **37**, 379.
Riis, P., and Wulff, H. (1960). *Acta Haematol.* **23**, 276.
Roszel, J. F. (1967). *Vet. Scope* **12**, 14.
Rusznyak, I., Foldi, M., and Szabo, G. (1967). "Lymphatics and Lymph Circulation." Pergamon Press, Oxford.
Shafer, W. H., Adams, R. D., and Calkins, E. (1962). *In* "A Syllabus of Laboratory Examinations in Clinical Diagnosis" (L. B. Page and J. C. Perry, eds.), pp. 265–291. Harvard Univ. Press, Cambridge, Massachusetts.
Smith, C. R., and Hamlin, R. L. (1965). *Proc. Am. Animal Hosp. Assoc.* p. 86.
Soderstrom, N. (1966). "Fine-Needle Aspiration Biopsy," pp. 55–58. Grune & Stratton, New York.
Spak, I. (1960). *Acta Chir. Scand.* Suppl. 261, 1–128.
Squire, R. A. (1965). *Am. J. Vet. Res.* **26**, 97.
Starling, E. H. (1894). *J. Physiol. (London)* **16**, 224.
Starling, E. H. (1896a). *Lancet* **I**, 1267.

Starling, E. H. (1896b). *J. Physiol. (London)* **19**, 312.

Stewart, P. B., and Burger, A. S. V. (1958). *J. Lab. Clin. Med.* **52**, 212.

Volkman, A. (1966). *J. Exptl. Med.* **124**, 241.

Vorburger, C. (1968). *Angiology* **19**, 362.

Wasserman, K., and Mayerson, H. S. (1951). *Am. J. Physiol.* **165**, 15.

Wilkinson, G. I. (1966). *In* "Current Veterinary Therapy" (R. W. Kirk, ed.), Vol. III, pp. 375–376. Saunders, Philadelphia, Pennsylvania.

Wilson, J. L., Herrod, C. M., Searle, G. L., Feichtmeir, T. V., Reilly, W. A., and Wallner, M. (1960). *Surgery* **48**, 766.

Wolfe, L. G., and Griesemer, R. A. (1966). *Pathol. Vet. (Basel)* **3**, 255.

Wolff, H. P., Bette, L., Blaise, H., Dusterdieck, G., Jahnecke, J., Kobayashi, T., Kruck, F., Lomner, D., and Schieffer, H. (1966). *Ann. N. Y. Acad. Sci.* **139**, 285.

Yamada, S. (1933). *Z. Ges. Exptl. Med.* **90**, 342.

9   # Use of Radioactive Isotopes in Veterinary Clinical Biochemistry

Jack R. Luick

I. INTRODUCTION

During the past decade great strides have been made in the development of techniques using radioactive isotopes for the diagnosis and therapy of many diseases. Although these techniques have largely resulted from the use of laboratory animals, their application in veterinary clinical medicine has been negligible. In contrast, radioisotopes have found widespread application in human medicine, particularly in the diagnosis and characterization of diseases such as thyroid, liver, kidney, and endocrine disorders, in the treatment and control of cancer, and in basic biochemical studies relating to the metabolism, digestion, and associated biokinetic phenomena

(Table I). In fact, since the by-product licensing program was initiated by the Atomic Energy Commission, more than 3500 licenses have been granted to medical institutions and private practitioners for this type of work.

In contrast, relatively few licenses have been requested by veterinary practitioners. The reason for this reluctance on the part of the veterinary profession to apply these newer techniques to the diagnosis and treatment of animal diseases is certainly not one of lack of interest. Rather it seems to hinge more on certain differences in veterinary medicine as compared with human medicine. These differences were considered by J. R. Holmes (1960b, 1962) in a series of short reviews on the application of radioactive isotopes in veterinary medicine. One can predict on the basis of these considerations that radioisotopes will not be used extensively by the veterinary practitioner in the immediate future. The only area which now seems feasible might

TABLE I   SOME DIAGNOSTIC PROCEDURES USING RADIOISOTOPES

Procedure	Isotopes and compound	Approximate dose
Thyroid function		
Uptake and excretion	^{131}I-sodium iodide	0.1–1.0 μCi/kg
Red cell uptake (*in vitro*)	^{131}I-triiodothyronine	0.01 μCi/ml blood
Conversion of iodide to thyroxine	^{131}I-sodium iodide	0.5–1.0 μCi/kg
Kidney function	^{131}I-hippuric acid	0.4 μCi/kg
	^{131}I-Diodrast	0.4 μCi/kg
Liver function	^{131}I-rose bengal	0.2 μCi/kg
Pernicious anemia	^{57}Co (or ^{60}Co)-vitamin B$_{12}$	0.01 μCi/kg
Hematology		
Cardiac output	^{131}I-serum albumin	0.2–0.3 μCi/kg
Blood volume	^{131}I-serum albumin	0.1–1.0 μCi/kg
Red cell mass and turnover	^{51}Cr-sodium chromate	1–3 μCi/kg
	^{51}Cr-glycine	2 μCi/kg
Myocardial blood flow	^{131}I-serum albumin	0.3 μCi/kg
Platelet turnover	^{35}S-sulfate	
Red blood cell formation	^{59}Fe-citrate	2 μCi/kg
Leukocyte studies	^{3}H-thymidine (*in vitro*)	2 μCi/ml (blood)
Globulin turnover	^{131}I-γ-globulin	1 μCi/kg
Copper–ceruloplasmin	^{64}Cu and ^{67}Cu (ionic)	6 μCi/kg (^{67}Cu)
Myocardial circulation	^{131}I-serum albumin,	
	^{131}I-Diodrast	0.03 μCi/kg
Hypertension	^{24}Na	0.06 μCi/kg
Digestion studies		
Iron absorption	^{59}Fe-citrate	0.015 μCi/kg
Water absorption	^{3}H-water	—
Albumin secretion	^{131}I-serum albumin	—
	(sheep)	5 μCi/kg
Fat digestion	^{131}I-triolein	0.3 μCi/kg
Fat absorption	^{131}I-oleic acid	0.3 μCi/kg
Phosphorus digestion	^{32}P-phosphate	10 μCi/kg
Calcium digestion	^{45}Ca-chloride	10 μCi/kg
Milk fever	^{45}Ca-chloride	10 μCi/kg
Acetonemia (ketosis)	^{14}C-organic compounds	10 μCi/kg
Rickets, ovine	^{32}P, ^{45}Ca-inorganic	10 μCi/kg

be the development of specialized radioisotope clinics in areas of high population density.

On the other hand, Luick (1965) has already called attention to the greatly expanded use of radioisotopes in clinical veterinary medicine at the institutional level. Radioisotope courses are now offered in a few veterinary schools, and veterinary clinicians are applying techniques developed with experimental animals and used in human medicine for the diagnosis and treatment of animal diseases.

As mentioned in Section II, persons who wish to use radioactive isotopes must comply with the licensing regulations of the Atomic Energy Commission. These regulations state in part that the applicant (for a license) must be qualified by training and experience to use the material for the purpose requested in a manner as to protect health and minimize danger to life or property. In practice, this requirement is usually met by completing a formal course in radioisotope technique. Hence, no mention will be made in this chapter of subjects taught in these basic courses. These subjects include: isotopy, characteristics of ionizing radiation, radiation measurements, methodology and instrumentation, dosimetry, biological effects, isotope procurement, radiation safety, and waste disposal.

II. LICENSING

Regulations governing the use of radioisotopes are listed in the Federal Register (Title 10, Chapter 1, part 30). Copies of this document and its amendments are available from the Atomic Energy Commission Isotopes Extension, Washington, D.C. Licenses for by-product materials are of two types: general and specific.

General licenses are effective without the filing of an application with the Atomic Energy Commission. In other words, any person may purchase "scheduled quantities" of radioisotopes provided he complies with the regulations governing usage, waste disposal, etc. The document noted above specifies the maximum amount of each isotope which may be purchased "license free" and in general these amounts would be adequate for most diagnostic procedures using small animals. However, two provisions of the general licensing requirements limit the usefulness of this type of license for private veterinary practitioners. First, the regulation states that no persons shall ". . . add, or direct the addition of, said scheduled items or quantities or any part thereof in any device, instrument, apparatus . . . intended for the use and diagnosis, treatment, or prevention of disease in human beings or animals or otherwise intended to affect the structure or any function of the body of human beings or animals."

Specific licenses are issued to named persons upon application filed pursuant to the regulations listed in the above-named document, and it seems most likely that all veterinarians working in private practice, in research laboratories, or in institutions, will be expected to comply with requirements governing special licensing. Although the requirements for obtaining a special license are rather rigorous, the advantages which accrue to the licensee are considerable. He may be authorized to purchase and use large quantities of a great number of radioisotopes not only for diagnosis and therapy but also for the research and development of new clinical techniques.

A recent publication by the United States Department of Agriculture (Meat Inspection Division Memorandum No. 270, March 10, 1959) specifies the condition under which meat containing radioactive isotopes may be used for human consumption. This memorandum states that, "meat from animals which have been treated with radioactive isotopes for experimental purposes will be considered wholesome and eligible to receive the marks of inspection, if otherwise acceptable, under the following conditions: if the radioactive material is not retained in the treated animal; or in the case of retained material, when decay of radioactivity of the residue has reduced the level of radiation to essentially that of normal background. The determination that essentially background radioactivity has been reached shall be made by a count on an ashed sample using an instrument capable of detecting activity 10% above the background of a similar sample from a control animal, to be measured in the same manner. Each organ and tissue such as muscle and bone intended to be used for food shall be separately tested in a like manner." This memorandum promises to stimulate the use of radioisotopes in large farm animals since, in establishing levels of acceptability for human consumption, it makes programs of research and development economically feasible.

III.   ROUTINE DIAGNOSTIC AND THERAPEUTIC PROCEDURES*

This section deals with procedures which are now considered to be routine applications of radioisotope technique in clinical medicine. Although these procedures were developed with laboratory animals, usually dogs, few have been applied to veterinary clinical medicine. In the discussion following the presentation of each idealized or typical procedure, references are made to the latest modifications and applications of the technique, especially as applied to veterinary medicine.

A. THYROID UPTAKE OF ^{131}I

The most widely used diagnostic procedure employing a radioisotope is undoubtedly the ^{131}I thyroid uptake test. This test is based on the well-established relation between the avidity of the thyroid gland for iodine and its functional state. Iodine is used by the gland in the synthesis of the hormones thyroxine (T_4) and triiodothyronine (T_3) which are, in turn, secreted into the blood stream for distribution to the tissues where they serve as key metabolic regulators. The rate at which the thyroid gland accumulates radioiodine from an administered dose and secretes labeled hormones to the blood stream are useful indexes of its function (Werner et al., 1950; Freedberg et al., 1952).

Of the several tests used for thyroid function, the direct measure of iodine uptake by the thyroid gland is by far the most popular. The estimation of the accumulation in the gland is usually made 24 hours after the oral administration of a tracer dose although there is evidence that shorter or longer time periods may be employed. The

*The author gratefully acknowledges the generous assistance of the Nuclear Chicago Corporation in the development of this section dealing with diagnostic and therapeutic applications of radioactive isotopes in clinical medicine. Dr. M. K. Yousef very kindly assisted in the revision of parts D and E.

test is relatively easy to perform and provides reliable information about the functional state in the majority of uncomplicated cases.

1. Procedure

a. Inject the radioiodine (1 μCi/kg body weight) as a solution diluted in saline. (Some clinicians prefer to dose orally either as a solution or as a precalibrated capsule.)

b. Set aside an identical dose of the iodine to be used later as a standard. Store the standard in a small lead shield; remove from the place of counting until it is required. With precalibrated solutions or capsules one standard may serve for a number of tests in which it is representative of the dose administered.

c. Determine the percent of the administered dose of radioiodine which has accumulated in the thyroid during the period 72 hours after dosing.

d. Estimate the uptake of radioiodine in the gland by external counting with a probe scintillation detector in which the scintillation crystal is covered by a $\frac{1}{16}$-in. thickness of lead to absorb low-energy scattered radiation. The procedure is to measure the radioactivity in the standard and then in the animal's thyroid. The uptake is the ratio of these two measurements. In order that reliable tests be obtained, precautions must be taken to measure the radioactivity at the same geometry in both instances.

e. Place the standard in a plastic phantom of the neck and position it accurately along the center line of the scintillation crystal with a rigid locating device at a distance of 25 cm from the end of the crystal. The phantom compensates for the average distance of the thyroid under the neck surface and provides a degree of absorption and scatter essentially equivalent to that of a structure in the neck.

f. Determine the radioactivity in the standard at the selected distance in units of counts per minute (cpm).

g. Determine the background count by placing a 4-in. $\times$ 4-in. $\times$ $\frac{1}{2}$-in. lead filter in front of the standard. Remove the standard and store in a lead shield at some distance from the detector.

h. Measure the radioactivity in the animal's thyroid at the same distance the standard was measured (see Fig. 1).

i. Measure the background count for the animal by placing the 4-in. square filter in front of the animal's thyroid gland.

j. Calculate the percent of the administered dose of radioiodine in the thyroid gland by the equation:

$$\text{Uptake } (\%) = \frac{\text{net cpm thyroid}}{\text{net cpm standard}} \times 100$$

2. Results and Discussion

Thyroid uptake studies have been reported for several species of animals generally encountered in veterinary medicine. These include dogs (Fredrickson et al., 1955; Kaneko et al., 1959; Lombardi et al., 1962), rabbits (Brown-Grant and Gibson, 1955), mink (Reineke et al., 1960), sheep (Hennemann et al., 1955), goats (Flamboe

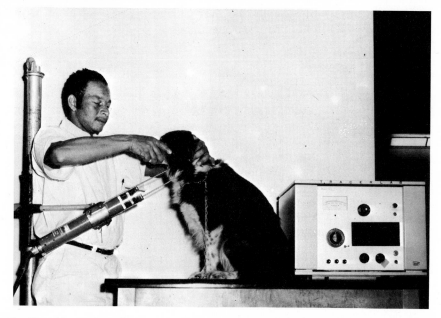

Fig. 1. Thyroid counting using a γ-sensitive sodium iodide crystal in a scintillation detector probe. (Courtesy of J. J. Kaneko.)

and Reineke, 1959), primates (Dowling *et al.*, 1961), dairy calves (Lodge *et al.*, 1957), and cattle (Pipes *et al.*, 1957; Swanson *et al.*, 1957). However, it seems that most of these studies will be of little direct value for the veterinary clinician since they emphasize basic research rather than establish criteria for diagnosis and therapy. Nevertheless, these interspecies studies of thyroid function are of considerable academic interest. The lack of an obvious correlation between rate of uptake of ^{131}I and either body size or metabolic rate is an interesting case in point. Maximum uptake occured at approximately 24 hours following dosing in man (Werner *et al.*, 1950) and mink (Reineke *et al.*, 1960). In contrast, maximum uptake occurred at 72 hours following injection of radioiodine in dogs (Kaneko *et al.*, 1959) and dairy cattle (Howes *et al.*, 1962; Pipes *et al.*, 1957).

a. STUDIES WITH NONRUMINANTS. Kaneko *et al.* (1959) used ^{131}I sodium iodide to establish a diagnostic test of thyroid function in the dog and applied this test to a number of dogs suffering from various thyroid diseases. Their results are based on the percentage of ^{131}I uptake at 72 hours postinjection and suggest the following diagnostic criteria: 0 to 10%, indicative of hypothyroidism; 11 to 40%, normal; 41 to 100%, indicative of hyperthyroidism. Similar values have recently been reported by Lombardi *et al.* (1962). Kaneko *et al.* (1959) also studied the effect of hypophysectomy and administration of thyrotropic hormone (TSH) on the ^{131}I uptake in dogs. Their results suggest a test based on ^{131}I before and after treatment with TSH which might be of value in differentiating primary hypothyroidism from pituitary hypothyroidism in dogs.

Brown-Grant and Gibson (1955) used the thyroid uptake test to calculate the thyroid blood clearance rate in rabbits. The normal rabbit cleared (on the average)

0.58 ml whole blood/min. The clearance rate of thyroid blood increased when the rabbits were treated with TSH and decreased following hypophysectomy. Treatment with either T_4 or cortisone also decrease thyroid blood clearance. Reineke et al. (1960) reported thyroidal iodine turnover, thyroxine secretion rate (TSR), and thyroactive iodinated casein utilization in mink. At 24 hours after the injection of 30 μCi of carrier-free inorganic iodine, ^{131}I, approximately 8.14% of the injected dose had accumulated in the thyroid glands. Thereafter the radioactivity in the thyroid gland decreased exponentially with a half-time of 3.48 days from which the "thyroid output rate" was calculated to be 19.9%/day. The thyroid output rate is presumably the relative secretion rate, i.e., the percent of the ^{131}I present in the thyroid gland which is secreted during a 24-hour period and should not be confused with the TSH.

b. STUDIES WITH RUMINANTS. Radioiodine has been used extensively to study the thyroid activity of ruminants, and methods for the in vivo uptake of ^{131}I have been published for cattle (Blincoe, 1953; Pipes et al., 1957), dairy heifers (Lodge et al., 1957), pigs (Sorensen, 1958; Seigneur et al., 1959), sheep (Henneman et al., 1952), and for dairy goats (Flamboe and Reineke, 1959). These studies have centered largely on the environmental and physiological factors which affect thyroid activity rather than on studies pertaining to veterinary clinical medicine, i.e., diagnosis and/or therapy. For example, studies on the effect of age, breed, pregnancy, lactation, and season of the year on thyroid secretion rates have been reported for sheep (Henneman et al., 1955), goats (Flamboe and Reineke, 1959), and dairy cattle (H. D. Johnson and Ragsdale, 1959; Pipes et al., 1959; Premachandra et al., 1958; Howes et al., 1962).

Studies on the effect of dietary iodine on thyroid uptake tests in sheep (Bustad et al., 1958), dairy calves (Lodge et al., 1958), and dairy cows (Swanson et al., 1957) suggest that nutritional or biochemical factors may alter results of this test significantly. Recently Sharpe (1961) reported that an antihistamine, p-bromdylamine maleate, inhibited ^{131}I uptake in humans. The results of these studies recall the work of Werner et al. (1950), who concluded that a single test of thyroid activity, no matter how precise, is not a completely reliable index of the state of its activity. In fact, one may even be misled when several functions of the gland are tested. They conclude that sound clinical judgment is still the final arbiter in the diagnosis of thyroid disease.

Several hormones have been reported to affect the thyroid uptake test. Pipes et al. (1958b) studied the effect of estrogen and progesterone on cattle and reported that their results indicated that the level of estrogen secreted in late pregnancy stimulated an increased secretion of T_4 and TSH during early lactation. Turner et al. (1961) reported that hydrocortisone tended to depress TSH and T_4 secretion in cattle, whereas Meticorten, a synthetic glucocorticoid, tended to stimulate the thyroid function in dairy cattle. Premachandra and Turner (1961) caused a milk hyperthyroidism in dairy cattle by administering exogenous T_4 which reduced the secretion of ^{131}I in the milk of these cows by 50% in the first 24-hours period. Singh et al. (1956) reported that ewes with high thyroid activity, as measured by the thyroid output (biological half-time), tended to produce faster-gaining twin lambs than ewes with low thyroid activity—an effect which the authors thought might be attributed to greater milk production.

c. GOITROGENS AND THE ^{131}I THYROID UPTAKE TEST. Goitrogens interfere with the utilization of iodine for T_4 synthesis. This phenomenon has been used to prevent the recycling of ^{131}I during thyroid uptake and thyroid secretion tests and has suggested to Pipes et al. (1958a) a technique for estimating the effectiveness of goitrogens in cattle. This technique involves the administration of ^{131}I iodide and the subsequent measurement of the rate of release of ^{131}I from the thyroid gland. The goitrogen is then fed, following which a downward trend in the slope of the "release rate" curve is noted. The sharpness of the break is a measure of the effectiveness of the goitrogen to prevent recycling of ^{131}I through the thyroid (and hence to inhibit thyroid hormone synthesis). Two goitrogens were tested: thiouracil and 6-methyl thiouracil. They proved to be equally effective in that 1 gm/100 lb body weight completely blocked the recycling of ^{131}I through the thyroid glands.

A similar technique has been used to detect minute amounts of giotrogenic residues in the tissues of various animals (Raun et al., 1958; Premachandra and Turner, 1960). The comparative uptake of ^{131}I by fetal and maternal sheep tissues and the possible relationship between fetal thyroid activity and the incidence of congenital goiter was reported by Wright and Sinclair (1959).

B. RED CELL UPTAKE OF ^{131}I-LABELED TRIIODOTHYRONINE

Thyroxine is firmly bound in the plasma to the T_4-binding globulin, a mucoprotein which migrates electrophoreticaly as an α-globulin. In the hyperthyroid state, the T_4 globulin is relatively saturated with T_4 in comparison with the euthyroid states where excess binding capacity exists. Triiodothyronine is more weakly bound to plasma proteins and will not displace T_4 from its binding site on the globulin. Also T_3 can be bound to the erythrocyte site, the amount reflecting the competition between this binding site and the plasma protein affinities for T_3.

In hyperthyroidism, the degree of the saturation of the plasma protein binding sites by T_4 decreases their availability for T_3, and in whole blood added T_3 is bound to a greater extent on the erythrocytes. Hamolsky et al. (1957) devised a method for estimating thyroid function based on the in vitro uptake by the erythrocytes of radioiodine-labeled T_3 added to a sample of human blood. In hyperthyroid states there is a greater uptake on the erythrocytes than in euthyroid states. The method is simple and offers a technique for estimating thyroid function which does not require the administration of radioactive materials to patients.

1. Procedure

a. Dilute ^{131}I-labeled T_3 in 0.9% NaCl to give a solution containing $10–120 \times 10^{-4}$ $\mu g/0.1$ ml. The radioiodine content should be in the range of $4 \times 10^{-2} \mu Ci$ to give good counting rates.

b. Draw 10 ml of blood from the patient who is in either the fasting or nonfasting state. Discharge the sample carefully into a bottle containing 0.1 ml of 40% potassium oxalate. Citrated or heparinized blood may also be used.

c. After adequate mixing, pipet out 3 ml samples of blood in duplicate into 10-ml Erlenmeyer flasks. Add 0.1 ml of ^{131}I-T_3 solution to each flask and mix by swirling.

d. Incubate the samples with shaking at 37°C for 2 hours.

e. At the end of the incubation period mix the samples well and pipet two 1-ml aliquots into test tubes which will fit into a scintillation well counter. Determine the hematocrit on another sample.

f. Count the samples.

g. After counting, centrifuge the tubes to pack the erythrocytes. Remove the supernatant plasma carefully and resuspend the cells in 10 ml of isotonic saline. Centrifuge and remove the supernatant saline carefully. Repeat the washing procedures four more times. Care should be used to avoid losing red blood cells in decanting the supernatant solutions.

h. Count the residual radioactivity in the erythrocyte fraction in a well counter.

i. Calculte the erythrocyte uptake by the formula:

$$\text{Erythrocytic uptake } (\%) = \frac{\text{net cpm in red blood cells from 1 ml blood}}{\text{net cpm in 1 ml whole blood}} \times 100$$

j. The values are arbitrarily corrected to a hematocrit of 100% by the formula:

$$\text{Erythrocyte uptake } (\%/100\% \text{ hematocrit}) = \frac{\text{erythrocyte uptake} \times 100}{\text{hematocrit}}$$

2. Results and Discussion

Hamolsky et al. (1957) reported the results of 376 red cells uptake tests on 296 human subjects. In 231 determinations on 209 euthyroid subjects, the values for the corrected erythrocyte uptakes ranged from 10.3 to 17.0% with an average of 13.9%. For 110 determinations on 67 hyperthyroid patients, the uptakes ranged from 16.4 to 34.1% with an average of 21.9%. There was some overlap in the two groups of values but 95.5% of all hyperthyroid uptakes were greater than 17% and 96.2% of euthyroid uptakes ranged below 16.0%. The test also has value in the diagnosis of hypothyroidism. In 35 determinations of 29 patients, the values ranged from 5.0 to 11.0%, averaging 9.3%. These values were essentially confirmed in a recent report by Ureles and Murray (1959).

As stated above, the determination of red cell uptake of ^{131}I-T$_3$ is simple and rapid. Furthermore, no radioactivity need be given to the patient since the test is conducted with a small blood sample in vitro. Hamolsky et al. claim that the test has the diagnostic accuracy of other standard thyroid tests and may be applicable when the other tests are not. It may be useful when following the course of therapy for hyperthyroidism or hypothyroidism.

Red cell uptake is decreased during normal pregnancy, after the administration of estrogen and following the administration of propylthiouracil in five of six cases of hyperthyroidism. Red cell uptake was increased in nephrosis, hepatitis, hepatic cirrhosis, and in extensive metastatic malignancy, and following the administration of Dicumarol (Hamolsky et al., 1957, 1959).

Hansard (1962) reported an evaluation of the red cell ^{131}I-labeled T$_3$ tests for measuring thyroid status in cattle, sheep, and swine; 4-ml samples of whole blood were incubated with T$_3$ for 4 hours at 37°C. Radioactivity was measured in whole blood and in the red cells after washing five times with ice-cold saline. Hansard concluded that the procedure offered possibilities where more tedious methods were not available and was applicable for rapid area surveys of thyroid status and for relative animal response measurements to thyroid treatment.

An interesting modification of the above technique was recently reported by Sterling and Tabachnik (1961). ^{131}I-labeled T_3 is added to a mixture of serum and IRA-400 anion exchange resin. The resin absorbs T_3 which is not bound to serum proteins. The mixture is counted, then the resin is washed three times with water and recounted. The authors reported an elevated resin uptake during thyrotoxicosis which diminished following treatment.

C. IODIDE-THYROID HORMONE CONVERSION RATIO

The rate at which radioiodine-labeled thyroid hormone is secreted into the blood stream after the administration of a tracer dose of radioiodine is related to the functional state of the gland. In hyperthyroids a greater amount of labeled hormone is found in the circulating plasma after 24 hours than is found in euthyroids. In order to estimate the amount of labeled hormone in the plasma in the presence of inorganic radioiodide which may be present, advantage is taken of a strong binding of T_4 to the plasma proteins. The hormonally active iodine is precipitated with the plasma proteins by agents such as trichloracetic acid. "Protein-bound iodine" ($[^{131}I]$ PBI) is not absorbed by anion exchange resins at pH's near neutrality under conditions in which inorganic iodide is removed from the plasma. Both of these phenomena are used in estimating the circulating labeled hormone.

Clark, et al. (1949) increased the sensitivity of the plasma-labeled $[^{131}I]$ PBI level as a measure of thyroid function by comparing it to the level of total radioactive iodine in the plasma. The latter is the sum of the $[^{131}I]$ PBI and inorganic iodide ^{131}I. They introduced the term "conversion ratio" for a given quantity of plasma.

$$\text{Conversion ratio} = \frac{[^{131}I] \text{ PBI}}{\text{total } ^{131}I} \times 100$$

Since hyperthyroids have a greater $[^{131}I]$ PBI than normals and a lower inorganic iodine ^{131}I in the plasma because of the increased avidity of the gland, the conversion ratio is higher in hyperthyroids than in euthyroids. The ratio is usually determined 24 hours after the administration of a tracer dose.

Because of the small percentage of the administered dose present in the circulating blood, a tracer dose of approximately 1 μCi ^{131}I/kg body weight is usually necessary if the conversion ratio is to be determined. To increase the number of counts per minute obtained in the $[^{131}I]$ PBI fraction, the precipitate from 4 ml of plasma can be countered.

1. Procedure for Trichloroacetic Acid Precipitation Method

a. Twenty-four hours after the administration of the tracer dose of ^{131}I, draw 10 ml of blood and discharge it into a tube containing EDTA or oxalate anticoagulant. Centrifuge and remove the plasma with a capillary pipet.

b. Pipet 2 ml plasma into the plastic tube. Count for 10 minutes in a scintillation well detector.

c. Add 2 ml more plasma to the plastic tube.

d. Add 4 ml of 14% trichloracetic acid; the first ml quickly, the last 3 ml in drops.

e. Mix the solution with the glass stirring rod until homogeneous; let solution sit a minute; then rinse stirring rod into the tube with a few milliliters of distilled water.

f. Centrifuge; remove the supernatant by inverting test tube quickly and allowing to drain for 1 minute.

g. Pipet 4 ml of 7% trichloracetic acid into the tube. Resuspend and precipitate until homogeneous, using the stirring rod. Centrifuge. Invert the tube and discard the supernatant.

h. Repeat the washing procedure twice.

i. Count the washed precipitate for 10 minutes in a well detector.

j. Calculate as follows:

$$\text{Conversion ratio (\%)} = \left(\frac{\text{net cpm in precipitate}}{2} + \text{net cpm in 2 ml plasma}\right) \times 100$$

2. Procedure for Anion Exchange Resin Method

a. Same as trichloracetic acid precipitation method.

b. Pipet 2 ml plasma into a plastic tube and count for 10 minutes in a scintillation well detector.

c. Prepare column:

i. Dampen filter paper with saline to prevent its floating.

ii. Fill with Ioresin (Abbott) or "PBI-Rezikit" (Squibb) until 2-cm columns are formed. Express liquid with bulb.

iii. Rinse with a 3-ml saline. Express excess liquid after gravity drained.

d. Pour plasma from plastic tube onto column. Allow to gravity drain into a plastic tube, then express excess.

e. Rinse the original plastic tube with a total of 3 ml saline: rinse down the side of the tube with 2 ml and then pour it onto column; pipet the remaining 1 ml into the original tube. Then pour onto the column until first aliquot has drained through. Express the column until dry.

f. Count filtrate for 10 minutes.

g. Calculate as follows:

$$\text{Conversion ratio, \%} = \left(\frac{\text{net cpm filtrate}}{\text{net cpm plasma}} \times \text{correction factor}\right) \times 100$$

h. The correction factor is a ratio of the efficiency of the counter for 2-ml volume and 5-ml volume in the plastic tube. It can be determined by counting 2 ml of a standard and then adding 3 ml of water to the tube and recounting.

3. Results and Discussion

Fields and Seed (1960) state that it is generally accepted that a conversion ratio greater than 35% at 24 hours after the dose indicates a thyrotoxic condition. The method does not yield results that can be used to distinguish the hypothyroid patient from the normal. Although most of the published studies have been made on humans, the recent report by Lombardi *et al.* (1962) is of particular interest to the veterinary clinician. These workers determined the [131I]PBI conversion ratio in dogs. Their results indicate that the production and release of thyroid hormone occurs more slowly in dogs than in man, and further, that dogs require relatively lower levels of thyroid hormone to maintain normal metabolism.

D. THYROIDAL 131I RELEASE RATE

The rate at which the thyroid activity in the thyroid gland decreases with time after maximum uptake is, of course, not a direct measure of the rate of 131I output, because the rate of fall in 131I content of the thyroid gland is determined partly by the reentry of 131I from the hormone catabolized in the tissues (Brown-Grant *et al.*, 1954). If the reentry rate is low, then the output rate is likely to be an index of thyroid activity. The *in vivo* thyroidal 131I release rate is found to be equivalent to the secretion of labeled thyroid hormones in dogs (Fredrickson *et al.*, 1955), rabbits (Brown-Grant and Gibson, 1956), rat (Wolff, 1951), cattle (Blincoe, 1953), and fowl (Biellier, 1955).

1. Procedure

a. Inject the radioiodine as a saline solution intraperitoneally.

b. Set aside an identical dose of the 131I to be used as a standard.

c. After 16 hours postinjection, count the thyroid region as described in the 131I uptake method of the animal once every 12 or 24 hours for a period of 3 to 4 days.

d. Plot the exponential loss of 131I (values corrected for background activity and expressed as percent dose) from the thyroid gland against time on semilogarithm paper. This slope or the semilogarithmic regression, exponent k, is used as an expression of thyroid activity.

e. The thyroidal 131I release rate (k) can be calculated from the equation

$$k = \frac{(\ln A_o - A_t)}{\Delta_t}$$

where A_0 is the theoretical 131I activity at zero time (obtain by extrapolation of the rectilinear curve), and A_t is the 131I activity at the last count.

2. Results and Discussion

The thyroidal 131I release rate has been determined in various species under different physiological and environmental conditions, i.e., in cattle (H. D. Johnson *et al.*, 1958), guinea pigs (Stevens *et al.*, 1953; D'Angelo, 1960), rabbits (Brown-Grant and Gibson, 1956; H. D. Johnson *et al.*, 1958), and rats (H. D. Johnson *et al.*, 1964, 1966). This technique seems to be reliable only under normal conditions. Fish *et al.* (1952) reported that the 131I release curve depends upon the iodine content of the diet and upon recirculation of 131I due to changes in extrathyroid iodine metabolism. Recently, Yousef and Johnson (1968b) concluded that results of the release rate technique should be interpreted with caution when animals are taken from their normal comfort environment. These workers found a significant change in the plasma–iodo compounds in rats exposed for a long period to high environmental temperatures.

E. Thyroxine Secretion Rate

There are at least two methods for estimation of TSR; both are "indirect" methods involving the use of radioiodine, ^{131}I, and/or ^{131}I-labeled T_4.

Underlying the "thyroxine substitution or replacement method" is the classical concept that the thyroid and hypophysis constitute a "feedback" mechanism in which blood level of the thyroid hormones is the main regular of the TSH secretion. The daily TSR is calculated to be equivalent to the amount of hormone which, when injected, prevents the release of ^{131}I from the thyroid gland.

1. Procedure

a. Inject ^{131}I; determine the maximum uptake and its subsequent release from the gland.

b. Block recycling of ^{131}I which is liberated from the metabolism of T_4 by a goitrogen (usually tapazole).

c. Inject exogenous T_4 in increasing dosages until the release of ^{131}I from the gland is blocked. (Usually this is accomplished when the count rate over the thyroid gland attains a plateau or a constant level.)

2. Results and Discussion

This method has been applied to rats (Reineke and Singh, 1955), poultry (Stahl and Turner, 1961), sheep (Brooks et al., 1962), goats (Flamboe and Reineke, 1959), dairy calves (Lodge et al., 1957), and dairy cows (Pipes et al., 1957). This method required special equipment for restraining the animals (similar to the one used in the uptake and release rate techniques) and for radiation detection. Also, it requires a rather long period of time, about 2 weeks, to complete one estimation. Another disadvantage is the daily injection of exogenous T_4, a practice which neglects the important consideration that a single dose of T_4 has a long biologically effective time (2–3 days) as measured by O_2 consumption (Yousef and Johnson, 1966) or by its effect on the radioactivity of blood (Pipes and Turner, 1956). This method has been recently criticized by Yousef and Johnson (1967) and by Heroux and Brauer (1965).

The "thyroxine degradation method" was developed for man (Sterling et al., 1954) and later applied to rats (Yousef and Johnson, 1968a) and cattle (Yousef and Johnson, 1967). This technique measures the rate of T_4 degradation and it is assumed that for the steady state, hormone synthesis and release equals hormone degradation. The T_4 degradation rate (or secretion rate) is calculated as the product of the thyroxine distribution space (TDS), plasma thyroxine (PT), and thyroxine turnover rate (k). The terminology and procedures are discussed in detail by Yousef and Johnson (1967, 1968a).

Using this method one may determine the TSR within 2–4 days with no need for any special equipment for restraining the animals or for the use of goitrogens. This is especially important as goitrogens have been shown to influence thyroid activity through direct action on the thyroid gland and on secretion of pituitary TSH (Florsheim *et al.*, 1966).

F. KIDNEY FUNCTION

The labeling with radioactive iodine of substances cleared by the kidneys has made possible an evaluation of the function of these organs by external counting with probe scintillation detectors. A number of compounds have been used for this purpose. The original labeled dye, ^{131}I-Diodrast (Sterling), is removed in part from the blood by the liver. This necessitates careful positioning of the probes to avoid including liver radioactivity in the test. This source of interference can be reduced greatly by preceding the radioactive Diodrast with a loading dose of 1 gm of nonradioactive ("cold") Diodrast to block liver clearance (Block and Burrows, 1960; Block *et al.*, 1960). Other labeled compounds, such as Miokon (Mallinckrodt), Hypaque (Winthrop), and Renografine (Squibb), have been used by some because they are not appreciably taken up by the liver. This gives the advantage of reducing the requirement for critical positioning of the probes and allows relatively wide-angle collimation without the necessity of X-ray localization of the kidneys. However, Winter and Taplin (1958) reported that these compounds are removed from the blood more slowly than Diodrast. This extends the time required for the test and reduces the sensitivity. Recently ^{131}I-labeled hippuric acid has been used with considerable success for kidney function tests. This compound is rapidly removed from the blood by the kidneys and little is taken up by the liver (Nordyke *et al.*, 1960; D. E. Johnson *et al.*, 1961).

Inspection of the pattern of recorded curves of radioactivity over each kidney has given information about the vascularity, parenchymal function, and potency of the excretory ducts. Two complete counting systems, each consisting of a collimated probe scintillation detector, count rate meter, and recorder make possible the study of the function of each kidney independently.

1. Procedure

a. See that the patient is placed in a comfortable position. Position the matched scintillation probes with flat field collimators parallel to each other at right angles to the back and centered over the kidneys. Connect the scintillation probes to rate meters and rectilinear recorders. The usual rate meter range is 5000 cpm with a time constant of 10 seconds. Operate the recorders at a paper speed of 12 in./hr.

b. Inject intravenously a dose of 0.4 μCi/kg body weight of radioiodine-labeled Diodrast or hippuric acid at the rate of 0.1 ml/sec using a solution containing 20 μCi/ml. When Diodrast is used, inject a loading dose of 1 gm of "cold" Diodrast prior to the labeled Diodrast to block liver uptake. Change the syringe and inject the labeled material.

c. Observe the appearance of radioactivity over the kidney area for 10 or 15 minutes after the injection of the labeled compound.

2. Results and Discussion

In the normal human being the radioactivity curve over each kidney can be resolved into three components (Winter, 1956). The first phase is a sharp rise which is completed in less than 1 minute. This represents the distribution of the radioactive substance through the kidney vascular bed and is termed the "vascular segment." In the following "secretory segment," the radioactivity continues to rise but at a slower rate as the dye is concentrated and excreted by the kidney. The radioactivity begins to decline as the dye passes into the urinary bladder during the "excretory phase."

In elderly individuals, or patients with vascular disease, the vascular segment is of small magnitude. In patients with absent or nonfunctioning kidneys, the vascular segment is diminished and a secretory segment is absent. The secretory segment is reduced with impairment of tubular function or the reduction of the total amount of kidney parenchyma. The excretory segment is absent and the radioactivity over the kidney area does not fall if there is an obstruction of the ureters. Typical response curves are shown in Fig. 2. A clinical evaluation of the Diodrast technique for evaluating kidney function has been published by Serrato et al. (1959).

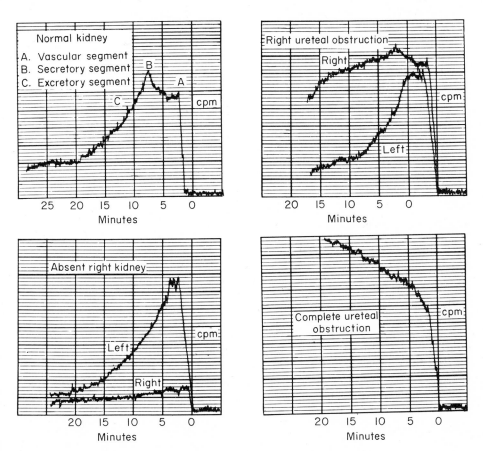

Fig. 2   Uptake and subsequent release of [131] I-Diodrast by human kidneys.

G. Liver Function Tests

Liver function tests based on the uptake and excretion of two dyes, rose bengal and Bromsulphalein, have been used for several years and in general, give excellent correlation with liver function (Nordyke and Blahd, 1959). The dyes are extracted from the blood by the hepatic polygonal cells and are then excreted via the bile duct into the intestine. Neither dye is taken up by the Kupffer cells of the reticuloendothelial system nor are they appreciably reabsorbed from the intestine following secretion in the bile. Dye excretion tests have found little application, however, in hepatic diseases accompanied by jaundice due to problems in spectrophotometry and the chance of further damaging the liver by large doses of dyes. These problems have been circumvented through the use of ^{131}I-labeled rose bengal. The radioactive (^{131}I) rose bengal is injected intravenously and the rate of uptake of the dye in the liver is measured with a collimated γ-scintillation detector probe and is registered graphically with a recording rate meter.

1. Procedure

a. Center the scintillation probe at right angles to the body and position so that γ-sensitive crystal "sees" liver tissue but not the gallbladder.

b. Inject 0.2–0.4 μCi ^{131}I rose bengal/kg body weight intravenously. The dose should contain 0.5–5.0 ml of dye.

c. Recordings are made continuously for periods up to 2 hours after injection.

2. Results and Discussion

Taplin et al. (1955) used rabbits in the first studies of ^{131}I-labeled rose bengal uptake and secretion. They stated that the test has several advantages over all other liver function tests. It measures polygonal cell function directly. This eliminates the necessity for counting blood samples. It registers the uptake and excretion of the dye graphically with time. Further, it can be used safely in the presence of biliary obstruction because of the minute quantities and low toxicity of the dye and it gives information on liver circulation and patency of the biliary tract. Lastly, the test appears to be many times more sensitive than the traditional, i.e., nonradioactive, tests.

Moertel and Owen (1958) measured "half-uptake times" and "half-excretion times" using a technique similar to that published earlier by Taplin et al. (1955). They reported that the uptake of ^{131}I rose bengal was slower in patients with hepatic disease than in normal patients but that a large overlap occurred between the two groups. They concluded that because of this lack of sensitivity, the radioactive rose bengal test could not be recommended for routine evaluation of hepatic function in nonjaundice patients. Several modifications and evaluations of the ^{131}I-rose bengal test have been reported subsequently.

Combes (1960) compared the ^{131}I-rose bengal test with the Bromsulphalein test and concluded that the ^{131}I-rose bengal test was suitable for measurement of hepatic blood flow. Westover et al. (1959) reported an interesting modification of Taplin's rose bengal test in which ^{131}I-labeled human serum albumin was used in conjunction with ^{131}I-labeled rose bengal. Their procedures lead to the calculation of the percent uptake per minute of rose bengal by liver cells—a function which could be used as an index of hepatic vascularity.

Mena *et al.* (1959) noted that although the rose bengal test is frequently within the normal range in patients suffering mild liver disease, Bromsulphalein could be used simultaneously to differentiate normal patients from those with mildly diseased livers.

Nordyke and Blahd (1958, 1959) noted that most efforts to use the original method of Taplin *et al.* (1955) were unsuccessful chiefly due to difficulties in external liver counting. These difficulties presumably arise because the scintillation probe "sees" a complex series of simultaneously occurring functions which include: dye uptake by the hepatic cells, blood flow through the liver, dye concentrations in hepatic blood and tissue, pooling of dye in the cholangioles, bile duct, and gallbladder, and excretion of dye into the intestine. They state further that each of these factors is dependent on the position of the patient, exercise, fever, and food ingestion. In addition, organ movement and difficulty in positioning the probe make it difficult to obtain reproducible curves. The authors propose a new method in which three wide-angle scintillation detectors are mounted as follows:

1. Horizontally against the head (reflects the level of radioactive dye in blood).
2. Anteriorly over the liver (measures uptake of dye by liver cells).
3. Perpendicularly over the lower left abdominal quadrant (reflects changes in the abdominal blood and intestinal lumen).

The authors state that biliary tract obstruction of any kind decreases the rate of accumulation of rose bengal in the intestine. Further, extrahepatic obstruction leads to a delayed arrival time of the dye in the intestine. In contrast, intrahepatic obstruction yields arrival times that are either normal or early.

The only application of the ^{131}I-rose bengal test directly applicable to clinical veterinary medicine has been reported by J. R. Holmes (1960a). First, 20 μCi of the radioiodinated dye was injected in four crossbred sheep which had been fed normally prior to the experiment and which were held in a metabolism cage with no anesthesia or sedative throughout the test. Then, hepatic uptake and secretion of the dye were traced on a recording rate meter equipped with a scintillation probe mounted over the liver. The test was conducted with normal sheep, sheep in which severe centrolobular necrosis had been induced by carbon tetrachloride, and in one case of biliary tract obstruction. The results of these tests are shown in Fig. 11 of Chapter 5, Volume I (Second edition). Holmes states that the test, or modifications of it, may be sufficiently sensitive to evaluate hepatic function in ruminants.

H. Cardiac Output

Cardiac output has been estimated for a number of years by the dye dilution technique. In this method, Evan's blue dye is injected intravenously and the pattern of appearance in arterial blood is followed by arterial sampling. The necessity for arterial puncture and the loss of blood during the procedure does not make the dye method suitable for the seriously ill patient in which cardiac output would often provide important information. A radioisotope technique has been described which makes it possible to estimate cardiac output by external measurement of

γ-radiation over the heart following intravenous injection of radioiodinated (^{131}I) serum albumin (Huff *et al.*, 1954, 1955; Pritchard *et al.*, 1955).

A probe scintillation detector is directed toward the aorta through tissue which has little intervening musculoskeletal blood. A solution of iodinated serum albumin (^{131}I) is administered and the passage of radioiodine through the heart is recorded with a rate meter and a chart recorder. Cardiac output can be calculated from the area under the curve and the blood volume.

1. Procedure (for Humans)

a. The patient is seated or reclining and at rest for 10 minutes before beginning the test.

b. Position the collimated probe scintillation counter on the chest in contact with the skin between the first and second ribs, or over the second rib at the parasternal line with the axis of the collimator making an angle of about 10° to the left side posteriorly. The rate meter time constant is set for 2 seconds and the range for 3000 cpm (the proper range for the rate meter may vary with the sensitivity of the scintillation counter used). The recorder is run at a paper speed of 180 in./hr.

c. Make a venipuncture with a 21-gauge needle using an empty syringe. When the blood is flowing freely, attach a syringe containing 100 μCi of ^{131}I-labeled human serum albumin in a volume of 1 ml. Inject the labeled albumin with a single continuous motion in 1 second.

d. To estimate blood volume:

i. At 10 minutes after the injection of the radioiodinated human serum albumin, draw a 10-ml blood sample from the opposite arm used for injection and discharge into a bottle containing anticoagulant.

ii. Mix the blood sample well and pipet 3 ml of the sample into a plastic tube for counting in a well scintillation detector.

iii. Prepare a diluted standard by pipetting 1 ml of the radioiodinated human serum albumin solution used for injection into a 100-ml volumetric flask and make to volume with saline. After mixing well, pipet 1 ml of the diluted standard into a 1-liter volumetric flask and make to volume with water. Pipet 3 ml of the final dilution into a plastic tube for counting in a well scintillation detector.

iv. Subtract the background counting rate from the count rate obtained for the blood sample and diluted standard. Blood volume may then be calculated from the formula:

$$\text{Blood volume (liters)} = \frac{\text{cpm in standard}}{\text{cpm in blood sample}} \times 100$$

e. The curve of radioactivity recorded by the counter should show a rapid rise which is completed in about 10 seconds, followed by an exponential decay in activity (see Fig. 3). The decay does not reach the baseline because of recirculation. The descending component of the curve can be extended to meet the baseline. Measure the area under the curve by planimetry or any other suitable method and determine the equilibrium radioactivity when mixing is complete. Calculate the cardiac output by the following method:

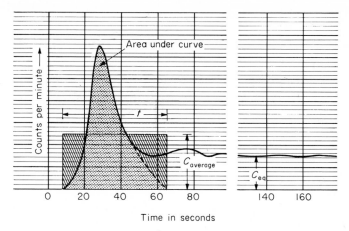

Fig. 3.   Tracing obtained with a scintillation detector positioned over the aorta and recording rate meter following intravenous injection of ^{131}I-labeled human serum albumin.

i. From the area under the curve, the average activity, C_{av} during the period of passage of radioiodinated serum albumin can be calculated.

$$C_{av} = \frac{area}{t}$$

ii. A comparison of C_{av} with the final activity when equilibrium has occurred (C_{eq}) gives the portion of the total blood volume (F') which has flowed through the heart during the time, t.

$$F' = \frac{C_{eq}}{C_{av}}$$

iii. To correct to liters per minute, the cardiac output calculated above must be multiplied by the blood volume and divided by the time, t.

$$F = \frac{C_{eq}}{C_{av}} \times \frac{blood\ volume}{t}$$

2.   Results and Discussion

Cardiac output was determined by Huff *et al.* (1954, 1955) following the injections of 100–200 μCi ^{131}I-labeled human serum albumin into dogs and humans. The results of their tests with 28 women indicated a cardiac output of 3.3 ±0.8 liters per minute per square meter body surface area. Similar experiments with 36 men gave 3.6 ±0.8 liters per minute per square meter body surface area. Huff and co-workers also measured cardiac output by the direct Fick method and reported close agreement between it and the *in vivo* radioisotope method. Pritchard *et al.* (1955) reported the results of a similar study in which they found that the cardiac output ranged from 1.7 to 8.3 liters/min. (Note: these values are not corrected for body surface area and hence cannot be compared directly with Huff's data.) Pritchard *et al.* (1955) also reported excellent correlation in all determinations of 3.5 liters/min or less and stated that these values were obtained with patients having cardiac failure with anemia.

Love and Burch (1958) published a method for estimating cardiac output which is based on the infusion of rubidium, ^{86}Rb. Cardiac output was calculated from the amount of isotope taken up by the tissue and the arteriovenous difference in radio-activity across that tissue. The authors state that this method could be used to measure plasma flow to any organ or tissue except brain. However, it would seem that the necessity and inconvenience of placing indwelling catheters into specific arteries and veins and the obtaining of repeated blood samples therefrom will prob-ably limit the application of this technique to experimental medicine.

Groom and Rowlands (1956) determined cardiac output, blood volume, and pul-monary circulation time of cats by injection of ^{32}P and measuring the radioactivity which flowed through a plastic tube placed in series with the carotid artery. Lastly, Sevelius and Johnson (1959) reported a modification of the ^{131}I-human serum albumin technique for measuring cardiac output in which they obtained a third peak in the heart curve tracing which they correlated with myocardial blood flow. This peak occurred on the down slope of the peak from the left heart chamber. The area under the curve was then used to calculate coronary blood flow. Forty-six normal patients gave values of 287 ± 107 ml/min. In contrast, 16 patients with myocardial infarction gave an average value of 149 ml/min.

I. Blood Volume Studies

Blood and plasma volume measurements are based on the dilution which takes place when a material is introduced into and becomes mixed with the total circulating blood. Until recently the most commonly employed technique for blood volume studies was the Evan's blue method. Unfortunately, this dye stains blood and tissue and therefore precludes immediate repetition of the test. Use of radioisotopes for these measurements eliminates this disadvantage.

The most commonly used radioisotope for blood and plasma volume studies is ^{131}I-labeled serum albumin. When given intravenously, the labeled material is quickly distributed throughout the blood. If a known volume of radioactive material is added to an unknown volume of blood and later, after mixing is complete, the same volume is withdrawn, the decrease in radioactivity will be directly proportional to the dilu-tion in the blood. Calculation is then easily made of the total blood volume (Aust *et al.*, 1951; Fields *et al.*, 1954).

Since the radioiodinated serum albumin is confined to the plasma, and the activity is not transferred to the red cells, it is possible to separate the plasma from the whole blood, count the plasma in exactly the same way, and thus have a measurement of the plasma volume. The time required for both determinations is about 30 minutes.

Red cell mass can be determined readily through the use of radiochromium (^{51}Cr)-tagged cells. Viable red blood cells are incubated in a test tube with ^{51}Cr-labeled sodium chromate of high specific activity in a Strumia solution (disodium citrate monohydrate 2.55 gm, citric acid 0.80 gm, dextrose 1.20 gm, in 100 ml solution). At room temperature, 90% of the ^{51}Cr can be bound in 30 minutes. The unbound chromate is reduced to trivalent chromium by ascorbic acid. The latter does not bind to red blood cells but is loosely bound to plasma proteins.

A measure sample of the labeled red cells is reinjected into the patient and another aliquot is used for a standard. In the latter, the plasma is removed and the cells are washed with isotonic saline to remove unbound chromium. This sample is then diluted for counting. At 20 and 30 minutes after injection, blood samples are withdrawn and the cells from a measured volume of blood separated and washed with saline. The activities of the standard and samples are measured in a well scintillation detector.

1. Procedure for Plasma Volume

a. Using sterile precautions, remove the radioiodinated serum albumin from the ampule and add to 10 ml of sterile saline in a sterile diluting bottle. Approximately 0.25 μCi ^{131}I/kg body weight will be needed for this determination. Mix well and fill a calibrated 5-cm^3 syringe with the diluted solution making sure that all air bubbles are expelled. (Note: the labeled albumin must be diluted just before use, since upon standing in dilute solution the radioiodine tends to dissociate from the albumin molecule.

b. Attach a new needle to the syringe and inject the contents of the syringe intravenously. The vein must be well cannulated since infiltration of the tissue with the solution invalidates the results and precludes repeating the test immediately.

c. Mixing may be assumed to be complete in 10 to 15 minutes. At that time, draw a 10-ml sample of blood from the arm not used for injection and discharge into a bottle containing dry oxalate anticoagulant.

d. Pipet 3 ml of blood into a test tube and measure the radioactivity in a well scintillation detector.

e. Preparation of the standard:

  i. Dilute 1 ml of labeled albumin solution administered to the patient to 500 ml in a volumetric flask with a 0.9% saline. Mix well by inversion.

  ii. Pipet 3 ml of the diluted standard into a test tube and measure the activity in a well scintillation detector.

f. Subtract the background counting rate of the well scintillation detector from the counting rate of the blood sample and the standard sample.

g. Calculate the blood volume from the formula:

$$\text{Blood volume (ml)} = \frac{\text{cpm in standard}}{\text{cpm blood sample}} \times 500 \times 5$$

h. *Plasma volume* may be determined as follows:

  i. Centrifuge the blood taken from the patient and obtain sample of plasma.

  ii. Pipet 3 ml of the plasma into a test tube and measure the activity in a well scintillation detector.

  iii. Subtract the background counting rate of the well scintillation detector from the counting rate of the plasma sample and the standard sample.

  iv. Calculate the plasma volume from the formula:

$$\text{Plasma volume (ml)} = \frac{\text{cpm in standard}}{\text{cpm plasma sample}} \times 500 \times 5$$

2. *Procedure for Red Cell Mass*

a. Draw 20 ml of blood and discharge carefully into a sterile siliconed bottle containing 10 ml of Strumia solution, mix, and add approximately 25 μCi of sodium chromate (^{51}Cr).

b. Incubate 30 minutes at room temperature. Add, by sterile syringe, 100 mg ascorbic acid in 1-ml solution (sterile and suitable for parenternal administration), mix, and allow to incubate 5 minutes.

c. Mix blood well in bottle and withdraw 20 ml into a sterile syringe. Weigh syringe rapidly on a triple beam balance to the nearest 0.01 gm.

d. Inject labeled blood through needle placed in vein with another syringe. Do not permit blood from the vein to flow back into the syringe containing labeled blood.

e. Reweigh empty syringe to the nearest 0.01 gm to determine weight of blood injected.

f. Draw a 10-ml blood sample from the opposite arm at 20 minutes after injection and discharge carefully into a blood bottle containing anticoagulant. Determine the hematocrit.

g. Preparation of standard:

i. Mix sample of labeled blood well and add approximately 5 ml to each of the two weighed centrifuge tubes.

ii. Reweigh tubes to determine the amount of blood in each sample.

iii. Centrifuge 10 minutes at 2000 rpm and carefully pour off plasma. Do not lose red cells.

iv. Add 10 ml of 9% sodium chloride to tubes and gently resuspend cells.

v. Centrifuge 10 minutes at 2000 rpm and carefully pour off supernatant.

vi. Repeat steps iv and v.

vii. Transfer washed cells to 100-ml volumetric flask with water. The cells will lyse during this procedure.

viii. Mix well and pipet 3 ml samples into glass tubes and count in a well scintillation detector.

h. Preparation of timed samples:

i. Mix blood samples well and pipet 5 ml into a centrifuge tube which will fit into a well scintillation detector.

ii. Carry out procedures iii and iv above.

iii. Count red cells in well scintillation detector.

i. Calculations:

$$\text{Total counts administered} = \frac{\text{wt of blood injected}}{\text{wt of standard blood}} \times \frac{100}{3} \times \text{net cpm standard}$$

$$\text{Red blood cell radioactivity (cpm/ml)} = \frac{\text{red blood cell sample net cpm}}{\text{(hematocrit) (vol. blood washed)}}$$

$$\text{Red blood cell mass} = \frac{\text{total counts administered}}{\text{red blood cell radioactivity (cpm/ml)}}$$

3. Results and Discussion

In one of the earliest applications of the ^{131}I-labeled human serum albumin techniques for measuring blood volume, Aust et al. (1951) noted close agreement with the traditional Evan's blue dye technique. In their method, Lugol's solution was administered to the patient at regular intervals starting 24 hours before injection of the radioiodine-labeled albumin to block thyroid uptake of ^{131}I which might be eluted from the tagged serum albumin.

Portman et al. (1952) used ^{131}I-labeled human serum albumin to measure the blood volume of ducks. Doses ranging from 0.5 to 0.9 μCi/kg body weight were injected into the leg veins of 42 ducks, and blood samples were taken at 15 minutes postinjection. They noted that the percent blood volume decreased as body weight increased. Klement et al. (1954) published a method for the simultaneous use of ^{131}I-albumin and ^{51}Cr-labeled red cells for blood volume studies with goats. Their results with four goats gave a mean red cell volume of 1.40% body weight and a mean plasma volume of 5.96% body weight.

Stahl and Dale (1958) determined the blood volumes of 17 dairy calves using the ^{51}Cr red cell technique. Simultaneous measurements with Evan's blue dye (T1824) were also made. The authors noted that the dye consistently gave higher blood volumes than the ^{51}Cr method. The authors also noted that the ^{51}Cr activity in red cells decreased steadily with time, suggesting that the zero time value should be used for calculating blood volume. (Zero time activity in the red cells was obtained by regressing the values of five samples taken at 20-minute intervals after injection of the tagged cell to zero time.) A similar study was conducted by Rapaport et al. (1956) with Nembutalized dogs. Shires et al. (1960) published an elaborate technique for the simultaneous measurement of plasma volume, extracellular fluid volume, and blood cell mass in man, utilizing ^{131}I-labeled human serum albumin, [34]SO_4, and ^{51}Cr-tagged red cells. The method required a single injection of the labeled materials and a single blood sample taken 15 minutes following injection. The radiosulfate technique for determining extracellular fluid volume in man and dogs was published earlier by Walser et al. (1953).

Blood volume can also be determined through the use of radiophosphorus (^{32}P-labeled red cells. The incubation procedures are similar to those used for the ^{51}Cr studies. Hansard et al. (1953) used this technique to measure the blood volume of sheep, swine, cattle, and burros, and a similar study was published by Collery and Keating (1958) using horses and donkeys. Finally, ^{59}Fe-labeled compounds have been used to measure blood volume and related hemodynamic phenomena in humans (Huff et al., 1951), swine (Jensen et al., 1956), and various ruminants (Baker and Douglas, 1957; Hansard et al., 1959).

J. Red Cell Survival Using Radiochromium (^{51}Cr)

Chromium-51-labeled cells may also be used for estimating the red cell survival (Strumia et al., 1955; Read, 1954). After labeling a sample of the patient's own cells as described previously, they are reinfused. A blood sample is taken at 24 hours to serve as a standard for comparison with subsequent samples taken at twice weekly intervals for about 2 weeks. The radiochromate label remains on the red cells until they are removed from the blood for destruction (except for a small amount of leaching which averages about 1% label present per day). The chromate released on destruction of the cells does not relabel other cells (Ebaugh *et al.*, 1953).

1. Procedure

a. Draw 10-ml blood samples twice weekly for 2 weeks and discharge carefully into blood bottles containing anticoagulant.

b. Obtain hematocrit of the blood for the standard solution and for each aliquot by centrifugation at 3000 rpm for 30 minutes in a Wintrobe tube.

c. Determine the radioactivity with a scintillation well counter using 3-ml aliquots of whole blood and plasma.

d. Determine ^{51}Cr activity per milliliter cells either by subtracting plasma activity from whole blood activity or by counting cells directly.

e. Correct all counting data for radioactive decay and calculate the "percentage surviving red cells" according to the formula:

$$\text{Surviving red cells (\%)} = \frac{\text{net cpm/ml red cells at time } t}{\text{net cpm/ml red cells at time } 0} \times 100$$

f. Plot percent surviving red cells on the ordinate axis of a semilogarithmic plot against time on the linear abscissa. Determine the ^{51}Cr half-time survival value.

g. Figure 4 shows typical values for red blood cell survival in humans using ^{51}Cr-tagged cells.

2. Results and Discussion

Marvin and Lucy (1957) studied the disappearance of ^{51}Cr-labeled erythrocytes in pigeons, ducks, and rabbits. Values cited for the time of 50% destruction are as

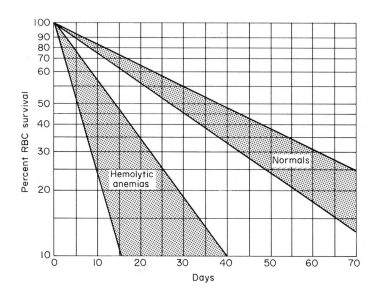

Fig. 4.   Red cell survival as determined by the ^{51}Cr technique.

follows: pigeons, 10.8 days; ducks, 12.5 days; rabbits, 19 days. More recently, Baker *et al.* (1961) used the ^{51}Cr red cell survival technique to study experimental anaplasmosis in Hereford cattle. They reported that the clearance curve consisted of two components during the first few days which they separated into a fast and a slow component by appropriate arithmetic means. The fast components presumably represented either an excess of ^{51}Cr in the cells, or the removal of nonviable labeled cells. The mean half-time value of the continuous (slow) component was 11.7 days with a range of 10.5–13.0 days. During the hemolytic crisis in splenectomized calves suffering from experimental anaplasmosis, the red cell survival time was reduced eight- to tenfold. In contrast, the production of hemoglobin was increased at a much slower rate. Thus the authors concluded that the major factor in the production of anemia in anaplasmosis was an acute extravascular hemolysis as suggested earlier by Hansard and Foote (1958).

Chromium-51-tagged red blood cells have also been used to study various experimentally induced (i.e., nutritional) anemias in swine (Bush *et al.*, 1956a,b), and the anemias observed in various ruminants suffering from acute parasitic gastroenteritis caused by trichostrongyloid parasites (Baker and Douglas, 1957; Baker *et al.*, 1959).

K.   RED CELL SURVIVAL USING ^{14}C-GLYCINE

Red cell survival has also been determined through the use of ^{14}C-labeled glycine. In this procedure, however, the isotope is injected intravenously and eventually labels 8 of the 34 carbon atoms of the porphyrin moiety of hemoglobin. The ^{14}C-specific activity of red cell hemin is determined at regular intervals over a period of several weeks. 2-^{14}C Glycine has been used to measure red cell survival in humans (Shemin and Rittenberg, 1946), rats (Kaplan and Zuelzer, 1950), swine (Bush *et al.*, 1955), horses (Cornelius *et al.*, 1960), and various zoo animals (Cornelius *et al.*, 1959a; Kaneko *et al.*, 1961a).

1. *Procedure*

a. Inject 2-^{14}C-glycine intravenously using approximately 20 μCi/kg body weight.

b. Withdraw 20 ml of venous blood at weekly intervals for erythrocyte counting and for the isolation and purification of the erythrocyte hemin.

c. Oxidize the hemin to CO_2 and prepare $BaCO_3$ planchettes for counting.

d. Plot the specific activity of hemin-^{14}C versus time. Calculate the probability of erythrocyte survival according to the methods described by Cornelius *et al.* (1959a) and plot on the same graph.

e. Determine the time after formation of the cell population at which one-half of the cells still survive. This value is referred to as the "median survival time" (Cornelius *et al.*, 1960).*

---

*Students and investigators are cautioned to examine carefully the terms and definitions used in this field before attempting to compare the published results of various investigators. For example, a cursory survey of the literature pertaining to the red cell survival showed the following terms now in use: "life span," "apparent life span," "average life span," "survival time," "mean survival time," "median survival time," "half survival time," "half-time," and "apparent half survival time."

2. Results and Discussion

Measurement of erythrocyte survival by the ^{14}C-glycine technique is claimed by Cornelius et al. (1959a) to obviate problems encountered in the ^{51}Cr and/or ^{59}Fe ferric citrate procedures. On the other hand, certain technical difficulties are encountered with the 2-^{14}C-glycine technique. First, the initial labeling of cells occur over a considerable time period. In the mule deer, for example, peak activity is not attained until nearly 50 days postinjection. Second, the decline in radio-activity in erythocyte hemin may be continuous or biphasic. This means that the specific activity in hemin must be determined over a period of several weeks. Third, the biochemical manipulations of each blood sample and the mathematical analysis of the data are obviously more tedious and time-consuming than the ^{51}Cr method.

Cornelius et al. (1959a) reported that the half-survival-time for erythrocytes of the mule deer and the springbok antelope were 95 and 80 days, respectively. In contrast, an aoudad sheep exhibited two separate populations of erythrocytes with half-survival-times of 65 and 170 days. In a similar study with sheep, Kaneko et al. (1961a) reported the following median survival times. Crossbred white-faced lambs, 94 days and 118 days; a Southdown lamb, 64 days; a Karakul ewe, 130 days; and a Bighorn sheep, 147 days. Median survival times for ^{14}C-labeled erythrocyte popula-tions in two Thoroughbred stallions was reported to be 140 and 150 days (Cornelius et al., 1960). Bush et al. (1955) reported the mean red cell survival time of growing swine to be 62 days. This work was confirmed by Jensen et al. (1956) using the [59]FE ferric chloride technique. Critical reviews of the methods for estimating red cell pro-duction and destruction have recently been published (Berlin et al., 1959; Stohlman, 1961).

Kaneko et al. (1961b) used the 2-^{14}C-glycine red cell survival technique to study the experimental molybdenosis in sheep. They observed two distinct plateaus in the specific activity time curves which they interpreted to reflect the existence of two separate populations of erythrocytes with different survival times. A similar biphasic curve had been observed earlier for the normal aoudad sheep (Cornelius et al., 1959a). In contrast, the normal sheep yields a curve with a single plateau.

Lastly, Kaneko (1963) used ^{59}Fe ferric citrate and 2-^{14}C-glycine-labeled red cells to study the erythrokinetics and iron metabolism of cows suffering from porphyria erythropoietica. These experiments showed that the median survival time of red blood cells in the porphyria erythropoietica cows was only one-fifth that of normal cows. In addition, the heme replacement rates and the red blood cell iron replacement rates in porphyria erythropoietica were approximately three times greater than in normal cows. Kaneko states that his results also indicate that an increased red cell replacement rate precedes the appearance of morpho-logical evidence of anemia in the peripheral blood of these cows.

L. MISCELLANEOUS STUDIES ON BLOOD AND CIRCULATION

1. Blood Proteins

Mills et al. (1961) used ^{131}I-labeled normal human γ-globulin to study the plasma disappearance time and the catabolic half-time of γ-globulin in patients suffering from amyloidosis and rheumatoid arthritis. Radioiodine, ^{131}I, has also been used to determine the globulin turnover in patients suffering from hypergammaglobuline-mia—multiple myeloma patients (Lippincott *et al.*, 1961). This technique involves direct whole-body counting through the use of a large γ-scintillation crystal, three photomultiplier tubes, and a 100-channel pulse height analyzer. In studies with ^{64}Cu and ^{67}Cu, Sternlieb *et al.* (1961) reported that no exchange occurred between ionic copper and copper-ceruloplasmin in patients suffering from Wilson's disease (excessive deposit of tissue copper). Whipple *et al.* (1955) used ^{60}Co-labeled vitamin B_{12} to study the role of that vitamin during the active regeneration of red cell stroma protein. Their results indicated that vitamin B_{12} is a factor of considerable importance during the first steps of stroma protein formation in the first few days of life of dog red cells.

Radioisotopes have been used to a limited extent to study the turnover of blood proteins in sheep and cattle. Campbell *et al.* (1961) injected ^{131}I-labeled plasma albumin into sheep in a study designed to elucidate the role which the passage of albumin into the small intestine might play in supplementing endogenous fecal protein secretion. Dixon *et al.* (1952, 1953) reported that serum albumin and γ-globulin in mature cattle "turned over" with a half-time of approximately 21 days.

Cornelius *et al.* (1959b) used 1-^{14}C-glycine to label the blood proteins of two lactating dairy cows. By following the change in ^{14}C specific activity with time, they calculated that the biological half-time of total serum protein was approximately 15 days, and, further, that the extravascular pool contained twice the quantity of exchangeable protein as the vascular pool. In a subsequent study Cornelius *et al.* (1962) used ^{131}I-labeled bovine serum albumin to measure albumin turnover and compartmentalization in normal and parasitized cattle. Turnover rates of albumin were similar in control calves and the majority of calves with heavy trichostrongylid infections. In addition this radioisotope technique enabled the investigators to demonstrate that parasitized calves had a higher rate of albumin catabolism and a lower rate of albumin synthesis than the control calves.

2. Hemodynamic Studies

Long and Cornell (1959) recently published an interesting technique using the radioisotope ^{85}Kr for detecting left to right circulatory shunts in dogs. Left to right circulatory shunts were constructed by an anastomosis of the left subclavian artery to the left pulmonary artery. In this study 30 μCi of ^{85}Kr was used. The early appearance of ^{85}Kr in the expired air (2 seconds) in dogs with circulatory shunts compared with 10 seconds for normal dogs indicated that the method might be useful in detecting left to right shunts in patients with congenital heart disease. In fact, they state that preliminary clinical experience using ^{85}Kr in patients with this disease has shown considerable promise. O'Meallie *et al.* (1960) used ^{131}I-labeled albumin to differentiate massive pericardial effusion from cardiac dilation in humans, and Dahl *et al.* (1961) noted the prolonged biological half-life of radiosodium (^{22}Na) in patients with essential hypertension. The latter state that their preliminary calculations indicate that the prolonged half-life resulted from a larger metabolic pool of sodium.

3. Blood Cell Studies

Kaneko et al. (1960) used tritium-labeled thymidine to study nucleic acid synthesis in normal and leukemic bovine leukocytes. They demonstrated that the DNA-synthesizing power of leukocytes in leukemic blood was higher than that in normal blood. Radiosulfur (^{35}S-sulfate) was used by Robinson et al. (1961) to determine the biological half-life of platelets in swine blood. Hjort et al. (1960) used ^{32}P-labeled diisopropylfluorophosphate ([^{32}P]DFP) to determine the reliability of a method for studying erythrokinetics using DFP. They demonstrated that ^{32}P was released from the cells during the first 1 to 3 days following infusion and concluded that this method for tagging red blood cells was unreliable, particularly in the early periods following infusion.

M. ^{60}Co-Vitamin B$_{12}$

Vitamin B$_{12}$ is absorbed from the gastrointestinal tract in the presence of an intrinsic factor elaborated by the gastric mucosa. Absorption may be followed after the oral administration of radiocobalt (^{60}Co)-labeled vitamin B$_{12}$ by estimation of the unabsorbed radioactivity in the feces, by measuring the radioactivity in the liver which acts as a temporary storage site after absorption, or by the method introduced by Schilling et al. (1955) in which the liver uptake is blocked by parental administration of a large dose of unlabeled vitamin B$_{12}$ and the urine is collected for 24 hours. In this case, the labeled vitamin absorbed from the intestinal tract is promptly excreted in the urine.

In the patient with pernicious anemia, lack of intrinsic factor prevents normal absorption of vitamin B$_{12}$ from the gastrointestinal tract. Following subtotal gastrectomy the absorption of vitamin B$_{12}$ may be low as in pernicious anemia. The administration of a dose of potent intrinsic factor prepared from hog's stomach will increase the absorption in subsequent tests in these two types of patients. In sprue, the absorption of vitamin B$_{12}$ is low and there is no improvement on administering intrinsic factor.

The amount of vitamin B$_{12}$ absorbed during the test also depends on the weight of the vitamin given. In general, there is an increase in the percent absorption as the dose is lowered. With doses of the order of 0.5 mg of vitamin B$_{12}$, patients with pernicious anemia, sprue, or an allied intestinal condition, excrete less than 4–5% of the administered dose in the urine in 24 hours. If the output is 10–12% or more, it is considered definite that the patient does not have pernicious anemia. Whenever it is desirable to differentiate between pernicious anemia and malabsorption due to other causes, it is recommended that the test be repeated 2 to 3 days later. At this time the patient is given a potent intrinsic factor preparation along with the labeled vitamin. If pernicious anemia is present, the patient will almost invariably show at least a twofold increase in percentage output and it may run as high as four to eight times as much. Such an increase will not occur in sprue or in cases where lack of absorption of vitamin B$_{12}$ is due to some cause other than the absence of intrinsic factor. In severely impaired kidney function, the excretion may be sufficiently reduced to invalidate the test.

1. Procedures (for Humans)

a. The patient should be in an overnight fasting state.

b. Administer 0.5 μCi of ^{60}Co-labeled vitamin B_{12} by mouth in 30 ml of solution. Rinse the cup in which the dose was administered several times and have the patient drink the washes.

c. Inject 1 mg of nonradioactive vitamin B_{12} subcutaneously or intramuscularly within 1 hour after administration of the oral dose.

d. Collect all urine excreted during the 24 hours following the administration of the labeled vitamin.

e. Measure the 24-hour urine volume and transfer 1 liter to a standard 1-liter polyethylene bottle with a screw cap. If the 24-hour volume is less than 1 liter, dilute to 1 liter before transferring to the bottle.

f. Position the bottle on a crystal of a well scintillation detector and count.

g. Measure a second sample of the ^{60}Co-labeled B_{12} administered to the patient into a liter volumetric flask and dilute to 1 liter with water. Measure 100 ml of the diluted standard into a second standard polyethylene screw cap bottle and dilute to 1 liter with water. This represents 10% of the dose administered diluted to the standard volume of 1 liter.

h. Position the standard of the crystal of a well scintillation detector and measure the activity.

i. Measure background in a water-filled polyethylene bottle positioned on top of the well detector.

j. Calculate the percent excretion by the formula:

$$\text{Excretion (\%)} = \frac{U \times 10 \times \text{net cpm urine}}{\text{net cpm standard}}$$

where U = liters of urine collected in 24 hours.

2. Results and Discussion

Evaluations of the ^{60}Co-vitamin B_{12} absorption tests have been published recently (I. H. Holmes and Bell, 1961; Germann, 1961), the latter concluding that the test is extremely valuable in the evaluation of patients with various gastrointestinal diseases. Cobalt-60 vitamin B_{12} has also been used to study pernicious anemia and various liver diseases including virus and serum hepatitis, hepatic cirrhosis, leukemic infiltration, obstructive jaundice, malignancies, schistosomiasis hypersplenism, and hepatomegaly (Glass, 1958; Glass and Mersheimer, 1958; Glass et al., 1958).

Tissue distribution studies of ^{60}Co-labeled B_{12} have been reported for the dog (Woods et al., 1958; Cooperman et al., 1960) and for man (Doscherholmen et al., 1960). Luhby et al. (1959) demonstrated that radioactive vitamin B_{12} was transferred across placental membranes and, further, that the biological half-life of the labeled vitamin was 2 months for both pups and the bitch during the postpartum period. These results were confirmed by Woods et al. (1960) who also showed that the pup receives vitamin B_{12} through milk when nursing. Prinz et al. (1959) used ^{58}Co- and ^{60}Co-labeled vitamin B_{12} to follow the absorption of the vitamin in normal and gastrectomized pigs. Their report includes a study of the effect of intrinsic factor, sorbose, homologs of the vitamin, and inorganic salts of cobalt on B_{12} absorption.

N. FAT DIGESTION AND ABSORPTION

Incomplete utilization of fat in the diet is a frequent accompaniment of diseases of the gastrointestinal tract. The poor utilization can be due to incomplete digestion of the fat due to a lack of emulsifying effect of bile or the lack of fat-splitting enzymes, chiefly those in the pancreatic secretion. In biliary obstruction or pancreatitis, there is an abnormally high fat content in the feces representing unabsorbed fat. Poor utilization may also be due to disturbances in the intestinal mucosa which prevent normal absorption of digested fat. In sprue the voluminous fatty stools are apparently due to this cause. Patients with gastrectomies and fast passage time of intestinal content may also have poor utilization of dietary fat.

Iodine-131 triolein, a fat, and ^{131}I-labeled oleic acid, the product of splitting triolein, are useful in evaluating fat digestion and absorption (Tannhauser and Stanley, 1949). The labeled triolein is administered as a capsule or emulsion in milk and its appearance in the blood stream is followed by making counts of the blood at intervals after ingestion of the fat. If the amount of ^{131}I which appears in the blood stream is low, ^{131}I-labeled oleic acid can be used to differentiate between poor digestion and impaired absorption as the cause. Poor digestion will not affect oleic acid absorption and a normal appearance curve in the blood is obtained. In patients with abnormalities of the intestinal mucosa or with fast passage time, the appearance of the labeled oleic acid in the blood stream will also be below normal limits.

A number of methods for administering the labeled fat, or oleic acid, have been proposed. It has long been recognized that the absorption of fat is strongly dependent on the manner in which it is fed. The original investigators used a 48% emulsion of peanut oil stabilized with Tween 80, as the vehicle for administration. Subsequent investigators have used emulsions in milk or capsules containing the labeled material (Isley *et al.*, 1958).

1. Procedure

a. Patients are fasted for 6 hours before the test. The test meal consists of one capsule containing 25 μCi of labeled triolein in a total volume of 0.5 ml peanut oil and three capsules each of 0.5 gm barium sulfate (X-ray grade). Give the patient 20 drops of Lugol's solution immediately after the test meal to block thyroid uptake of the radioiodine released during the metabolism of the fat.

b. Obtain blood samples at 4, 5, and 6 hours. Fluoroscope patients at 3 hours to make sure of gastric emptying and to confirm the dissolution of the capsules. Collect feces for 48 hours. There is no restriction of food after the last blood sample is obtained.

c. Appearance of radioactivity:

i. Draw 3-ml samples of blood and discharge into plastic tubes for radioassay in a well scintillation detector.

ii. Determine the radioactivity administered by making a 1:1000 dilution of one of the capsules containing an identical amount of labeled triolein in petroleum ether and counting 3 ml of the diluted standard in a well detector. Dilution may be made by breaking a capsule into 10 ml petroleum ether and dissolving the triolein. A 1:100 dilution of this solution in petroleum ether can then be made.

iii. Calculate the total amount of radioactivity in the patient's blood volume from the following formula which assumes that the blood volume is 7% of the body weight:

$$^{131}I \text{ in total blood volume } (\%) = \frac{\text{sample cpm} \times 70 \times \text{body wt (kg)}}{\text{standard cpm} \times 1000}$$

d. Fecal radioactivity:

i. Collect the feces in a standard container.

ii. Position a probe scintillation detector 30 cm from the top surface of the sample container and measure the radioactivity.

iii. In the same type of container, and in the same way, count a 100-grain homogeneously distributed standard solution containing an amount of radioactivity equal to that ingested by the patient.

iv. Calculate the percent of the administered dose excreted in the sample of feces from the data:

$$\text{Fat excreted } (\%) = \frac{\text{fecal cpm}}{\text{standard cpm}} \times 100$$

2. Results and Discussion

In normal subjects the peak blood radioactivity occurs approximately 3–4 hours after the administration of ^{131}I-labeled triolein. The peak values of circulating ^{131}I are approximately 14–15% of the dose administered in normal subjects. Normally, excretion of ^{131}I occurs by way of the kidneys with 3–4% being excreted in the feces over a 3- to 4-day period. In patients having gastrointestinal disease, blood levels of radioactivity rise slowly and reach peak levels of only 4–7%.

The average radioactivity in the feces of normal subjects is about 1.2%. The maximum in normal subjects is 3.5%. Patients having malabsorption syndromes usually show a 12–20% excretion but may have as high as 80% excretion. If the excreted radioactivity is high, the test may be repeated 3 or 4 days later using an equivalent dosage of ^{131}I-labeled oleic acid.

If the patient has a malabsorption syndrome, as indicated by low blood levels of radioactivity, or high radioactivity level in the feces, the basic defect may be due either to a lack of pancreatic enzymes or to a functional disturbance in the intestine (Kaplan et al., 1958; Beres et al., 1957). If the patient shows normal levels of radioactivity in the blood or feces after the administration of ^{131}I-oleic acid, the malabsorption defect originates in the pancreas since ^{131}I-oleic acid is absorbed by the intestine without the aid of pancreatic enzymes. If the second test employing radioleic acid again shows low blood activity or high fecal activity, the basic absorption defect is in the intestine.

Primary pancreatic insufficiency may be due to pancreatitis or carcinoma of the pancreas. Reduced absorption of radioleic acid may be due to Whipple's disease (intestinal lipodystrophy), regional enteritis, ulcerative colitis, or cirrhosis of the liver (see Fig. 5).

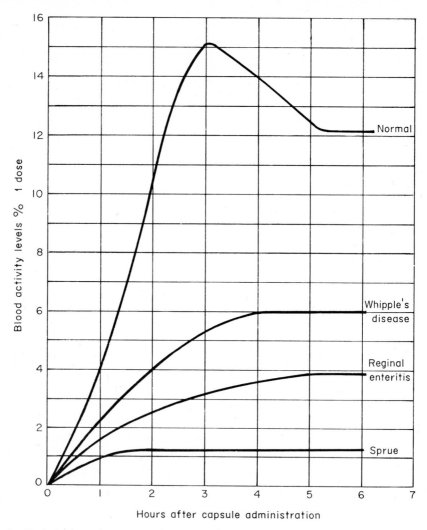

Fig. 5. Typical absorption curves of human patients after the ingestion of a capsule containing ^{131}I-triolein.

Michaelson *et al.* (1960) studied the absorption of ^{131}I-labeled fat in normal dogs. Following an 18-hour fast 50 μCi of ^{131}I-triolein were administered to each dog. The authors concluded from the rate of appearance of ^{131}I in blood that young dogs seemed to have a longer gastric emptying time than old dogs. Within 2 hours after the ingestion of a fat meal, intestinal absorption and distribution in blood were practically complete. Rosenthall (1961) recently described a technique which might be used as a rapid screening method for the ^{131}I absorption tests. This technique obviates the necessity of repeated venipunctures and the counting of several blood samples following the administration of oral ^{131}I-triolein. A γ-scintillation detector is positioned to detect the rate of appearance of ^{131}I as it passes through the vascular bed in the head. Rosenthall noted the existence of a linear relationship between head counting and the number of μCi of ^{131}I in the blood. According to his procedure, a "head count" is made 3 hours after the oral administration of ^{131}I-triolein at which time it can be determined whether or not fat absorption is normal.

Lastly, Van Handel and Zilversmit (1958) used ^{131}I- and ^{14}C-labeled fat and fatty acids in a critical study of the limitations of the use of ^{131}I-labeled fat in metabolic experiments. They noted that the distribution of ^{131}I-fatty acids in tissue neutral fat was similar to that of ^{14}C-fatty acids. However, in the liver, ^{14}C-fatty acids was incorporated into phospholipids, whereas ^{131}I-fatty acids were not. The authors concluded that because of this difference, ^{131}I-labeled oleic acid has a limited use in metabolic experiments.

O. Miscellaneous Absorption and Digestion Studies

Owen et al. (1954) described a method using ^{51}Cr-labeled erythrocytes for the detection of gastrointestinal hemorrhage. The ^{51}Cr-labeled red cells were injected intravenously, and the appearance of radiochromium in feces was used to determine quantitatively the amount of blood passing into the gut by gastrointestinal bleeding. Roche and Peréz-Jiménez (1959) studied the intestinal loss and reabsorption of iron in severe hookworm infections of humans using radiochromium (^{51}Cr) and radioiron (^{59}Fe). They noted that although 3–21 mg of iron was secreted into the intestine daily through bleeding, 44% of this iron was subsequently reabsorbed. Yonehiro et al. (1958) used ^{59}Fe ferrous citrate to develop a method which could be used to detect ulcerated lesions of the alimentary tract and "silent" cancers of the mucous membranes of the gastrointestinal tract. Saylor and Finch (1953) used two isotopes of iron (^{55}Fe administered orally and ^{59}Fe-labeled plasma injected intravenously) to determine quantitatively iron absorption in rats. They noted that rats with bone marrow damage, hemolytic anemia, turpentine abscesses, and elevated iron stores showed a diminished absorption of iron. Lastly, Van Hoek and Conrad (1961) used a whole-body liquid scintillation counter to study iron absorption in man. They noted that following the ingestion of 1 μCi ^{59}Fe-citrate, iron-deficient humans absorbed approximately three times the amount of radioiron as did iron-replete humans.

A method for studying the digestive absorption of water in humans suffering from cirrhosis of the liver using orally administered deuterium oxide and intravenously injected tritiated water has recently been published by Laine-Boszormenyi and Fallot (1960). The blood clearance and tissue distribution of intravenously administered colloidal radiogold has been followed by Sheppard et al. (1951) and Ganz and Brucer (1958). Steenberg (1959), following the uptake and loss of orally administered ^{131}I to dairy cows, noted that the urinary loss was quantitatively more important than that via milk secretion.

P. Skeletal Metabolism and Related Diseases

A large number of radioisotopes have been used to study diseases of the skeleton, particularly those associated with rickets and dysfunction of the parathyroid glands. Radiostrontium, ^{85}Sr, and radiocalcium, ^{45}Ca, have been used to study osteoporosis, Paget's disease, and disorders of the parathyroid glands (Rich et al., 1961; Dow and Stanbury, 1960).

Bone-seeking radioisotopes have also been used to study metabolic diseases of farm animals. For example, Boda and Cole (1954) demonstrated that the hypocalcemia associated with parturient paresis (milk fever) in dairy cows could be prevented by feeding low-calcium: high-phosphorus diets before calving. Luick et al. (1957a) used radiocalcium, ^{45}Ca, to study this phenomenon and reported that the cows on the milk fever preventive diet utilized calcium less efficiently than cows on high-calcium diets; a greater response was noted in the decrease in absorption of dietary calcium than in the increased secretion of metabolic fecal calcium. In a subsequent report, Luick et al. (1957b) demonstrated that cows fed low-calcium, high-phosphorus diets had larger reservoirs of skeletal calcium than cows fed high-calcium, low-phosphorus diets. Since they had found earlier that the low-calcium, high-phosphorus cows were in negative calcium balance, the authors concluded that the larger stores of mobilizable calcium must have accrued at the expense of stable bone calcium.

Radiocarbon (^{14}C-acetate), radiophosphorus (^{32}P), and radiocalcium (^{45}Ca) were used to study an outbreak of spontaneous rickets in young lambs (Luick, unpublished). The radioautographs in Fig. 6 were obtained from the right and left femurs of a rachitic lamb injected with inorganic ^{45}Ca. They show how calcium is selectively deposited at the site of a spontaneous fracture. Radiophosphorus has also been used to study the secretion of phosphate into cow's milk (Kleiber et al., 1948), the turnover of tissue phosphate in cows (Kleiber et al. 1950), and the mobility of the skeletal phosphate of lactating dairy cows (Black et al., 1953). Smith et al. (1951, 1952) used ^{32}P-phosphate to study the time distribution of intravenously injected phosphorus in swine and sheep tissues. Radiophosphorus has also been used as a tracer to determine sites of absorption and secretion of phosphate within the digestive tract of swine, sheep, and dairy cattle (Smith et al., 1955a,b, 1956).

A radioisotope of magnesium, ^{28}Mg, has become available for biological research. Although this isotope has a relatively short physical half-life (23.3 hours), Simesen et al. (1962) used it in dairy cattle to determine for the first time the true digestibility of dietary magnesium and the loss of metabolic magnesium in the feces (the latter has also been called endogenous fecal magnesium). Similar studies were reported earlier for the digestibility of calcium (Visek et al., 1952, 1953; Hansard et al., 1954; Luick et al., 1957a) and phosphorus (Kleiber et al., 1951; Lofgreen et al., 1952; Lofgreen and Kleiber, 1953; Luick and Lofgreen, 1957). Radiomagnesium, ^{28}Mg, has also been used to study hypomagnesemia (grass tetany), the exchange of maternal and fetal magnesium, and the magnesium turnover of dairy cows and calves (Simesen and Luick, unpublished).

Q. RADIOISOTOPE SCANNING

Bone structures and organs, such as the stomach, gallbladder, and lungs, which can be filled with fluids that are opaque to X rays, may be "seen" by the radiologist through conventional X-ray techniques. However, many glands and other soft tissues cannot be filled with or will not absorb opaque media, and thus cannot be made to show up on a radiograph. Fortunately, among the latter glands and tissues, there are some which will absorb or concentrate specific drugs which can be labeled with radioisotopes. A "picture" can then be made of the radiation emitted from the area in which the radioactive material has been localized. Dark areas on the "picture"

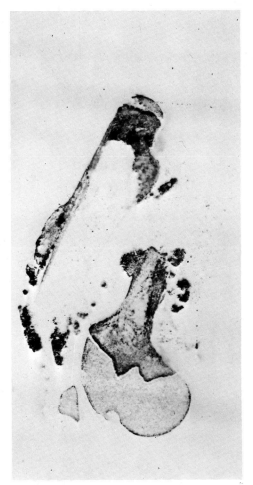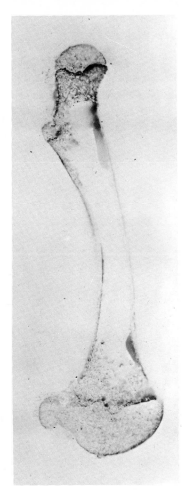

Fig. 6.   Calcium-45 radioautogram of the right and left femurs of a young lamb with spontaneous rickets. Note how calcium is selectively deposited at the site of the fracture. (Luick, unpublished.)

correspond to a part of the organ which has absorbed an appreciable amount of the administered material, while a light area represents tissues which have taken on little or none of the radioactive material. Thus, the "picture" can be interpreted in the same manner as the radiograph where the tissue in which the contrast medium has concentrated is differentiated from the surrounding tissue because it absorbs a greater percentage of the X rays (Fig. 7).

1.   Procedure

a. Administer a tracer dose of an isotopically labeled compound to the patient and allow sufficient time to elapse to insure that the radioisotope has accumulated in the organ being studied.

b. Position the scanner over the patient so that the scintillation detector is directly over the organ. A motor-driven mechanical system moves the collimated

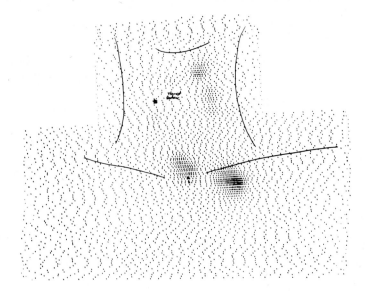

Fig. 7. Postoperative papillary carcinoma of thyroid metastasis shown as a scan following dosage with radioiodine, [131]I.

scintillation detector back and forth in stepwise sweeps over the organ area and the intensity of irradiation is measured at regular intervals along the tract.

c. Record the radiation intensity at frequent intervals either by means of a mechanical or an electrical stylus or by a light beam which briefly illuminates one spot on a photographic film.

2.   Results and Discussion

Although radioisotope scanning techniques for the localization of tumors have been developed only recently, they have already been used to demonstrate the size, position, and configuration of normal and diseased organs. Several examples are listed in Table II. Thyroid scanning and liver scanning are now done routinely in some large clinics and remarkable accuracy has been achieved. For example, Bender and Blau (1959), using the ^{131}I-rose bengal procedure, reported they had correctly diagnosed 90% of patients having tumors of the liver. In 102 patients with brain tumors, 73% were accurately localized through the use of ^{131}I-octoiodofluorescein (Tocus et al., 1962).

Bender and Blau (1959) point out that since radioisotope scanning is a diagnostic screening procedure, the instrument must be capable of resolving small differences in the radioisotope content between the target and nontarget tissues. More important, counting efficiency should be as high as possible to minimize the amount of radioisotope required for the scan. Highest resolution and counting efficiency are now being achieved through the use of large sodium iodide crystals equipped with focusing collimators. Few applications of this very promising diagnostic technique have been published as yet in the field of veterinary medicine.

TABLE II   APPLICATIONS OF RADIOISOTOPE SCANNING

Organ of tissue "scanned"	Radioisotope and compound	Reference
Liver	^{198}Au-colloidal gold	Donato et al. (1959)
	^{131}I-rose bengal	Bender and Blau (1959)
Spleen	^{51}Cr-red blood cells	Winkelman et al. (1960)
Pancreas	^{75}Se-selenomethionine	Blau and Manske (1961)
	^{65}Zn-amino acids	Greenlaw et al. (1962)
Lymph nodes	Colloidal gold (^{198}Au)	Sage and Gozun (1958)
Bone tumors, fractures, and repair	^{85}Sr (inorganic)	Fleming et al. (1961)
Brain tumors	^{131}I-human serum albumin	Planiol (1959), McAfee and Taxdal (1961)
	^{131}I-octoiodofluorescein	Tocus et al. (1962)
	^{74}As and ^{64}Cu positron-annihilation	Mundinger (1960)
Thyroid	^{131}I-iodide	Groesbeck (1959a,b)
	^{125}I-iodide	Endlich et al. (1962)
Heart (myocardium)	^{86}Rb	Carr et al. (1962)

R. THERAPY

Radioisotopes are used extensively in human medicine to irradiate and destroy rapidly growing tissues. Several examples are listed in Table III. In contrast, therapy through the selective deposition of a radioisotope is practically unknown in the field of veterinary medicine today. The only noteworthy exception appears to be the radiation of skin tumors by means of ^{90}Sr β-ray applicator (Friedell et al., 1951). Strontium-90 applicators, or probes, are usually wand-shaped and may contain 100 mCi or more of radiostrontium which is deposited as a point source at the tip of the probe. A typical probe has been reported to deliver 5200 rep/min over an active surface area of 0.8 cm^2 (Wheat et al., 1954). β-Ray therapy with an ^{90}Sr probe has

TABLE III   SOME USES OF RADIOISOTOPES IN THERAPEUTIC MEDICINE

Tissue/organ	Isotope and compound
Eye tumors	^{32}P-sodium phosphate
Brain tumors	^{131}I-serum albumin
Brain tumors	^{74}As-sodium arsenate
Thyroid tumors	^{124}I- and ^{131}I-sodium iodide
Hyperthyroidism	^{131}I-sodium iodide
Intracavitary irradiation	^{198}Au-gold colloid
Prostatic tumors	^{198}Au-gold colloid
Prostatic tumors	^{51}Cr-colloid chromic phosphate
Polycythemia vera	^{32}P-sodium phosphate
Bladder carcinoma	^{182}Ta wire
Corneal epithelioma	^{90}Sr probe
Skin tumors	^{90}Sr probe
Uterine carcinoma	Colloidal ^{198}Au

been used successfully by veterinarians to treat various ocular diseases of cattle, horses, and dogs (Catcott *et al.*, 1953; Wheat *et al.*, 1954). The technique has also been used to treat adenomas of the anal area, epithelioma of the skin, nasal ulceration, senile warts on dogs, and warts on cow teats (Dalton, 1958). Radiocobalt, ^{60}Co, has also been used to treat ocular carcinoma in cattle. The isotope is deposited on needles or on nylon thread which are, in turn, placed adjacent to or in the tumor tissue. Banks (1956) states that the technique is as effective as other types of radiation for the treatment of ocular carcinoma. The use of radioisotopes in therapeutic medicine, especially as applied to man, was briefly reviewed by J. R. Holmes (1960b, 1962). A more comprehensive discussion of radioisotope therapy technique may be found in Fields and Seed (1960) and in Schwiegk and Turba (1961).

REFERENCES

Aust, J. B., Chou, S. N., Marvin, J. F., Brackney, E. L., and Moore, G. E. (1951). *Proc. Soc. Exptl. Biol. Med.* **77**, 514.
Baker, N. F., and Douglas, J. R. (1957). *Am. J. Vet. Res.* **18**, 295.
Baker, N. F., Cook, E. F., Douglas, J. R., and Cornelius, C. E. (1959). *J. Parasitol.* **45**, 643.
Baker, N. F., Osebold, J. W., and Christensen, J. F. (1961). *Am. J. Vet. Res.* **22**, 590.
Banks, W. C. (1956). *North Am. Vet.* **37**, 114.
Bender, M. A., and Blau, M. (1959). *Proc. IAEA/WHO Seminar Med. Radioisotope Scanning, Vienna, 1959* p. 31. I.A.E.A., Vienna.
Beres, P., Wenger, J., and Kirsner, J. B. (1957). *Gastroenterology* **32**, 1.
Berlin, N. I., Waldmann, T. A., and Weissman, S. M. (1959). *Physiol. Rev.* **39**, 577.
Biellier, H. V. (1955). Ph.D. Thesis, University of Missouri, Columbia, Missouri.
Black, A. L., Kleiber, M., Smith, A. H., and Ralston, N. P. (1953). *Proc. Soc. Exptl. Biol. Med.* **82**, 248.
Blau, M., and Manske, R. F. (1961). *J. Nucl. Med.* **2**, 102.
Blincoe, C. (1953). *Nucleonics* **22**, 70.
Block, J. B., and Burrows, B. A. (1960). *J. Lab. Clin. Med.* **56**, 463.
Block, J. B., Hine, G. J., and Burrows, B. A. (1960). *J. Lab. Clin. Med.* **56**, 110.
Boda, J. M., and Cole, H. H. (1954). *J. Dairy Sci.* **37**, 360.
Brooks, J. R., Pipes, G. W., and Ross, C. V. (1962). *J. Animal Sci.* **21**, 414.
Brown-Grant, K., and Gibson, J. G. (1955). *J. Physiol. (London)* **127**, 328.
Brown-Grant, K., and Gibson, J. G. (1956). *J. Physiol. (London)* **131**, 52.
Brown-Grant, K., Harris, G. W., and Reichlin, S. (1954). *J. Physiol. (London)* **126**, 1.
Bush, J. A., Berlin, N. I., Jensen, W. N., Brill, A. B., Cartwright, G. E., and Wintrobe, M. M. (1955). *J. Exptl. Med.* **101**, 451.
Bush, J. A., Jensen, W. N., Ashenbrucker, H., Cartwright, G. E., and Wintrobe, M. M. (1956a). *J. Exptl. Med.* **103**, 161.
Bush, J. A., Jensen, W. N., Athens, J. W., Ashenbrucker, H., Cartwright, G. E., and Wintrobe, M. M. (1956b). *J. Exptl. Med.* **103**, 701.
Bustad, L. K., Warner, D. E., and Kornberg, H. A. (1958). *Am. J. Vet. Res.* **19**, 893.
Campbell, R. M., Cuthbertson, D. P., Mackie, W., McFarlane, A. S., Phillipson, A. T., and Sudsaneh, S. (1961). *J. Physiol. (London)* **158**, 113.
Carr, E. A., Jr., Beierwaltes, W. H., Wegst, A. V., and Bartlett, J. D., Jr. (1962). *J. Nucl. Med.* **3**, 76.
Catcott, E. J., Tharp, V. L., and Johnson, L. E. (1953). *J. Am. Vet. Med. Assoc.* **122**, 172.
Clark, D. E., Moe, R. H., and Adams, E. E. (1949). *Surgery* **26**, 331.
Collery, L., and Keating, J. (1958). *Vet. Record* **70**, 216.
Combes, B. (1960). *J. Lab. Clin. Med.* **56**, 538.
Cooperman, J. M., Luhby, A. L., Teller, D. N., and Marley, J. F. (1960). *J. Biol. Chem.* **235**, 191.
Cornelius, C. E., Kaneko, J. J., and Benson, D. C. (1959a). *Am. J. Vet. Res.* **20**, 917.
Cornelius, C. E., Black, A. L., and Kleiber, M. (1959b). *Am. J. Vet. Res.* **20**, 44.

Cornelius, C. E., Kaneko, J. J., and Benson, D. C. (1960). *Am. J. Vet. Res.* **21**, 1123.
Cornelius, C. E., Baker, N. F., Kaneko, J. J., and Douglas, J. R. (1962). *Am. J. Vet. Res.* **23**, 837.
Dahl, L. K., Smiley, M. O., Silver, L., and Sparagen, S. C. (1961). *Nature* **192**, 267.
Dalton, P. J. (1958). *Vet. Record* **70**, 233.
D'Angelo, S. A. (1960). *Federation Proc.* **19**, 4; Suppl. 5, 51.
Dixon, F. J., Talmadge, D. W., Maurer, P. H., and Deichmiller, M. P. (1952). *J. Exptl. Med.* **96**, 313.
Dixon, F. J., Mauer, P. H., and Deichmiller, M. P. (1953). *Proc. Soc. Exptl. Biol. Med.* **83**, 287.
Donato, L., Beachini, M. F., and Panichi, S. (1959). *Proc. IAEA/WHO Seminar Med. Radioisotope Scanning, Vienna, 1959* p. 87. I.A.E.A., Vienna.
Doscherholmen, A., Finley, P. R., and Hagen, P. S. (1960). *J. Lab. Clin. Med.* **56**, 547.
Dow, E. C., and Stanbury, J. B. (1960). *J. Clin. Invest.* **39**, 885.
Dowling, J. T., Hutchinson, D. L., Hindle, W., and Kleeman, C. R. (1961). *J. Clin. Endocrinol. Metab.* **21**, 779.
Ebaugh, F. G., Emerson, C. P., and Ross, J. F. (1953). *J. Clin. Invest.* **32**, 1260.
Endlich, H., Harper, P., Beck, R., and Lathrop, K. (1962). *Am. J. Roentgenol., Radium Therapy Nucl. Med.* **87**, 148.
Fields, T., and Seed, L. (1960). "Clinical Use of Radioisotopes. A Manual of Technique." Year Book Publ., Chicago, Illinois.
Fields, T., Kaplan, E., and Terrill, M. (1954). *J. Lab. Clin. Med.* **43**, 332.
Fish, W. A., Carlin, H., and Hickey, F. C. (1952). *Endocrinology* **51**, 282.
Flamboe, E. E., and Reineke, E. P. (1959). *J. Animal Sci.* **18**, 1135.
Fleming, W. H., McIlraith, J. D., and King, E. R. (1961). *Radiology* **77**, 635.
Florsheim, W. H., Corcorran, N. L., and Rudko, P. (1966). *Federation Proc.* **25**, 617.
Fredrickson, D. S., Ganong, W. F., and Hume, D. M. (1955). *Proc. Soc. Exptl. Biol. Med.* **89**, 416.
Freedberg, A. S., Chamovita, D. L., and Kurland, G. S. (1952). *Metab., Clin. Exptl.* **1**, 26.
Friedell, H. L., Thomas, C. I., and Krohmer, J. S. (1951). *Am. J. Roentgenol. Radium Therapy* **65**, 232.
Ganz, A., and Brucer, M. (1958). *J. Lab. Clin. Med.* **52**, 20.
Germann, D. H. (1961). *Am. J. Roentgenol., Radium Therapy Nucl. Med.* **85**, 59.
Glass, G. B. J. (1958). *J. Lab. Clin. Med.* **52**, 875.
Glass, G. B. J., and Mersheimer, W. L. (1958). *J. Lab. Clin. Med.* **52**, 860.
Glass, G. B. J., Boyd, L. J., and Ebin, L. (1958). *J. Lab. Clin. Med.* **52**, 849.
Greenlaw, R. H., Strain, W. H., Callear, T. E., Dubilier, L. D., and Strain, S. C. (1962). *J. Nucl. Med.* **3**, 47.
Groesbeck, H. P. (1959a). *Cancer* **12**, 1.
Groesbeck, H. P. (1959b). *Cancer* **12**, 6.
Groom, A. C., and Rowlands, S. (1956). *J. Physiol. (London)* **132**, 5p.
Hamolsky, M. W., Stein, M., and Freedberg, A. S. (1957). *J. Clin. Endocrinol. Metab.* **17**, 33.
Hamolsky, M. W., Golodetz, A., and Freedberg, A. S. (1959). *J. Clin. Endocrinol. Metab.* **19**, 103.
Hansard, S. L. (1962). *J. Animal Sci.* **21**, 282.
Hansard, S. L., and Foote, L. E. (1958). *Federation Proc.* **17**, 478.
Hansard, S. L., Butler, W. O., Comar, C. L., and Hobbs, C. S. (1953). *J. Animal Sci.* **12**, 402.
Hansard, S. L., Comar, C. L., and Plumlee, M. P. (1954). *J. Animal Sci.* **13**, 25.
Hansard, S. L., Foote, L. E., and Dimopoullos, G. T. (1959). *J. Dairy Sci.* **42**, 1970–1976.
Henneman, H. A., Griffin, S. A., and Reineke, E. P. (1952). *J. Animal Sci.* **11**, 794.
Henneman, H. A., Reineke, E. P., and Griffin, S. A. (1955). *J. Animal Sci.* **14**, 419.
Heroux, O., and Brauer, R. (1965). *J. Appl. Physiol.* **20**, 597.
Hjort, P. F., Paputchis, H., and Cheney, B. (1960). *J. Lab. Clin. Med.* **55**, 416.
Holmes, I. H., and Bell, R. E. (1961). *Can. Med. Assoc. J.* **84**, 79.
Holmes, J. R. (1960a). *Cornell Vet.* **50**, 308.
Holmes, J. R. (1960b). *Can. Vet. J.* **2**, 179 and 348.
Holmes, J. R. (1962). *Vet. Bull.* **32**, 65–72.
Howes, J. R., Feaster, J. P., and Hentges, J. F., Jr. (1962). *J. Animal Sci.* **21**, 210.
Huff, R. L., Elminger, P. J., Garcia, J. F., Oda, J. M., Cockrell, M. C., and Lawrence, J. H. (1951). *J. Clin. Invest.* **30**, 1514.
Huff, R. L., Feller, D. D., and Bogardus, G. M. (1954). *J. Clin. Invest.* **33**, 944.
Huff, R. L., Feller, D. D., Judd, O. J., and Bogardus, G. M. (1955). *Circulation Res.* **3**, 564.

Isley, J. K., Jr., Sanders, A. P., Baylin, G. J., Ruffin, J. M., Singleton, W. W., Anlyan, W. G., and Sharpe, K. W. (1958). *Gastroenterology* **35**, 482.

Jensen, W. N., Bush, J. A., Ashenbrucker, H., Cartwright, G. E., and Wintrobe, M. M. (1956). *J. Exptl. Med.* **103**, 145.

Johnson, D. E., Taplin, G. V., Dore, E. K., and Hayashi, J. (1961). *J. Nucl. Med.* **2**, 8.

Johnson, H. D., and Ragsdale, A. C. (1959). *J. Dairy Sci.* **42**, 1821.

Johnson, H. D., Ragsdale, A. C., and Cheng, C. S. (1958). *Missouri, Univ., Agr. Expt. Sta., Res. Bull.* **648**.

Johnson, H. D., Kibler, H. H., and Silsby, H. (1964). *Gerontologia* **9**, 18.

Johnson, H. D., Ward, M. W., and Kibler, H. H. (1966). *J. Appl. Physiol.* **21**, 689.

Kaneko, J. J. (1963). *Ann. N.Y. Acad. Sci.* **104**, 689.

Kaneko, J. J., Tyler, W. S., Wind, A. P., and Cornelius, C. E. (1959). *J. Am. Vet. Med. Assoc.* **135**, 516.

Kaneko, J. J., Tyler, W. S., Theilen, G. H., and Schalm, O. W. (1960). *Am. J. Vet. Res.* **21**, 230.

Kaneko, J. J., Cornelius, C. E., and Heuschele, W. P. (1961a). *Am. J. Vet. Res.* **22**, 683.

Kaneko, J. J., Cornelius, C. E., and Baker, N. F. (1961b). *Proc. Soc. Exptl. Biol. Med.* **107**, 924.

Kaplan, E., and Zuelzer, W. W. (1950). *J. Lab. Clin. Med.* **36**, 511.

Kaplan, E., Edidin, B. D., Fruin, R. C., and Baker, L. A. (1958). *Gastroenterology* **34**, 901.

Kleiber, M., Smith, A. H., and Ralston, N. P. (1948). *Federation Proc.* **8**, 86.

Kleiber, M., Smith, A. H., and Ralston, N. P. (1950). *J. Gen. Physiol.* **33**, 525.

Kleiber, M., Smith, A. H., Ralston, N. P., and Black, A. L. (1951). *J. Nutr.* **45**, 253.

Klement, A. W., Ayer, D. E., and McIntyre, D. R. (1954). *Proc. Soc. Exptl. Biol. Med.* **87**, 81.

Laine-Boszormenyi, M., and Fallot, P. (1960). *Intern. J. Appl. Radiation Isotopes* **7**, 233.

Lippincott, S. W., Cohn, S. H., Hamel, H., Fine, S., and Korman, S. (1961). *J. Clin. Invest.* **40**, 697.

Lodge, J. R., Lewis, R. C., and Reineke, E. P. (1957). *J. Dairy Sci.* **40**, 209.

Lodge, J. R., Lewis, R. C., Reineke, E. P., and McGilliard, L. D. (1958). *J. Dairy Sci.* **41**, 641.

Lofgreen, G. P., and Kleiber, M. (1953). *J. Animal Sci.* **12**, 366.

Lofgreen, G. P., Kleiber, M., and Luick, J. R. (1952). *J. Nutr.* **47**, 571.

Lombardi, M. H., Comar, C. L., and Kirk, R. W. (1962). *Am. J. Vet. Res.* **23**, 412.

Long, R. T. I., and Cornell, W. P. (1959). *Proc. Soc. Exptl. Biol. Med.* **101**, 836.

Love, W. D., and Burch, G. E. (1958). *J. Lab. Clin. Med.* **52**, 515.

Luhby, A. L., Cooperman, J. M., and Donnenfeld, A. M. (1959). *Proc. Soc. Exptl. Biol. Med.* **100**, 214.

Luick, J. R. (1965). *Am. J. Vet. Res.* **26**, 566.

Luick, J. R., and Lofgreen, G. P. (1957). *J. Animal Sci.* **16**, 201.

Luick, J. R., Boda, J. M., and Kleiber, M. (1957a). *J. Nutr.* **61**, 597.

Luick, J. R., Boda, J. M., and Kleiber, M. (1957b). *Am. J. Physiol.* **189**, 483.

Luick, J. R., Unpublished studies.

McAfee, J. G., and Taxdal, D. R. (1961). *Radiology* **77**, 207.

Marvin, H. N., and Lucy, D. D. (1957). *Acta Haematol.* **18**, 239.

Mena, I., Kivel, R., Mahoney, P., Mellinkoff, S. M., and Bennett, L. R. (1959). *J. Lab. Clin. Med.* **54**, 167.

Michaelson, S. M., El-Tamami, M. Y., Thomson, R. A. E., and Howland, J. W. (1960). *Am. J. Vet. Res.* **21**, 364.

Mills, J. A., Calkins, E., and Cohen, A. C. (1961). *J. Clin. Invest.* **40**, 1926.

Moertel, C. G., and Owen, C. A., Jr. (1958). *J. Lab. Clin. Med.* **52**, 902.

Mundinger, F. (1960). *Medicamundi* **7**, 127.

Nordyke, R. A., and Blahd, W. H. (1958). *J. Lab. Clin. Med.* **51**, 565.

Nordyke, R. A., and Blahd, W. H. (1959). *J. Am. Med. Assoc.* **170**, 1159.

Nordyke, R. A., Tubis, M., and Blahd, W. H. (1960). *J. Lab. Clin. Med.* **56**, 438.

O'Meallie, L. P., Love, W. D., and Burch, G. E. (1960). *J. Lab. Clin. Med.* **56**, 933.

Owen, C. A., Jr., Bollman, J. L., and Grindlay, J. H. (1954). *J. Lab. Clin. Med.* **44**, 238.

Pipes, G. W., and Turner, C. W. (1956). *Missouri, Univ., Agr. Expt. Sta., Res. Bull.* **617**.

Pipes, G. W., Premachandra, B. N., and Turner, C. W. (1957). *J. Dairy Sci.* **40**, 340.

Pipes, G. W., Premachandra, B. N., and Turner, C. W. (1958a). *J. Animal Sci.* **17**, 227.

Pipes, G. W., Premachandra, B. N., and Turner, C. W. (1958b). *J. Dairy Sci.* **41**, 1387.

Pipes, G. W., Premachandra, B. N., and Turner, C. W. (1959). *J. Dairy Sci.* **42**, 1606.

Planiol, T. (1959). *Proc. IAEA/WHO Seminar Med. Radioisotope Scanning, Vienna, 1959*. p. 189. I.A.E.A., Vienna.

Portman, O. W., McConnell, K. P., and Rigdon, R. H. (1952). *Proc. Soc. Exptl. Biol. Med.* **81**, 599.

Premachandra, B. N., and Turner, C. W. (1960). *J. Animal Sci.* **19**, 1181.

Premachandra, B. N., and Turner, C. W. (1961). *J. Dairy Sci.* **44**, 2035.

Premachandra, B. N., Pipes, G. W., and Turner, C. W. (1958). *J. Dairy Sci.* **41**, 1609.

Prinz, W., Hill, H., and Heinrich, H. C. (1959). *Zentr. Veterinaermed.* **6**, 605.

Pritchard, W. H., MacIntyre, W. J., and Moir, J. W. (1955). *J. Lab. Clin. Med.* **46**, 939.

Rapaport, E., Hiroshi, K., Haynes, P. W., and Dexter, L. (1956). *Am. J. Physiol.* **185**, 127.

Raun, N., Cheng, E., Raun, A., Balloun, S., and Homeyer, P. (1958). *J. Animal Sci.* **17**, 1227.

Read, R. C. (1954). *New Engl. J. Med.* **150**, 1021.

Reineke, E. P., and Singh, O. N. (1955). *Proc. Soc. Exptl. Biol. Med.* **88**, 203.

Reineke, E. P., Travis, H. F., and Kifer, P. E. (1960). *Am. J. Vet. Res.* **21**, 862.

Rich, C., Ensinck, J., and Fellows, H. (1961). *J. Clin. Endocrinol. Metab.* **21**, 611.

Robinson, G. A., Bier, A. M., and McCarter, A. (1961). *Brit. J. Haematol.* **7**, 271.

Roche, M., and Peréz-Giménez, M. E. (1959). *J. Lab. Clin. Med.* **54**, 49.

Rosenthall, L. (1961). *Radiology* **76**, 251.

Sage, H. H., and Gozun, B. V. (1958). *Proc. Soc. Exptl. Biol. Med.* **97**, 895.

Saylor, L., and Finch, C. A. (1953). *Am. J. Physiol.* **172**, 372.

Schilling, R. F., Clatanoff, D. V., and Korst, D. R. (1955). *J. Lab. Clin. Med.* **45**, 926.

Schwiegk, H., and Turba, F., eds. (1961). "Radioactive Isotopes in Physiology, Diagnostics and Therapy," Vols. I and II. Springer, Berlin.

Seigneur, L. J., Test, L. D., and Bustad, L. K. (1959). *Am. J. Vet. Res.* **20**, 14.

Serrato, M., Grayhack, J., and Earle, D. P. (1959). *A.M.A. Arch Internal Med.* **103**, 851.

Sevelius, G., and Johnson, P. C. (1959). *J. Lab. Clin. Med.* **54**, 669.

Sharpe, A. R., Jr. (1961). *J. Clin. Endocrinol. Metab.* **21**, 739.

Shemin, D., and Rittenberg, D. (1946). *J. Biol. Chem.* **166**, 627.

Sheppard, C. W., Jordan, G., and Hahn, P. F. (1951). *Am. J. Physiol.* **164**, 345.

Shires, T., Williams, J., and Brown, F. (1960). *J. Lab. Clin. Med.* **55**, 776.

Simesen, M. G., and Luick, J. R. Unpublished study.

Simesen, M. G., Lunaas, T., Rogers, T. A., and Luick, J. R. (1962). *Acta Vet. Scand.* **3**, 75.

Singh, O. N., Henneman, H. A., and Reineke, E. P. (1956). *J. Animal Sci.* **15**, 625.

Smith, A. H., Kleiber, M., Black, A. L., Edick, M., Robinson, R., and Heitman, H., Jr. (1951). *J. Animal Sci.* **10**, 893.

Smith, A. H., Kleiber, M., Black, A. L., Luick, J. R., Larson, R. F., and Weir, W. C. (1952). *J. Animal Sci.* **11**, 638.

Smith, A. H., Kleiber, M., Black, A. L., and Luick, J. R. (1955a). *J. Nutr.* **57**, 497.

Smith, A. H., Kleiber, M., Black, A. L., and Baxter, C. F. (1955b). *J. Nutr.* **57**, 507.

Smith, A. H., Kleiber, M., Black, A. L., and Lofgreen, G. P. (1956). *J. Nutr.* **58**, 95.

Sorensen, P. H. (1958). "Radioisotopes in Scientific Research," Vol. III. Pergamon Press, Oxford.

Stahl, P. R., and Dale, H. E. (1958). *Am. J. Physiol.* **193**, 244.

Stahl, P. R., and Turner, C. W. (1961). *Poultry Sci.* **40**, 239.

Steenberg, K. (1959). *Acta Agr. Scand.* **9**, 198.

Sterling, K., and Tabachnik, M. (1961). *J. Clin. Endocrinol. Metab.* **21**, 456.

Sterling, K., Lashof, J. C., and Man, E. B. (1954). *J. Clin. Invest.* **33**, 1031.

Sternlieb, I., Morell, A. G., Tucker, W. D., Greene, M. W., and Scheinberg, I. H. (1961). *J. Clin. Invest.* **40**, 1834.

Stevens, C. E., D'Angelo, S. A., Paschkis, K. E., Cantarow, A., and Sunderman, F. W. (1953). *J. Clin. Endocrinol. Metab.* **13**, 872.

Stohlman, F., Jr. (1961). *Acta Radiol.* **56**, 189.

Strumia, M. M., Taylor, L., Sample, A. B., Colwell, L. S., and Dugan, A. (1955). *Blood* **10**, 429.

Swanson, E. W., Lengemann, F. W., and Monroe, R. A. (1957). *J. Animal Sci.* **16**, 318.

Tannhauser, S. J., and Stanley, M. M. (1949). *Trans. Assoc. Am. Physicians* **62**, 245.

Taplin, G. V., Meredith, O. M., Jr., and Kade, H. (1955). *J. Lab. Clin. Med.* **45**, 665.

Tocus, E. C., Okita, G. T., Evans, J. P., and Mullan, S. (1962). *Cancer* **15**, 153.

Turner, C. W., Pipes, G. W., and Premachandra, B. N. (1961). *J. Dairy Sci.* **44**, 163.

Ureles, A. I., and Murray, M. (1959). *J. Lab. Clin. Med.* **54**, 178.

Van Handel, E., and Zilversmit, D. B. (1958). *J. Lab. Clin. Med.* **52**, 831.

Van Hoek, R., and Conrad, M. E., Jr. (1961). *J. Clin. Invest.* **40**, 1153.

Visek, W. J., Barnes, L. L., and Loosli, J. K. (1952). *J. Dairy Sci.* **35**, 783.

Visek, W. J., Monroe, R. A., Swanson, E. W., and Comar, C. L. (1953). *J. Nutr.* **50**, 23.

Walser, M., Seldin, D. W., and Grollman, A. (1953). *J. Clin. Invest.* **32**, 299.

Werner, S. C., Hamilton, H. B., Leifer, E., and Goodwin, L. (1950). *J. Clin. Endocrinol.* **10**, 1054.

Westover, J. I., Greenfield, M. A., and Norman, A. (1959). *J. Lab. Clin. Med.* **54**, 174.

Wheat, J. D., Black, A. L., Hage, T. J., and Rhode, E. A. (1954). *J. Am. Vet. Med. Assoc.* **125**, 357.

Whipple, G. H., Robscheit-Robbins, F. S., and Bale, W. F. (1955). *J. Exptl. Med.* **102**, 725.

Winkelman, J. W., Wagner, H. N., McAfee, J. G., and Mozley, J. M. (1960). *Radiology* **75**, 465.

Winter, C. C. (1956). *J. Urol.* **76**, 182

Winter, C. C., and Taplin, G. V. (1958). *J. Urol.* **79**, 573.

Wolff, J. (1951). *Endocrinology* **48**, 284.

Woods, W. D., Hawkins, W. B., and Whipple, G. H. (1958). *J. Exptl. Med.* **108**, 1.

Woods, W. D., Hawkins, W. B., and Whipple, G. H. (1960). *J. Exptl. Med.* **112**, 431.

Wright, E., and Sinclair, D. P. (1959). *New Zeland J. Agr. Res.* **52**, 933.

Yonehiro, E. G., Root, H. D., Perry, J. F., Jr., Marvin, J. F., and Wangensteen, O. H. (1958). *Proc. Soc. Exptl. Biol. Med.* **98**, 339.

Yousef, M. K., and Johnson, H. D. (1966). *J. Animal Sci.* **25**, 150.

Yousef, M. K., and Johnson, H. D. (1967). *J. Animal Sci.* **26**, 1108.

Yousef, M. K., and Johnson, H. D. (1968a). *Endocrinology* **82**, 353.

Yousef, M. K., and Johnson, H. D. (1968b). *Nature* **217**, 5124.

Author Index

Numbers in italics refer to the pages on which the complete references are listed.

A

Aalund, O., 96, *107*
Abbrecht, P. H., 87, *107*
Abrams, R., 115, *147*
Abt, D., 138, *148*
Adam, A., 170, *177*
Adamesteau, I., 216, *230*
Adams, A. P., 81, *107*
Adams, E. E., 280, *308*
Adams, P. H., 5, *58*
Adams, R. D., 260, *269*
Aebi, H., 168, *176*
Aggeler, P. M., 186, *203*
Ailhaud, G., 135, *147*
Alami, Samih, Y., 191, *203*
Albritton, E. C., 95, 97, *107*
Alexander, B., 193, *203*, *204*
Alexander, R. S., 15, *59*
Ali, M. A., 16, *56*
Aliminosa, L., 29, *60*
Alkjaersig, N., 192, *204*
Allen, A. C., 11, *56*
Allen, R. C., 190, *205*
Allen, R. S., 120, 127, *150*
Allen, W. M., 140, 145, *151*
Alpen, E. L., 28, *56*
Alpers, D. H., 126, 127, 131, *147*
Altamirano, M., 115, *147*
Althausen, T. L., 10, *57*
Altman, P. L., 97, *107*, 257, *269*
Alvarado, F., 127, 128, 131, *147*, *148*
Ames, A., 209, 216, *230*, *231*
Amrousi, S. E., 97, *108*, 216, 217, *232*, 235, 236, 237, 238, 242, *252*
Amunden, M. A., 189, *205*
Anand, R. S., 97, *107*
Andersen, S. B., 145, *148*, *151*
Anderson, G. F., 190, *203*
Anderson, J. C., 114, *148*

Anderson, N. V., 142, *148*
Anderson, P. J., 171, 172, 174, *175*
Anderson, R. R., 33, 39, *56*, *58*
Andersson, B., 74, *107*
Andreev, P. P., 233, 240, 248, *252*
Anlyan, W. G., 300, *310*
Annegers, J. H., 141, *150*
Anstadt, G. L., 145, *149*
Archer, R. K., 187, 201, *203*
Archibald, J. A., 186, *205*, 244, *252*
Archibald, R. M., 29, *59*
Arias, I. M., 39, *57*
Arkina, R., 226, *231*
Ascari, E., *203*, *204*
Aschbacher, P. W., 96, *107*
Asheim, A., 33, *56*
Ashenbrucker, H., 293, 295, 296, *308*, *310*
Asmundson, V. S., 156, 167, 168, 169, *175*, *176*
Aso, Y., 136, *150*
Astorga, G., 248, *252*, *253*
Astrup, P., 81, *107*
Athens, J. W., 295, *308*
Aukland, K., 5, *56*
Auricchio, S., 126, *148*
Aust, J. B., 290, 293, *308*
Austin, W. G., 216, *231*
Ayer, D. E., 293, *310*
Ayyoub, N. I., 137, *151*

B

Bachrach, W. H., 115, *148*
Backus, P. L., *230*
Baeder, D. H., 251, *253*
Bahlmann, J., 20, *56*
Bahn, R. C., 26, *57*
Baines, A. D., 19, *56*
Bajusz, E., 171, *175*
Baker, J. R., 156, *176*

313

Subject Index

N

O

T